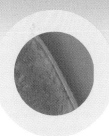

Medical Terminology Simplified

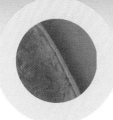

THIRD EDITION

Barbara A. Gylys, MEd, CMA-A

Professor Emerita
College of Health and Human Services
University of Toledo
Toledo, Ohio

Regina M. Masters, BSN, RN, CMA, MEd

Nursing Clinical Coordinator
School of Nursing
Owens Community College
Toledo, Ohio

Medical Terminology Simplified

A Programmed Learning Approach by Body Systems

F.A. DAVIS COMPANY • Philadelphia

This user-friendly text takes a programmed learning approach and offers users the freedom to learn medical terminology at their own pace.

What's *Inside...*

**The pages of Medical Terminology Simplified:
A Programmed Learning Approach by Body Systems, 3rd Edition**

Chapter Objectives
to give students goals to achieve for each chapter (see page 195)

Pronunciations
with all terms

Includes Suffixes
and their meanings

More Organized,
easily identified headings

Word Elements highlighted throughout the chapter to provide combining forms, word meaning, and analysis (see page 196)

Abbreviations
and their meanings for common terms
(see page 237)

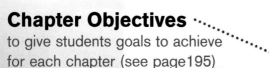

Abbreviations	Meaning	Abbreviations	Meaning
Ba	barium	GTT	glucose tolerance test
BaE, BE	barium enema	HCl	hydrochloric acid
cm	centimeter	IBD	inflammatory bowel disease
CT scan, CAT scan	computed tomography scan	IVC	intravenous cholangiography
Dx	diagnosis	UGI	upper gastrointestinal
EGD	esophagogastroduodenoscopy	UGIS	upper gastrointestinal series
ERCP	endoscopic retrograde cholangiopancreatography	US	ultrasonography, ultrasound
FBS	fasting blood sugar		
OTHER ABBREVIATIONS RELATED TO THE DIGESTIVE SYSTEM			
BM	bowel movement	HBV	hepatitis B virus
cm	centimeter	PE	physical examination
GI	gastrointestinal	RUQ	right upper quadrant
HAV	hepatitis A virus		

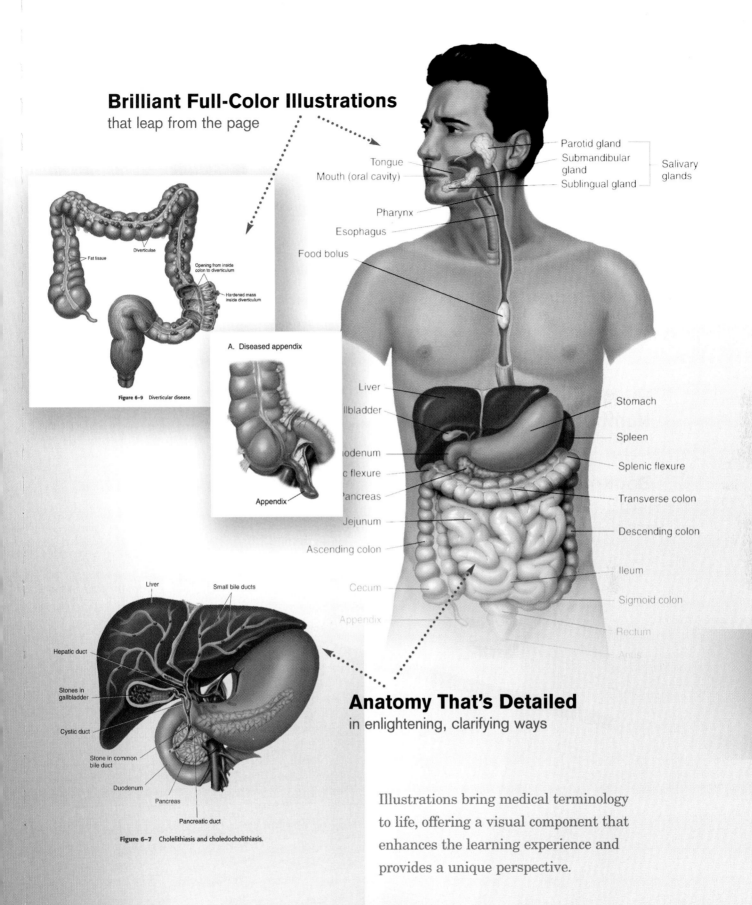

Brilliant Full-Color Illustrations
that leap from the page

Tongue
Mouth (oral cavity)

Parotid gland
Submandibular gland
Sublingual gland

Salivary glands

Pharynx
Esophagus
Food bolus

Diverticulae
Fat tissue
Opening from inside colon to diverticulum
Hardened mass inside diverticulum

Figure 6–9 Diverticular disease.

A. Diseased appendix

Liver
llbladder
iodenum
c flexure
ancreas
Jejunum
Ascending colon
Cecum
Appendix

Stomach
Spleen
Splenic flexure
Transverse colon
Descending colon
Ileum
Sigmoid colon
Rectum
Anus

Appendix

Liver
Small bile ducts
Hepatic duct
Stones in gallbladder
Cystic duct
Stone in common bile duct
Duodenum
Pancreas
Pancreatic duct

Figure 6–7 Cholelithiasis and choledocholithiasis.

Anatomy That's Detailed
in enlightening, clarifying ways

Illustrations bring medical terminology
to life, offering a visual component that
enhances the learning experience and
provides a unique perspective.

...A Unique Blend of Words and Art

The Programmed Learning Approach

encourages students to write out the medical terminology to reinforce learning and increase retention

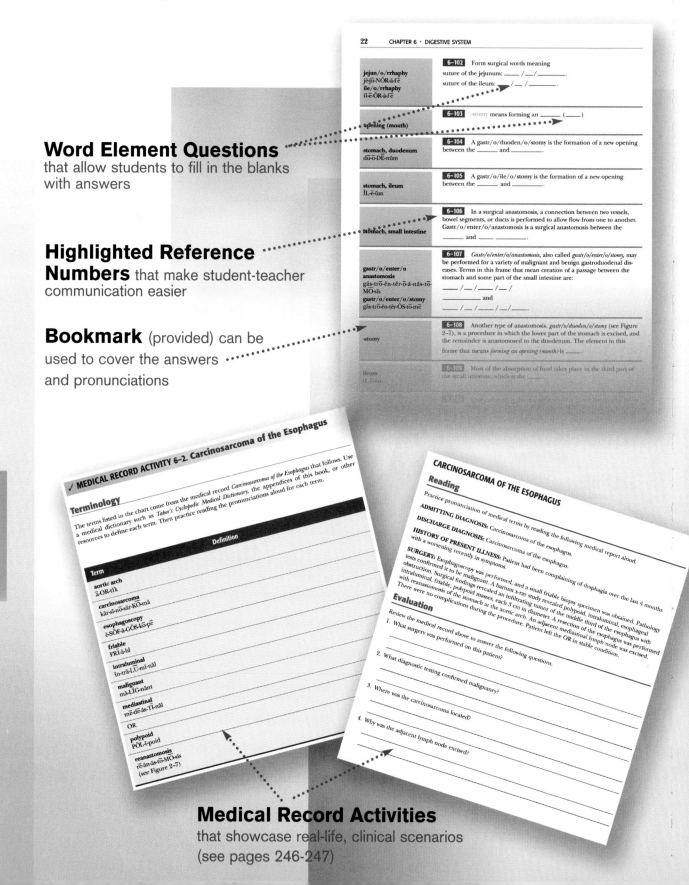

Word Element Questions

that allow students to fill in the blanks with answers

Highlighted Reference Numbers that make student-teacher communication easier

Bookmark (provided) can be used to cover the answers and pronunciations

Medical Record Activities

that showcase real-life, clinical scenarios (see pages 246-247)

Worksheets Containing Exercises and Activities
are featured in each chapter, to help track progress and
review for quizzes and tests (see pages 210 and 242)

Packages available with **Interactive Medical
Terminology 2.0** on CD-ROM. Designed to be
used in tandem with the text, this interactive software
helps students master medical terminology. IMT 2.0
includes:

- Nearly 1,200 test items
- Choice of basic or advanced
  testing modes
- Interactive exercises such as
  crossword puzzles, word drag-
  and-drop, and word scrambles
- Comprehensive score
  reporting for each exercise

F.A. Davis Company
1915 Arch Street
Philadelphia, PA 19103
www.fadavis.com

Copyright © 2005 by F.A. Davis Company

Printed in the United States of America

Last digit indicates print number: 10 9 8 7 6 5 4 3 2

Acquisitions Editor: Andy McPhee
Developmental Editor: Julie Munden
Art and Design Manager: Joan Wendt

As new scientific information becomes available through basic and clinical research, recommended treatments and drug therapies undergo changes. The author(s) and publisher have done everything possible to make this book accurate, up to date, and in accord with accepted standards at the time of publication. The author(s), editors, and publisher are not responsible for errors or omissions or for consequences from application of the book, and make no warranty, expressed or implied, in regard to the contents of the book. Any practice described in this book should be applied by the reader in accordance with professional standards of care used in regard to the unique circumstances that may apply in each situation. The reader is advised always to check product information (package inserts) for changes and new information regarding dose and contraindications before administering any drug. Caution is especially urged when using new or infrequently ordered drugs.

Library of Congress Cataloging-in-Publication Data

Gylys, Barbara A.
  Medical terminology simplified : a programmed learning approach by body systems/Barbara A. Gylys, Regina M. Masters.—3rd ed.
    p. ; cm.
  Includes index.
  ISBN 10: 0-8036-1254-0   ISBN 13: 978-0-8036-1254-9
  1. Medicine—Terminology—Programmed instruction.
  [DNLM: 1. Terminology—Programmed Instruction. W 15 G996m 2005] I. Masters, Regina M., 1959-II. Title.
  R123. G935 2005
  610′.1′4—dc22

                                                                                2005002868

This book is dedicated with love

■ ■ ■ ■ ■

to my best friend, colleague,
and husband, Julius A. Gylys

and

to my children,
Regina Maria
and Julius A., II

and

to Andrew,
Julia, Caitlin, Anthony,
and Matthew

—Barbara Gylys

to my mother, best friend,
mentor, and co-author,
Barbara A. Gylys

and

to my father, Julius A. Gylys

and

to my husband, Bruce Masters,
and my children, Andrew,
Julia, and Caitlin, all of
whom have given me continuous
encouragement and support.

—Regina Masters

Acknowledgments

The third edition of *Medical Terminology Simplified* was greatly improved by comments that the authors received from the many users of previous editions—both educators and students. Though there are too many people to acknowledge individually, we are deeply grateful to each one. As in the past, the editorial and production staffs at F.A. Davis have inspired, guided, and shaped this project.

- Andy McPhee, Acquisitions Editor, who provided the overall design and layout for the third edition. Although he doesn't quite acknowledge his talents, he was instrumental in helping the authors design a wide variety of pedagogical devices within the text to aid students in their learning activities and to help instructors plan course work and presentations. These teaching aids are described in the "Supplemental Teaching Aids" section of the Preface.
- **Susan Rhyner, Manager of Creative Development,** whose expertise and care are evident in the quality of support staff she selected for the third edition. We are especially grateful that she was on board for the developing stages of the textbook. We will remember her continued support of this project and thank her for "planting a few seeds of creativity" that are evident in both the textbook and Activity Pack.
- **Margaret Biblis, Publisher,** who once again provided "behind-the-scenes" efforts that are evident in the quality of the finished product.
- **Julie Munden, Developmental Editor,** who systematically and meticulously read the manuscript, helping it along at every stage. Her patience, creativity, and untiring assistance and support during this project were greatly appreciated, and the authors are grateful for all of her help.
- **Anne Rains, Artist,** who developed high-quality illustrations throughout the textbook. Her ability to capture in line and color the words and concepts envisioned by the authors is outstanding. The authors wish to acknowledge her artistic talents and thank her for being a part of this project.

We also acknowledge and thank our exceptionally dedicated publishing partners who helped guide and shape this large project:

- Robert Butler, Production Manager
- Mimi McGinnis, Managing Editor
- Joan Wendt, Art and Design Manager
- Jack Brandt, Illustrations Specialist
- Kirk Pedrick, Senior Developmental Editor, Electronic Publishing
- Frank Musick, Associate, Electronic Publishing
- Melissa Reed, Assistant Editor of Development
- Kimberly Harris, Administrative Assistant.

We thank my former colleague, James A. Van Fleet, PhD, Professor Emeritus of The University of North Carolina, for editing the Spanish appendix.

In addition, we also extend our deepest gratitude to the following students:

- Julia M. Masters, pre-med student at Miami University in Miami, who worked through the entire final copy of the textbook, evaluated the question bank, assisted in the audio recording template, and provided detailed suggestions for improving the textbook.
- Andrew R. Masters, student at Miami University in Oxford, Ohio, who also worked through the final copy of the text and provided invaluable feedback to the authors.

Last, we extend our sincerest gratitude to Neil Kelly, Director of Sales, and his staff of sales representatives, whose continued efforts have undoubtedly contributed to the success of this textbook.

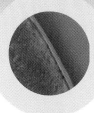

Reviewers

We were very fortunate to have a knowledgable and hard-working panel of reviewers, whose forthright criticisms and helpful suggestions added immeasurably to the quality of the final text. The review panel for the third edition included:

Lisa Morris Bonsall, RN, MSN, CRNP
Independent Clinical Consultant
West Chester, Pennsylvania

Peg Calvert
Assistant Professor and Academic
Coordinator of Clinical Education
Department of Physical Therapy
Saint Francis University
Loretto, Pennsylvania

John Clouse, MSR, RT(R)
Associate Professor
Department of Radiography
Owensboro Community College
Owensboro, Kentucky

Collette Bishop Hendler, RN, BS, CCRN
Clinical Leader, Intensive Care Unit
Abington Memorial Hospital
Abington, Pennsylvania

Cindy Konrad, RN, MS
Associate Professor
Health Management Department
Ferris State University
Big Rapids, Michigan

Marie L. Kotter, PhD, MS, BS
Professor and Chairperson
Health Sciences
Weber State University
West Ogden, Utah

Kay A. Nave, CMA/MRT
Program Director, Medical Assisting
Program
Medical Department
Hagerstown Business College
Hagerstown, Maryland

Karen R. Snipe, CPhT, AS, BA, MAEd
Coordinator, Pharmacy Technician Program
Allied Health Department
Trident Technical College
Charleston, South Carolina

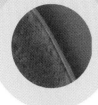

Preface

The third edition of *Medical Terminology Simplified: A Programmed Learning Approach by Body Systems* continues to reflect current trends and new approaches to teaching medical terminology. It remains a self-instructional book that can also be used in the traditional lecture and classroom environment. The organization and pedagogical devices of this text are designed to help you learn medical terminology easily and quickly. Use the teaching tools provided and you will find the more active you are in your studies, the better you learn and the more enjoyable the language of medicine becomes.

All of the enhancements and new material in the third edition are constructed to make learning easier and at the same time improve retention. One of the most outstanding features of this edition is the extraordinary collection of all-new, visually outstanding, full-color illustrations. They are extremely useful as you learn the association of medical terms to anatomy, physiology, pathology, and medical treatments of the human body. All of the artwork is designed to present precise and well-composed depictions of medical terms in action. Full color in the figures enables you to see a true representation of the body system, pathological condition, and operative procedure.

The most effective method of learning medical terminology is to understand the terms in their appropriate relationship to the human body. This includes having an understanding of anatomy and physiology, the types of treatments used to cure various disorders, and the disease processes of the human body—all of which are covered in this textbook.

Another new feature of the third edition is the omission of possessive forms of all eponyms (names of diseases or disorders named after someone). For instance, we've changed *Bowman's capsule* to *Bowman capsule, Cushing's syndrome* to *Cushing syndrome,* and *Parkinson's disease* to *Parkinson disease.* Many medical dictionaries, as well as the American Association for Medical Transcription and the American Medical Association, support these changes. The third edition also contains updated, comprehensive lists of medical abbreviations and their meanings, including a "do not use" abbreviations list mandated by the Joint Commission on Accreditation of Healthcare Organizations.

In addition, all outdated medical terms have been replaced with the most recent, state-of-the-art terms. To develop a contemporary teaching-and-learning package, the authors have implemented a number of insightful suggestions from numerous educators and students. Each body system chapter was updated to include:

- Newly developed objectives at the beginning of each chapter help you understand what is essential in the chapter. The reviews and activities are linked directly to these objectives, so you can better evaluate your competency in each area. If you have not mastered a certain area, you might use the objectives as a study instrument to help you improve your understanding of the chapter.
- Each chapter has a newly designed and more effective preview of word elements, along with a section review and competency verification to ensure maximum retention of medical terms.
- *Listen-and-Learn* audio CD exercises will help you master the pronunciation, spelling, and meanings of selected medical terms. Learning the key terms is most effective

when used with the audio recordings that accompany the textbook. The audio recordings can also be used to begin developing transcription skills.

- An enhanced pathology section, as well as a newly developed diagnostic and therapeutic section, will help you learn the clinical application of these new terms.
- Flash card activities are included throughout the textbook. The cards present a quick and effective way to review medical word elements and their meanings.
- Pronunciations are now included for medical records terminology, including many more pronunciations throughout each chapter. In addition, more than 200 terms from the Medical Records activities are now online. Visit the Listen and Learn Online! section for this book at www.fadavis.com/gylys/simplified to hear these terms.

Teaching and Learning Package

A substantial number of supplemental teaching aids are available free of charge to instructors who adopt the third edition of *Medical Terminology Simplified*. These supplementary teaching materials are designed to aid students in their learning activities and to help instructors plan course work and presentations. After these supplements are integrated into course content, instructors will find that the various supplements provide a sound foundation for learning and help guarantee a full program of medical terminology excellence for all of your students.

Instructor's Resource Disk

The Instructor's Resource Disk (IRD) features new and familiar teaching aids, created to make your teaching job easier and more effective than ever. The supplemental teaching aids on the IRD can be used in various educational settings- traditional classroom, distance learning, or independent studies. The IRD consists of an Activity Pack, *three* PowerPoint® presentations, and a Brownstone computerized test bank, a powerful test-generation program.

Activity Pack: Your Instructional Resource Kit

The Activity Pack* provides instructional support for using the textbook. It contains an abundance of information and resources to help students retain what they have learned in a given chapter. It will also help you plan course work and presentations. These supplementary materials include:

- *Question Bank.* The questions and answers in this section are taken from the *Brownstone Computerized Test Bank* found elsewhere on the IRD. The multiple-choice questions here offer only a small sample of the more than 700 test items available in the Brownstone test bank. Besides multiple-choice questions, the test bank also includes short answer and vocabulary questions. These items are available for every chapter in the text. A special feature of the multiple-choice questions is that they emulate the testing format used on many allied health national board examinations. This helps your students become better qualified to answer those types of questions.
- *Anatomical Illustrations.* This new feature for each body system will help your students reinforce their understanding of anatomical structures introduced in the chapter. A template is provided for each illustration so you can use the illustration as a review exercise or testing device.
- *Suggested Course Outlines.* Course outlines are included to help you determine a comfortable pace and plan the best method of covering the material presented.

---

*Activity Pack: Your Instructional Resource Kit is available in hard copy on request for those who adopt the textbook.

- *Practical, Clinical, and Research Activities.* A variety of newly-developed practical, clinical, and research application activities are included in this edition. These activities integrate a clinical connection as a solid reinforcement of content. Feel free to select activities you deem suitable for your course and decide whether an activity is to be completed independently, with peers, or as a group project. The clinical connection exercises help your students understand how medical terms are used in clinical discussions.

The practical application activities reinforce the spelling, pronunciation, and application of medical terminology in chart notes. Last, the research application activities will help your students understand the important role medical terminology plays in medical research. Included in this section are research projects related to the health-care industry. Your students will have an opportunity to hone their research skills by completing oral or written projects. These projects are also useful as an introductory element for exploring and then becoming members of professional organizations. A class visit to a meeting of a professional organization's local chapter can help students understand the significance of developing research skills and how they affect the profession. An evaluation template for research projects can be found in the Activity Pack.

- *Community and Internet Resources.* This section contains updated and expanded resources that offer a rich supply of technical journals, community organizations, and Internet resources to supplement classroom, internet, and oral and written projects.
- *Supplemental Medical Record Activities.* In addition to updating the medical record activities from the previous edition, we've added supplemental activities for each of body system chapter. As in the textbook, these medical record activities use common clinical scenarios to show how medical terminology is used in the clinical area to document patient care. Activities for terminology, pronunciation, and medical record analyses are provided for each medical record, along with an answer key (in the Activity Pack). In addition, each medical record focuses on a specific medical specialty. These records can be used for group activities, oral reports, medical coding activities, or individual assignments. The medical records are designed to reinforce and enhance terminology presented in the textbook.
- *Crossword Puzzles.* These fun, educational activities are included for each body system chapter. They're designed to reinforce material covered in the chapter and can be used individually or in a group activity. They can also be used to provide extra credit or "just for fun." An answer key is included for each puzzle.
- *Terminology Answer Keys.* In response to requests we've received from instructors like you, this section provides the answers to the *Terminology* activities in the medical records sections of the textbook. This added feature provides instructional support in using the textbook and assists the instructor in correcting terminology assignments.
- *Master Transparencies.* The transparency pages offer large, clear, black-and-white medical illustrations from selected figures in the text and have been chosen for their value as a testing device in reinforcing lecture information. They are perfect for making overhead transparencies or anatomical test questions and are provided for each body system.

PowerPoint Presentations

This edition of *Simplified* contains not one but *three* PowerPoint presentations for your use:

- *Lecture Notes* provides an outline-based presentation for each body system chapter. It consists of a chapter overview, the main functions and structures of the body system, and selected pathology, vocabulary, and procedures for each. Full-color illustrations from the textbook are included.
- *Illus-Station* contains most illustrations from the text, with one illustration per slide.
- *Med TERMinator* is an interactive presentation in which key terms from a chapter swoop into view each time the presenter clicks the mouse. You can ask students to say

the term aloud, define the term, identify the suffix, prefix, combining form, or combining element in each term, or provide other feedback before advancing to the next term.

Brownstone Electronic Test Bank

An updated, powerful Brownstone test bank allows you to create custom-generated or randomly-selected tests in a printable format from more than 700 multiple-choice, short answer, and matching test items. The program requires Windows 95, Windows 98, or Windows NT and is available for Macintosh on request.

Audio CDs

Two audio CDs are included free of charge in each textbook. These audio CDs contain *Listen-and-Learn* exercises designed to strengthen spelling, pronunciation, and meanings of selected medical terms. They include pronunciation and spelling exercises for each body system chapter. The exercises provide continuous reinforcement of correct pronunciation, spelling, and usage of medical terms.

The audio CDs can also be used for students in beginning transcription courses. Medical secretarial and medical transcription students can use the CDs to learn beginning transcription skills by typing each word as it is pronounced. After the words are typed, spelling can be corrected by referring to either the textbook or a medical dictionary such as *Taber's Cyclopedic Medical Dictionary*.

Interactive Medical Terminology 2.0

Interactive Medical Terminology 2.0 (IMT), a powerful interactive CD-ROM program, comes with the text, depending on which version you've chosen. IMT is a competency-based, self-paced, multimedia program that includes graphics, audio, and a dictionary culled from *Taber's Cyclopedic Medical Dictionary*, 19th edition. Help menus provide navigational support. The software comes with numerous interactive learning activities, including:

- word-building and word-breakdown activities
- drag-and-drop anatomical exercises
- word search puzzles
- word scrambles
- crossword puzzles.

The exercises throughout are designed at a 90% competency level, providing immediate feedback on student competency. Students can also print their progress as they go along. The CD-ROM is especially valuable as a distance-learning tool because it provides evidence of student drill and practice in various learning activities.

Taber's Cyclopedic Medical Dictionary

The world-famous *Taber's Cyclopedic Medical Dictionary* is the recommended companion reference for this book. Most of the terms in the third edition of *Simplified* may be found in *Taber's*. In addition, *Taber's* contains etymologies for nearly all main entries presented in this textbook.

How to Use This Book

This self-instructional book is designed to provide you with skills to learn medical terminology easily and quickly. The following distinctive features are included in this learning package:

- The programmed learning approach presents a word-building method for developing a medical vocabulary in an effective and interesting manner. It can be used in a traditional classroom setting or with an instructor for independent study.
- The workbook-text format is designed to guide you through exercises that teach and reinforce medical terminology.
- Numerous activities in each unit are designed to enable you to be mentally and physically involved in the learning process. With this method you not only understand but also remember the significant concepts of medical word building.
- You learn by active participation. You write answers in response to blocks of information, complete section review exercises, and analyze medical reports. After the review exercises, reinforcement frames will direct you—if you are not satisfied with your level of comprehension—to go back and rework the corresponding informational frames.
- You can make flash cards for the word elements in the chapter. Use the flash cards to reinforce your retention of word elements. First, compile the flash cards for the word elements included in the review you are completing, and review those elements. Then complete and correct the review. Follow this procedure each time you are ready to complete a review. The flash cards can also be used before you complete the Chapter Review exercises at the end of each chapter.
- The *Listen-and-Learn* exercises provide reinforcement of pronunciation, definitions, and spelling practice of medical terms.
- Pronunciation keys for all medical words are included in the frame answer boxes. The pronunciation guidelines on the inside front cover of this book show you how to interpret the keys.
- The appendices are useful for study, review, and reference as you begin your career in the allied health field.

Appendix A: Glossary of Medical Word Elements contains alphabetical lists of medical word elements with corresponding meanings.

Appendix B: Answer Key provides answers to labeling and chapter exercises.

Appendix C: Diagnostic and Therapeutic Procedures includes diagnostic and therapeutic procedures used to establish a diagnosis and determine treatment.

Appendix D: Drug Classifications provides information on prescription and nonprescription agents used for the treatment of various medical conditions.

Appendix E: Abbreviations lists commonly used medical abbreviations and their meanings.

Appendix F: Medical Specialties provides a summary and description of medical specialties.

Appendix G: Spanish Translations is a newly developed appendix of English-Spanish vocabulary and phrases relevant to each body system or medical specialty. It is intended to help health-care providers who do not speak Spanish but who encounter Spanish-speaking patients.

We hope you enjoy and profit from *Medical Terminology Simplified*. We also trust that this book makes learning the language of medicine an exciting and rewarding process. Keep in mind that learning medical terminology will be a valuable instrument in which you can interact more effectively in the health care environment.

Barbara A. Gylys
Regina M. Masters

Contents at a Glance

Chapter 1
Introduction to Programmed Learning and Medical Word Building   1

Chapter 2
Body Structure   23

Chapter 3
Integumentary System   59

Chapter 4
Respiratory System   99

Chapter 5
Cardiovascular and Lymphatic Systems   143

Chapter 6
Digestive System   195

Chapter 7
Urinary System   255

Chapter 8
Reproductive Systems   301

Chapter 9
Endocrine and Nervous Systems   357

Chapter 10
Musculoskeletal System   411

Chapter 11
Special Senses: The Eyes and Ears   463

Appendices

A p p e n d i x   A
Glossary of Medical Word Elements   **497**

A p p e n d i x   B
Answer Key   **505**

A p p e n d i x   C
Diagnostic and Therapeutic Procedures   **539**

A p p e n d i x   D
Drug Classifications   **547**

A p p e n d i x   E
Abbreviations   **551**

A p p e n d i x   F
Medical Specialties   **559**

A p p e n d i x   G
Spanish Translations   **563**

I n d e x   **575**
Pronunciation Guidelines   **Inside Front Cover**
Rules for Plural Suffixes   **Inside Back Cover**

ımed Learning and Medical Word Building   1

3

ιs   15
16
17
19
minutive Suffixes   19

22

27
ody   27

35

37

drants   41
ons   42
4   46

stic, and Therapeutic Terms   47

gnostic, and Therapeutic Terms Review   52

ummary   54

Word Elements Review   56
Chapter 2 Vocabulary Review   58

Chapter 3
Integumentary System   59

Objectives   59
Word Elements   61
    Section Review 3–1   63
Skin   64
Accessory Organs of The Skin   70
    Section Review 3–2   74
Combining Forms Denoting Colors   75
Cells   75
Other Related Terms   78
    Section Review 3–3   81
Abbreviations   82
Pathological, Diagnostic, and Therapeutic Terms   82
    Pathological   82
    Diagnostic   86
    Therapeutic   86
    Pathological, Diagnostic, and Therapeutic Terms Review   87
    Primary and Secondary Lesions Review   89
Medical Record Activities   90
    Medical Record Activity 3–1 Compound Nevus   90
    Medical Record Activity 3–2 Psoriasis   92
Chapter Review   94
    Word Elements Summary   94
    Word Elements Review   96
Chapter 3 Vocabulary Review   98

Chapter 4
Respiratory System   99

Objectives   99
Word Elements   101
    Section Review 4–1   104
Respiratory System   104
    Upper Respiratory Tract   104
    Section Review 4–2   110
    Lower Respiratory Tract   111
    Section Review 4–3   125
Abbreviations   126
Pathological, Diagnostic, and Therapeutic Terms   126
    Pathological   126
    Diagnostic   129
    Therapeutic   129
    Pathological, Diagnostic, and Therapeutic Terms Review   131
Medical Record Activities   133
    Medical Record Activity 4–1 Papillary Carcinoma   133
    Medical Record Activity 4–2 Lobar Pneumonia   135
Chapter Review   137
    Word Elements Summary   137
    Word Elements Review   140
Chapter 4 Vocabulary Review   142

C h a p t e r   5
Cardiovascular and Lymphatic Systems   143

Objectives   143
Word Elements   145
   Section Review 5–1   147
Cardiovascular System   148
   Walls of the Heart   148
   Circulation and Heart Structures   150
   Blood Flow Through The Heart   154
   Heart Valves   159
   Section Review 5–2   161
   Conduction Pathway of The Heart   162
   Cardiac Cycle and Heart Sounds   164
Lymphatic System   169
Word Elements   170
   Section Review 5–3   171
   Section Review 5–4   175
Abbreviations   176
Pathological, Diagnostic, and Therapeutic Terms   177
   Pathological   177
   Cardiovascular System   177
   Lymphatic System   178
   Diagnostic   179
   Cardiovascular System   179
   Lymphatic System   180
   Therapeutic   180
   Cardiovascular System   180
   Pathological, Diagnostic, and Therapeutic Terms Review   182
Medical Record Activities   184
   Medical Record Activity 5–1 Myocardial Infarction   184
   Medical Record Activity 5–2 Cardiac Catheterization   186
Chapter Review   188
   Word Elements Summary   188
   Word Elements Review   190
Chapter 5 Vocabulary Review   193

C h a p t e r   6
Digestive System   195

Objectives   195
Word Elements   196
   Section Review 6–1   199
Oral Cavity, Esophagus, Pharynx, and Stomach   199
   Section Review 6–2   210
   Word Elements   211
   Section Review 6–3   213
Small and Large Intestine   213
   Section Review 6–4   224
Word Elements   225
   Section Review 6–5   226
Accessory Organs of Digestion: Liver, Gallbladder, and Pancreas   226
   Section Review 6–6   236
Abbreviations   237

Pathological, Diagnostic, and Therapeutic Terms   238
  Pathological   238
  Diagnostic   240
  Therapeutic   241
  Pathological, Diagnostic, and Therapeutic Terms Review   242
Medical Record Activities   244
  Medical Record Activity 6–1 Rectal Bleeding   244
  Medical Record Activity 6–2 Carcinosarcoma of The Esophagus   246
Chapter Review   248
  Word Elements Summary   248
  Word Elements Review   251
Chapter 6 Vocabulary Review   254

C h a p t e r   7
Urinary System   255

Objectives   255
Word Elements   257
  Section Review 7–1   259
Kidneys   259
  Section Review 7–2   266
Ureters, Bladder, Urethra   267
  Section Review 7–3   275
Nephron Structure   276
  Section Review 7–4   286
Abbreviations   287
Pathological, Diagnostic, and Therapeutic Terms   287
  Pathological   287
  Diagnostic   288
  Therapeutic   289
  Pathological, Diagnostic, and Therapeutic Terms Review   290
Medical Record Activities   291
  Medical Record Activity 7–1 Cystitis   291
  Medical Record Activity 7–2 Benign Prostatic Hypertrophy   293
Chapter Review   295
  Word Elements Summary   295
  Word Elements Review   298
Chapter 7 Vocabulary Review   300

C h a p t e r   8
Reproductive Systems   301

Objectives   301
Female Reproductive System   301
Word Elements   303
  Section Review 8–1   306
  Internal Structures   306
  Section Review 8–2   316
  External Structures   317
  Breasts   319
  Section Review 8–3   325
Male Reproductive System   326
Word Elements   327
  Section Review 8–4   329
  Section Review 8–5   337
Abbreviations   338

Pathological, Diagnostic, and Therapeutic Terms   338
   Pathological   338
   Female Reproductive System   338
   Male Reproductive System   340
   Sexually Transmitted Diseases   341
   Diagnostic   341
   Female Reproductive System   341
   Male Reproductive System   343
   Therapeutic   344
   Female Reproductive System   344
   Male Reproductive System   344
   Pathological, Diagnostic, and Therapeutic Terms Review   345
Medical Record Activities   347
   Medical Record Activity 8–1 Postmenopausal Bleeding   347
   Medical Record Activity 8–2 Bilateral Vasectomy   349
Chapter Review   351
   Word Elements Summary   351
   Word Elements Review   354
Chapter 8 Vocabulary Review   356

C h a p t e r   9
Endocrine and Nervous Systems   357

Objectives   357
Endocrine System   357
Word Elements   359
   Section Review 9–1   361
   Hormones   361
   Table 9–1 Hormones   363
   Pituitary Gland   364
   Table 9–2 Pituitary Hormones   368
   Thyroid Gland   369
   Table 9–3 Thyroid Hormones   371
   Section Review 9–2   373
   Parathyroid Glands   374
   Table 9–4 Parathyroid Hormone   374
   Adrenal Glands   375
   Table 9–5 Adrenal Hormones   376
   Pancreas (Islets of Langerhans)   378
   Table 9–6 Pancreatic Hormones   379
   Pineal and Thymus Glands   381
   Ovaries and Testes   381
   Section Review 9–3   383
Nervous System   384
Word Elements   385
   Section Review 9–4   387
   Section Review 9–5   391
Abbreviations   392
Pathological, Diagnostic, and Therapeutic Terms   393
   Pathological   393
   Endocrine System   393
   Nervous System   394
   Diagnostic   395
   Endocrine System   395
   Nervous System   395

Therapeutic   396
Pathological, Diagnostic, and Therapeutic Terms Review   397
Medical Record Activities   399
Medical Record Activity 9–1 Diabetes Mellitus   399
Medical Record Activity 9–2 Cerebrovascular Accident   401
Chapter Review   403
Word Elements Summary   403
Word Elements Review   406
Chapter 9 Vocabulary Review   408

Chapter 10
Musculoskeletal System   411

Objectives   411
Skeletal System   411
Word Elements   413
Section Review 10–1   416
Structure and Function of Bones   416
Section Review 10–2   423
Joints   424
Combining Forms Related to Specific Bones   425
Fractures and Repairs   428
Vertebral Column   429
Section Review 10–3   434
Muscular System   435
Word Elements   436
Section Review 10–4   438
Table 10–1 Types of Movements Produced by Muscles   440
Section Review 10–5   442
Abbreviations   443
Pathological, Diagnostic, and Therapeutic Terms   443
Pathological   443
Bones and Joints   443
Spinal Disorders   444
Muscular Disorders   446
Diagnostic   447
Therapeutic   447
Pathological, Diagnostic, and Therapeutic Terms Review   449
Medical Record Activities   451
Medical Record Activity 10–1 Degenerative, Intervertebral Disk Disease   451
Medical Record Activity 10–2 Rotator Cuff Tear, Right Shoulder   453
Chapter Review   456
Word Elements Summary   456
Word Elements Review   459
Chapter 10 Vocabulary Review   461

Chapter 11
Special Senses: The Eyes and Ears   463

Objectives   463
The Eye   463
Word Elements   464
Section Review 11–1   466
The Ear   473
Word Elements   474
Section Review 11–2   475
Section Review 11–3   479

Abbreviations   480
Pathological, Diagnostic, and Therapeutic Terms   480
   Pathological   480
   The Eye   480
   The Ear   482
   Diagnostic   483
   The Eye   483
   The Ear   484
   Therapeutic   484
   The Eye   484
   The Ear   485
   Pathological, Diagnostic, and Therapeutic Terms Review   486
Medical Record Activities   488
   Medical Record Activity 11–1 Retinal Detachment   488
   Medical Record Activity 11–2 Otitis Media   490
Chapter Review   492
   Word Elements Summary   492
   Word Elements Review   494
Chapter 11 Vocabulary Review   495

Appendices

A p p e n d i x   A
Glossary of Medical Word Elements   497

A p p e n d i x   B
Answer Key   505

A p p e n d i x   C
Diagnostic and Therapeutic Procedures   539

A p p e n d i x   D
Drug Classifications   547

A p p e n d i x   E
Abbreviations   551

A p p e n d i x   F
Medical Specialties   559

A p p e n d i x   G
Spanish Translations   563

I n d e x   5 7 5
Pronunciation Guidelines   Inside Front Cover
Rules For Plural Suffixes   Inside Back Cover

Introduction to Programmed Learning and Medical Word Building

OBJECTIVES

Upon completion of this chapter, you will be able to:

■ Learn medical terminology by using the programmed learning technique.

■ Identify and define the four elements that are used to build medical words.

■ Analyze and define the various parts of a medical term.

■ Apply the rules learned in this chapter to pronounce medical words correctly.

■ Apply the rules learned in this chapter to write the singular and plural forms of medical words.

Instructions

In the first few pages, you will learn the most efficient use of this self-instructional programmed learning approach.

First remove the sliding card and cover the left-hand answer column with it.

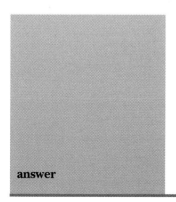

1-1   This text is designed to help you learn medical terminology effectively. The principal technique used throughout the book is known as programmed learning, which consists of a series of teaching units called *frames*.

Each frame presents information and calls for an answer on your part. When you complete a sentence by writing an answer on the blank line, you are learning information by using the programmed learning technique.

A frame consists of a block of information and a blank line. The purpose

answer   of the blank line is to write an _____.

1-2 Slide the card down in the left column to see the correct answer. After you correct the answer, read the next frame.

answer

1-3 It is important to keep the left-hand answer column covered until you write your _____.

learning

1-4 Several methods are employed in this book to help you master medical terminology, but the main technique used is called programmed _____.

answer(s)

1-5 After you write your answer, it is important to verify it is correct. To do this, compare your answer with the one listed in the left-hand answer column.

To obtain immediate feedback on your responses, you must verify your _____.

Study the frames in sequence because each frame builds on the previous one. Words are reviewed and repeated throughout the book to reinforce your learning. Consequently, you do not need to memorize every word that is presented.

one

1-6 The number of blank lines in a frame determines the number of words you write for your answer. Review the number of blank lines in Frame 1–5. It has _____ blank line(s). Therefore, the answer requires one word.

two

lines

1-7 A frame that requires two answers will have _____ blank _____.

1-8 In some frames, you will be asked to write the answer in your own words. In these instances, there will be one or more blank lines across the entire frame.

List at least two reasons why you want to learn medical terminology. Keep these objectives in mind as you work through the book.

_____

_____

Do not look at the answer column before you write your response and do not move ahead in a chapter. Progress in developing a medical vocabulary depends on your ability to learn the material presented in each frame.

frame

1-9 Completing one frame at a time is the most effective method of learning. To achieve your goal of learning medical terminology, complete one _____ at a time.

back	**1-10** Whenever you make an error, it is important to go back and review the previous frame(s). You need to determine why you wrote the wrong answer before proceeding to the next frame. You may always go _____ and review information you have forgotten. Just remember do not look ahead.
correct, check, *or* verify	**1-11** Do not be afraid to make a mistake. In programmed learning, you will learn and profit by your mistakes if you correct them immediately. Always _____ your answer immediately after you write it.
answer	**1-12** Because accurate spelling is essential in medicine, correct all misspelled words immediately. Do this by comparing your answer with the one in the left-hand _____ column.
correctly *or* accurately	**1-13** In medicine, it is important to spell correctly. Correct spelling can be a crucial component in determining the validity of evidence presented in a malpractice lawsuit. A physician can lose a lawsuit because of misspelled words that result in a misinterpreted medical record. To provide correct information, medical words must be spelled _____ in a medical record.

Medical Word Elements

A medical word consists of some or all of the following elements: *word root, combining form, suffix,* and *prefix.* How you combine these elements and whether all or some of them are present in a medical word determine the meaning of a word. The purpose of this chapter is to help you learn to identify these elements and use them to form medical terms.

suffix, prefix	**1-14** The four elements that are used to build a medical word are the word root, combining form, _____, and _____.
elements *or* parts	**1-15** Medical terminology is not difficult to learn when you understand how the *elements* are combined to form a word. To develop a medical vocabulary, you must understand the _____ that form medical words.

Word Roots

A *word root* is the main part or foundation of a word; all medical words have at least one word root.

teach	**1-16** In the words **teach**er, **teach**es, **teach**ing, the word root is _____.
speak	**1-17** In the words **speak**er, **speak**s, **speak**ing, the word root is _____.

1-18 Identify the roots in the following words:

Word	Root
reader	_____
spending	_____
playful	_____

read
spend
play

A word root may be used alone or combined with other elements to form another word with a different meaning.

ALERT

1-19 Review the following examples to see how roots are used alone or with other elements to form words.

The meaning of each term in the right-hand column is also provided.

Root as a Complete Word	Root as a Part of a Word
alcohol	**alcohol**ism condition marked by impaired control over alcohol use
sperm	**spermi**cide agent that kills sperm
thyroid	**thyroid**ectomy excision of the thyroid gland

1-20 Throughout the book, a slash is used to separate word elements, as shown in the following examples. Identify the word root in these examples:

alcohol alcohol/ic _____

dent dent/ist _____

lump lump/ectomy _____

insulin insulin/ism _____

gastr gastr/itis _____

1-21 In medical words, the root usually indicates a body part. For

cardi example, the root in cardi/al, cardi/ac, and cardi/o/gram is _____ and it means heart.

1-22 You will find that the roots in medical words are usually derived from Greek or Latin words. Some examples are **dent** in the word dent/ist, **pancreat** in the word pancreat/itis, and **dermat** in the word dermat/o/logist.

	Underline the roots in the following words:
dent/al DĔN-tăl **pancreat**/itis păn-krē-ă-TĪ-tĭs **dermat**/o/logist dĕr-mă-TŎL-ō-jĭst	**dent**/al **pancreat**/itis **dermat**/o/logist

	1-23 In Frame 1–22, the root **dent** means tooth, **pancreat** means
part	*pancreas,* and **dermat** means *skin.* All three roots indicate a body _____.

Combining Forms

A *combining form* is created when a word root is combined with a vowel. This vowel is usually an **o.** The vowel has no meaning of its own, but enables two word elements to be linked.

	1-24 Like the word root, the combining form is the basic foundation on which other elements are added to build a complete word. In this text, a combining form will be listed as word root/vowel, such as **dent/o** and **gastr/o.** A word root + a vowel (usually an **o**) forms a new element known as a
combining form	_____ _____.

	1-25 The combining form in therm/o/meter is _____ / __;
therm/o gastr/o	the combining form in gastr/o/scope is _____ / ____.

	1-26 **gastr/o** is an example of the word element called a
combining form gastr, o	_____ _____. The root in **gastr/o** is _____; the combining vowel is ____.

	1-27 List the combining vowel in each of the following elements:
o o o	**arthr/o** ____ **phleb/o** ____ **lith/o** ____

	1-28 Underline the word root in the following combining forms:
therm/o **abdomin**/o **nephr**/o	**therm**/o **abdomin**/o **nephr**/o

1-29 Use the combining vowel **o** to change the following roots to combining forms, and separate the elements with a slash.

Root	Combining Form (Root + Vowel)
cyst	_____
arthr	_____
leuk	_____
gastr	_____

cyst/o

arthr/o

leuk/o

gastr/o

1-30 Usually the combining vowel is an **o,** although other vowels may be encountered occasionally.

The combining vowel is usually an _____.

o

1-31 Instead of joining the two word roots **speed** and **meter** directly, the combining vowel **o** is attached to the root to form the word speed/o/meter. The vowel has no meaning of its own, but enables two elements to be connected to each other.

Use the combing vowel to build medical terms below. Therm/o/meter is an example that is completed for you.

Word Root	Suffix		Medical Term
therm	-meter	becomes	therm/o/meter
dermat	-logy	becomes	_____ / ___ / _____
encephal	-graphy	becomes	_____ / ___ / _____
neur	-logy	becomes	_____ / ___ / _____

therm/o/meter
thĕr-MŎM-ĕ-tĕr

dermat/o/logy
dĕr-mă-TŎL-ō-jē

encelphal/o/graphy
ĕn-sĕf-ă-LŎG-ră-fē

neur/o/logy
nū-RŎL-ō-jē

1-32 The words in Frame 1–31 are easier to pronounce because the word roots are linked with the combining vowel **o.** To make a word easier to pronounce, attach a combining _____ to the word root.

vowel

1-33 Even though you may or may not know the meaning of the words in this unit, you already have started to learn the word-building system by identifying the basic _____ of a medical word.

elements *or* parts

1-34 Using the word-building system will help you build an extensive medical vocabulary and also understand the meaning of medical terms.

By identifying the basic elements of a medical word, you are on your way to learning _____ terminology using the word-building system.

medical

1-35 In the word dermat/o/logy, the root is _____ ;
the combining form is _____ / ___ .

dermat

dermat/o

A combining form is used to link a root to another root to form a compound word. This holds true even if the next root begins with a vowel, as in *gastr/o/enter/itis.*

o	**1-36**　In the word gastr/o/enter/itis, the roots **gastr** *(stomach)* and **enter** *(intestine)* are linked together with the combining vowel _____.
leuk, cyt **-penia**	**1-37**　The roots in leuk/o/cyt/o/penia are _____ and _____. The suffix is _____.
leuk/o, cyt/o	**1-38**　Identify the combining forms in leuk/o/cyt/o/penia: _____ / _____ and _____ / _____.
electr/o, cardi/o	**1-39**　List the combining forms in electr/o/cardi/o/gram: _____ / _____ and _____ / _____.
back	**1-40**　You are now using the programmed learning method. If you are experiencing difficulty writing the correct answers, go back to Frame 1–1 and rework the frames. To master material that has been covered, you can always go _____ to review the frames.

Throughout the frames, word roots and combining forms that stand alone are in **bold,** suffixes that stand alone are preceded by a hyphen, and prefixes are followed by a hyphen.

Suffixes

A *suffix* is a word element located at the end of a word. Substituting one suffix for another suffix changes the meaning of the word. In medical terminology, a suffix usually indicates a procedure, condition, disease, or part of speech.

suffix	**1-41**　The element at the end of a word is called the _____.
play/er **read/er** **speak/er**	**1-42**　**Play, read,** and **speak** are complete words and also roots. Add the suffix -er (meaning *one who*) to each root to modify its meaning. **Play** becomes _____ / _____. **Read** becomes _____ / _____. **Speak** becomes _____ / _____.

	1-43 By attaching the suffix -er *(one who)* to **play, read,** and **speak,** we create nouns that mean the following:
	Play/er means one who plays.
one who	Read/er means _____ _____ reads.
one who	Speak/er means _____ _____speaks.

	1-44 By changing the suffix -er to -able *(capable of being)*, we create adjectives that mean the following:
capable of being	Play/able means _____ _____ _____ played.
capable of being	Speak/able means _____ _____ _____ spoken.
capable of being	Read/able means _____ _____ _____ read.

 A combining form (root + **o**) links a suffix that begins with a consonant.

1-45   Change the following roots to combining forms and link them with suffixes that begin with a consonant. Then practice pronouncing the terms aloud by referring to the pronunciations in the left-hand answer column.

	Word Root	**Suffix**		**Medical Term**
scler/o/derma sklĕr-ō-DĔR-mă	**scler**	-derma	becomes	_____ / ____ / _____
mast/o/dynia măst-ō-DĬN-ē-ă	**mast**	-dynia	becomes	_____ / ____ / _____
arthr/o/plasty ĂR-thrō-plăs-tē	**arthr**	-plasty	becomes	_____ / ____ / _____

 A word root links a suffix that begins with a vowel.

1-46   Link the following roots with suffixes, each of which begins with a vowel. Then practice pronouncing the terms aloud by referring to the pronunciations in the left-hand answer column.

	Word Root	**Suffix**		**Medical Term**
tonsill/itis tŏn-sĭl-Ī-tĭs	**tonsill**	-itis	becomes	_____ / _____
gastr/ectomy găs-TRĔK-tō-mē	**gastr**	-ectomy	becomes	_____ / _____
arthr/itis ăr-THRĪ-tĭs	**arthr**	-itis	becomes	_____ / _____

root, suffix	**1–47** Changing the suffix modifies the meaning of the word. In the word dent/al, **dent** is the word _____ and -al is the _____.

-ist **-al**	**1–48** A dent/ist is a specialist in teeth. Dent/al means pertaining to teeth. Simply changing the suffix has given the word a new meaning. The suffix in dent/ist is _____. It means specialist. The suffix in dent/al is _____. It means pertaining to or relating to.

hyphen	**1–49** Throughout the book, whenever a suffix stands alone, it will be preceded by a hyphen, as in -oma *(tumor)*. The hyphen indicates another element is needed to transform the suffix into a complete word. A suffix that stands alone will be preceded by a _____ .

A L E R T

Pronouncing medical words correctly in a clinical setting is crucial because mispronunciations can result in incorrect medical interpretations and treatments. In addition, misspelled terms in a medical report may become a legal issue. Learning how to pronounce and spell medical terms is a matter of practice. To familiarize yourself with medical words, make it a habit to pronounce a word aloud each time you see the pronunciation listed. Also, use the audio CD-ROM, *Listen and Learn,* to hear pronunciations of terms in the *Listen and Learn* sections (beginning in Chapter 3) of this book.

dent/<u>ist</u> DĔN-tĭst **arthr/o/<u>centesis</u>** ăr-thrō-sĕn-TĒ-sĭs **polyp/<u>oid</u>** PŎL-ē-poyd **angi/<u>oma</u>** ăn-jē-Ō-mă **gastr/<u>ic</u>** GĂS-trĭk **nephr/<u>itis</u>** nĕf-RĪ-tĭs **scler/o/<u>derma</u>** sklĕr-ō-DĔR-mă	**1–50** Underline the suffixes in the following words: **dent/ist** **arthr/o/centesis** **polyp/oid** **angi/oma** **gastr/ic** **nephr/itis** **scler/o/derma**

arthr/o, scler/o **dent, polyp, angi,** **gastr, nephr**	**1–51** The element preceding a suffix can be either a word root or a combining form. Review Frame 1–50 and identify the following. The combining forms that precede the suffixes: _____ / ____ and _____ / ____. The roots that precede the suffixes: _____, _____, _____, _____, _____.

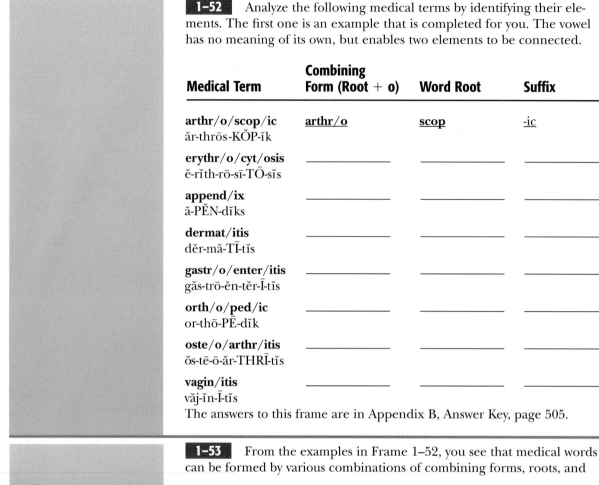

1-52 Analyze the following medical terms by identifying their elements. The first one is an example that is completed for you. The vowel has no meaning of its own, but enables two elements to be connected.

Medical Term	Combining Form (Root + o)	Word Root	Suffix
arthr/o/scop/ic ăr-thrōs-KŎP-ĭk	arthr/o	scop	-ic
erythr/o/cyt/osis ĕ-rĭth-rō-sī-TŌ-sĭs	_____	_____	_____
append/ix ă-PĔN-dĭks	_____	_____	_____
dermat/itis dĕr-mă-TĪ-tĭs	_____	_____	_____
gastr/o/enter/itis găs-trō-ĕn-tĕr-Ī-tĭs	_____	_____	_____
orth/o/ped/ic or-thō-PĒ-dĭk	_____	_____	_____
oste/o/arthr/itis ŏs-tē-ō-ăr-THRĪ-tĭs	_____	_____	_____
vagin/itis văj-ĭn-Ī-tĭs	_____	_____	_____

The answers to this frame are in Appendix B, Answer Key, page 505.

1-53 From the examples in Frame 1–52, you see that medical words can be formed by various combinations of combining forms, roots, and

suffixes   _____.

Three Rules of Word Building

Rule 1: A word root links a suffix that begins with a vowel.
Rule 2: A combining form (root + **o**) links a suffix that begins with a consonant.
Rule 3: A combining form (root + **o**) links a root to another root to form a compound word. This holds true even if the next root begins with a vowel.

1-54 **Rule 1:** In the following examples, use a word root to link suffixes that begin with a vowel.

Word Root	Suffix	Medical Term
leuk	-emia	becomes _____ / _____
cephal	-algia	becomes _____ / _____
gastr	-itis	becomes _____ / _____
append	-ectomy	becomes _____ / _____

leuk/emia
loo-KĒ-mē-ă
cephal/algia
sĕf-ă-LĂL-jē-ă
gastr/itis
găs-TRĪ-tĭs
append/ectomy
ăp-ĕn-DĔK-tō-mē

1-55 **Rule 2:** In the following examples, use a combining form (root + **o**) to link the suffixes that begin with a consonant.

Word Root	Suffix		Medical Term
gastr	-scope	becomes	_____ / ___ / _____
men	-rrhea	becomes	_____ / ___ / _____
angi	-rrhexis	becomes	_____ / ___ / _____
ureter	-lith	becomes	_____ / ___ / _____

gastr/o/scope
GĂS-trō-skōp
men/o/rrhea
měn-ō-RĒ-ă
angi/o/rrhexis
ăn-jē-ō-RĔK-sĭs
ureter/o/lith
ū-RĒ-tĕr-ō-lĭth

1-56 **Rule 3:** Use a combining form to link a root to another root to form a compound word. This holds true even if the next root begins with a vowel.

In the following two examples, apply the rule, "Use a combining form (root + **o**) to link a root to another root to form a compound word."

oste + chondr + itis becomes

_____ / ___ / _____ / _____.

oste + chondr + oma becomes

_____ / ___ / _____ / _____.

In the following two examples, apply the rule, "Use a combining form (root + **o**) to link a root to another root to form a compound word. This holds true even if the next root begins with a vowel.

oste + arthr + -itis becomes

_____ / ___ / _____ / _____.

gastr + enter + itis becomes

_____ / ___ / _____ / _____.

oste/o/chondr/itis
ŏs-tē-ō-kŏn-DRĪ-tĭs

oste/o/chondr/oma
ŏs-tē-ō-kŏn-DRŌ-mă

oste/o/arthr/itis
ŏs-tē-ō-ăr-THRĪ-tĭs

gastr/o/enter/itis
găs-trō-ĕn-tĕr-Ī-tĭs

word root

1-57 Would you use a *word root* or a *combining form* as a link to the following suffixes: -algia, -edema, and -uria? _____ _____

1-58 Refer to the three rules of word building on page 10 to complete frames 1–58 to 1–62.

Form a word with **cardi** and -gram:

_____ / ___ / _____
(root)   (suffix)

Summarize the rule that applies in this frame.

Rule 2: _____

_____

cardi/o/gram
KĂR-dē-ō-grăm

Rule 2: A combining form (root + o) links a suffix that begins with a consonant.

carcin/oma
kăr-sĭ-NŌ-mă

Rule 1: A word root links a suffix that begins with a vowel

1-59 Form a word with **carcin** and -oma:

_____/_____
  (root)   (suffix)

Summarize the rule that applies in this frame.

Rule 1: _____

_____

_____

enter/o/cyst/o/plasty
ĕn-tĕr-ō-SĬS-tō-plăs-tē

Rule 3: A CF links a root to another root to form a compound word
Rule 2: A CF links a suffix that begins with a consonant.

1-60 Complete the following frames to reinforce the three rules of word building on page 10.

Build a medical word with enter + cyst + plasty:

_____ / _____ / _____ / _____ / _____.

Summarize the word building rules that apply in forming the above term. Use CF to denote combining form.

Rule 3: _____

_____

Rule 2: _____

_____

leuk/o/cyt/o/penia
loo-kō-sī-tō-PĒ-nē-ă

Rule 3: A CF links a root to another root to form a compound word.
Rule 2: A CF links a suffix that begins with a consonant.

1-61 Build a medical word with leuk + cyt + penia:

_____ / _____ / _____ / _____ / _____.

Summarize the word building rules that apply in forming the above term. Use CF to denote combining form.

Rule 3: _____

_____

Rule 2: _____

_____

erythr/o/cyt/osis
ĕ-rĭth-rō-sī-TŌ-sĭs

Rule 3: A CF links a root to another root to form a compound word.
Rule 1: A word root links a suffix that begins with a vowel.

1-62 Build a medical word with erythr + cyt + osis:

_____ / _____ / _____ / _____.

Summarize the word building rules that apply in forming the above term. Use CF to denote combining form.

Rule 3: _____

_____

Rule 1: _____

_____

root, suffix	**1-63** You may or may not already know the meaning of the suffixes listed in this chapter. It is not necessary for you to know what they mean yet. These terms and definitions are reviewed in later chapters. What is important now is that you understand how to identify the component parts (prefix, root, combining form, suffix) of a word. For example, in the term pancreat/itis, **pancreat** is the _____; -itis is the _____.
suffix	**1-64** Suffixes that indicate a part of speech are known as *grammatical suffixes*. A medical term can be changed from a noun to an adjective simply by changing the suffix. To modify the part of speech of a word, you change the _____.
pertaining to, relating to **specialist** **condition**	**1-65** See if you can define the following grammatical suffixes. If needed, refer to Appendix A, Glossary of Medical Word Elements. gastr/ic _____ dent/ist _____ pneumon/ia _____

Prefixes

A *prefix* is a word element located at the beginning of a word. Substituting one prefix for another prefix changes the meaning of the word. The prefix usually indicates a number, time, position, or negation. Many prefixes found in medical terminology also are found in the English language.

micro/cyte MĪ-krō-sīt	**1-66** In the term *macro/cyte,* macro- is a prefix meaning *large;* -cyte is a suffix meaning *cell.* A *macro/cyte* is a large cell. Change the prefix macro- to micro- *(small).* Now form a word meaning a small cell: _____ / _____
-al **post-** **nat**	**1-67** Post/nat/al refers the period after birth. Identify the elements that mean pertaining to, relating to: _____. after, behind: _____. birth: _____.
pre/nat/al prē-NĀ-tl	**1-68** Use pre- *(before)* to build a word meaning pertaining to (the period) before birth: _____/_____/_____.

prefix	**1-69** A word element located at the beginning of a word is a _____.

ALERT

Throughout the subsequent frames in this book, prefixes that stand alone are in pink, word roots and combining forms that stand alone are **bold**, and suffixes that stand alone are blue.

intra- **post-** **peri-** **pre-**	**1-70** Intra/muscul/ar, post/nat/al, peri/card/itis, and pre/operative are medical terms that contain prefixes. Determine the prefix in this frame that means in, within: _____ after: _____ around: _____ before, in front of: _____
prefix **root** **suffix**	**1-71** Whenever a prefix stands alone, it will be identified with a hyphen after it, as in hyper-, and will be highlighted pink. When it is part of a word, the prefix will not be highlighted, but a slash will separate it from the next element, as in hyper/tension. Analyze hyper/insulin/ism by identifying the elements. hyper- is a _____. **insulin** is a _____. -ism is a _____.
prefixes	**1-72** Hypo-, intra-, super-, and homo- are examples of word elements called _____.
post/operative pōst-ŎP-ĕr-ă-tĭv **after**	**1-73** Pre/operative designates the time before a surgery. By changing the prefix, you alter the meaning of the word. Build a word that designates the time after surgery. _____ / _____ Can you guess what post- in post/operative means? _____
post-, after **after**	**1-74** You will recognize many prefixes in medical terms because they are the same ones found in the English language. In the term post/mortem, the prefix is _____ and means _____. Post/mortem means _____ death.

pre- **before, before**	**1-75** In the term pre/mature, the prefix is _____ and means _____. Pre/mature means _____ maturity.	

Some words, such as mature and sex, also are used as suffixes. Examples are pre/mature and uni/sex. Other words might consist of just a prefix and a word root, as in pre/test and dis/charge.

1-76 Use the following word roots with the adjective ending -al to form words that mean *pertaining to*. The first word is an example that is completed for you.

Word Root	Medical Word	Meaning
rect	rect/al	pertaining to the rectum
dent	_____ / ____	_____ the teeth
gastr	_____ / ____	_____ the stomach
intestin	_____ / ____	_____ the intestines

dent/al, pertaining to
DĔN-tăl
gastr/al, pertaining to
GĂS-trăl
intestin/al, pertaining to
ĭn-TĔS-tĭn-ăl

Combinations of four elements are used to form medical words. These four elements are the *word root, combining form, suffix,* and *prefix.* Some words also can be used as suffixes. Other words may consist of just a prefix and a word root.

Pronunciation Guidelines

Although the pronunciation of medical words usually follows the same rules that govern the pronunciation of English words, some may be difficult to pronounce when first encountered. Selected terms in this book include phonetic pronunciation. In addition, pronunciation guidelines can be found on the inside front cover of this book. Use it whenever you need help with the pronunciation of medical words. Locate and study the pronunciation guidelines before proceeding with Section Review 1–1.

Review the pronunciation guidelines (located in the inside front cover of this book). Use it as reference when needed.

Underline one of the items within the parentheses to complete the sentence.

1. The diacritical mark ˘ is called a (breve, macron).
2. The diacritical mark ‾ is called a (breve, macron).
3. The macron (‾) above a vowel is used to indicate (short, long) vowel pronunciations.
4. The breve (˘) above a vowel is used to indicate the (short, long) vowel pronunciations.
5. When *pn* is in middle of a word, pronounce (only *p, n, pn*). Examples are ortho*pn*ea, hyper*pn*ea.
6. The letters *c* and *g* have a (hard, soft) sound before other letters. Examples are *c*ardiac, *c*ast, *g*astric, *g*onad.
7. When *pn* is at the beginning of a word, pronounce (only *p, n, pn*). Examples are *pn*eumonia, *pn*eumo-toxin.
8. When *i* is at the end of a word (to form a plural), it is pronounced like (*eye, ee*). Examples are bronch*i*, fung*i*, nucle*i*.
9. For *ae* and *oe*, only the (first, second) vowel is pronounced. Examples are burs*ae*, pleur*ae*, r*oe*ntgen.
10. When *e* and *es* form the final letter or letters of a word, they are often pronounced as (combined, separate) syllables. Examples are syncop*e*, systol*e*, appendi*ces*.

Competency Verification: Check your answers in Appendix B, Answer Key, page 506. If you are not satisfied with your level of comprehension, review the pronunciation guidelines (on the inside front cover of this book) and retake the review.

Correct Answers _____ × 10 = _____% Score

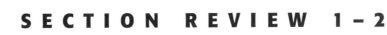

SECTION REVIEW 1–2

Identify the basic elements of each word in the appropriate box. Write the suffix first. Then write the element(s) in the first part(s) of the word. Lastly, write the element in the middle of the word. Remember, it is not important for you to know the meaning of the words in this chapter, but you should understand how to divide them into their basic elements. The first word is an example that is completed for you.

Medical Word and Meaning	Prefix	Combining Form(s) (root + vowel)	Word Root(s)	Suffix
BASIC ELEMENTS OF A MEDICAL WORD				
1. **peri / dent / al** around teeth pertaining to, relating to (pĕr-ĭ-DĔN-tăl)	*peri-*		*dent*	*-al*
2. **ab / norm / al** away normal, pertaining to, from usual relating to (ăb-NŌR-măl)				
3. **hepat / itis** liver inflammation (hĕp-ă-TĪ-tĭs)				
4. **supra / ren / al** above kidney pertaining to, relating to (soo-pră-RĒ-năl)				
5. **trans / vagin / al** through, vagina pertaining to, across relating to (trăns-VĂJ-ĭn-ăl)				
6. **gastr / o / intestin / al** stomach intestine pertaining to, relating to (găs-tr ō-ĭn-TĔS-tĭ-năl)				
7. **macro / cephal / ic** large head pertaining to, relating to (măk-rō-sĕf-ĂL-ĭk)				
8. **ren / o / pathy** kidney disease (rē-NŎP-ă-thē)				

(Continued)

		Basic Elements of a Medical Word *(Continued)*		
MEDICAL WORD AND MEANING	**PREFIX**	**COMBINING FORM(S) (ROOT + VOWEL)**	**WORD ROOT(S)**	**SUFFIX**
9. **therm/o/meter** heat instrument to measure (thēr-MŎM-ĕ-tĕr)				
10. **hepat/o/megaly** liver enlargement (hĕp-ă-tō-MĔG-ă-lē)				
11. **sub/stern/al** under, sternum pertaining to, below relating to (sŭb-STĔR-năl)				
12. **hypo/insulin/ism** under, insulin condition below, deficient (hī-pō-ĬN-sū-lĭn-ĭzm)				
13. **gastr/o/enter/o/pathy** stomach intestine disease (găs-trō-ĕn-tĕr-Ŏ-pă-thē)				
14. **arteri/o/scler/ osis** artery hardening abnormal condition (ăr-tē-rē-ō-sklĕ-RŌ-sĭs)				
15. **hypo/derm/ic** under, skin pertaining to, below, relating to deficient (hī-pō-DĔR-mĭk)				

Competency Verification: Check your answers in Appendix B, Answer Key, page 506. If you are not satisfied with your level of comprehension, review the terms in the table and retake the review.

Correct Answers _____ × 6.67 = _____% Score

SECTION REVIEW 1 – 3

Use the basic elements in Appendix B, Answer Key, Section Review 1–2, page 512, to form words, but first cover the left column, "Medical Word and Meaning." The first word is an example that is completed for you.

1. *peridental* _____
2. _____
3. _____
4. _____
5. _____
6. _____
7. _____
8. _____
9. _____
10. _____
11. _____
12. _____
13. _____
14. _____
15. _____

Competency Verification: Check your answers in Appendix B, Answer Key, page 507. If you are not satisfied with your level of comprehension, review the terms in the table and retake the review.

Correct Answers _____ × 6.67 = _____% Score

Adjective, Noun, and Diminutive Suffixes

Adjective and noun suffixes are attached to roots to indicate a part of speech; diminutive suffixes form a word designating a smaller version of the object indicated by the word root. Many of these suffixes are the same as those used in the English language. The adjective, noun, and diminutive suffixes are summarized below.

Suffix	Meaning	Word Analysis
ADJECTIVE		
-ac	pertaining to, relating to	cardi/ac (KĂR-dē-ăk): pertaining to the heart *cardi:* heart
-al		umbilic/al(ŭm-BĬL-ĭ-kăl): pertaining to the navel *umbilic:* umbilicus, navel
-ar		muscul/ar(MŬS-kū-lăr): pertaining to muscle *muscul:* muscle
-ary		pulmon/ary(PŬL-mō-nĕ-rē): pertaining to the lungs *pulmon:* lung
-eal		esophag/eal (ē-sŏf-ă-JĒ-ăl): pertaining to the esophagus *esophag:* esophagus
-ic		hepat/ic (hĕ-PĂT-ĭk): pertaining to the liver *hepat:* liver
-ical*		neur/o/log/ical (noor-ō-LŎJ-ĭk-ăl): pertaining to the study of nerves *neur/o:* nerve *log:* study of
-ile		pen/ile (PĒ-nĭl): pertaining to the penis *pen:* penis
-ior		anter/ior (ăn-TĬR-ē-or): pertaining to the front *anter:* anterior, front
-ous†		cutane/ous (kū-TĀ-nē-ŭs): pertaining to the skin *cutane:* skin
-tic		acous/tic (ă-KOOS-tĭk): pertaining to hearing *acous:* hearing
NOUN		
-esis	condition	di/ur/esis (dī-ū-RĒ-sĭs): abnormal secretion of large amounts of urine *di-:* double; *ur:* urine
-ia		pneumon/ia (nū-MŌ-nē-ă): infection of the lung usually caused by bacteria, viruses, or other pathogenic organisms *pneumon:* air, lung
-ism		hyper/thyroid/ism (hī-pĕr-THĪ-royd-ĭzm): condition characterized by overactivity of the thyroid gland *hyper-:* excessive, above normal *thyroid:* thyroid gland

Suffix	Meaning	Word Analysis
-iatry	medicine; treatment	pod/iatry (pō-DĪ-ă-trē): specialty concerned with treatment and prevention of conditions of the human foot *pod:* foot
-ist	specialist	dermat/o/log/ist‡ (dĕr-mă-TŎL-ō-jĭst): physician who specializes in treating skin disorders *dermat/o:* skin *log:* study of
DIMINUTIVE		
-y	condition, process	neur/o/path/y (nū-RŎP-ă-thē): any disease of the nerves *neur/o:* nerve *path:* disease
-icle	small, minute, little	ventr/icle (VĔN-trĭk-l): small cavity, as of the brain or heart *ventr:* belly, belly side
-ole		arteri/ole (ăr-TĒ-rē-ăl): minute artery; an arteriole is a terminal artery continuous with the capillary network *arteri:* artery
-ule		ven/ule (VĔN-ūl): tiny vein continuous with a capillary *ven:* vein

*-ical is a combination of -ic and -al.
†-ous also means composed of, producing.
‡when log + -ist is combined, it forms a new suffix -logist.

Plural Suffixes

Because many medical words have Greek or Latin origins, there are a few unusual rules you need to learn to change a singular word into its plural form. When you begin learning these rules, you will find that they are easy to apply. You also will find that some English word endings have been adopted for commonly used medical terms. When a word changes from a singular to a plural form, the suffix of the word is the part that changes. A summary of the rules for changing a singular word into its plural form is located on the inside back cover of this book. Use it to complete Section Review 1–4 below and whenever you need help forming plural words.

SECTION REVIEW 1 – 4

Write the plural form for each of the following words and state the rule that applies. The first word is an example that is completed for you.

Singular	Plural	Rule
1. sarcoma săr-KŌ-mă	sarcomata	Retain the *ma* and add *ta*
2. thrombus THRŎM-bŭs		
3. appendix ă-PĔN-dĭks		
4. diverticulum dī-vĕr-TĬK-ū-lŭm		
5. ovary Ō-vă-rē		
6. diagnosis dī-ăg-NŌ-sĭs		
7. lumen LŪ-mĕn		
8. vertebra VĔR-tĕ-bră		
9. thorax THŌ-răks		
10. spermatozoon spĕr-măt-ō-ZŌ-ŏn		

Competency Verification: Check your answers in Appendix B, Answer Key, page 507. If you are not satisfied with your level of comprehension, review the rules for changing a singular word into its plural form (on inside back cover of this book) and retake the review.

Correct Answers _____ × 10 = _____% Score

Body Structure

The human body consists of several levels of structure and function (see Figure 2–1). Each higher level incorporates the structures and functions of the previous level. The *cellular level* is the smallest structural and functional unit of the body. Groups of cells that perform a specialized function form the *tissue layer*. Groups of tissue that perform a specific function form the *organ level*, and groups of organs that are interconnected or that have similar or interrelated functions form the *system level*. Finally, the collection of body systems makes up the most complex level, the *organism level*—a human being.

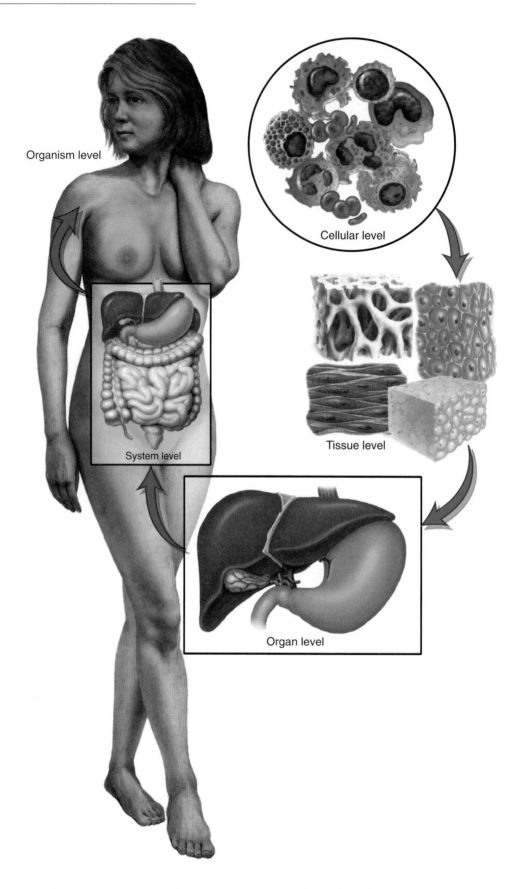

Organism level

Cellular level

Tissue level

System level

Organ level

Figure 2-1   Levels of structural organization of the human body shown from the basic unit of structure, the cellular level, to the most complex, the organism level.

Word Elements

This section introduces combining forms related to the basic structural units of the body and those that describe a particular location in the body. Key suffixes also are summarized in the following table. Other word elements are defined in the right-hand column as needed. Review the table, and pronounce each word in the word analysis column aloud before you begin to work the frames.

Word Element	Meaning	Word Analysis
COMBINING FORMS		
BASIC STRUCTURAL UNITS		
chondr/o	cartilage	chondr/oma (kŏn-DRŌ-mă): tumor composed of cartilage *-oma:* tumor
cyt/o	cell	cyt/o/meter (sī-TŎM-ĕ-ter): instrument for counting and measuring cells within a specified amount of fluid, such as blood, urine, or cerebrospinal fluid *-meter:* instrument for measuring
hist/o	tissue	hist/o/lysis (hĭs-TŎL-ĭ-sĭs): separation, destruction, or loosening of tissue *-lysis:* separation; destruction; loosening
nucle/o	nucleus	nucle/ar (NŪ-klē-ăr): pertaining to a cellular, atomic, or anatomical nucleus *-ar:* pertaining to, relating to
LOCATION		
anter/o	anterior, front	anter/ior (ăn-TĬR-ē-or): toward the front of the body, organ, or structure *-ior:* pertaining to, relating to
caud/o	tail	caud/ad (KAW-dăd): toward the tail; in a posterior direction *-ad:* toward
dist/o	far, farthest	dist/al (DĬS-tăl): pertaining to a point farthest from the center, a medial line or the trunk; opposed to proximal *-al:* pertaining to, relating to
dors/o	back (of body)	dors/al (DŌR-săl): pertaining to the back or posterior of the body *-al:* pertaining to, relating to
infer/o	lower, below	infer/ior (ĭn-FĒ-rē-or): toward the undersurface of a structure; underneath; beneath *-ior:* pertaining to, relating to
later/o	side, to one side	later/al (LĂT-ĕr-ăl): pertaining to the side *-al:* pertaining to, relating to
medi/o	middle	super/medi/al (soo-pĕr-MĒ-dē-ăl): above the middle of any part *super-:* upper, above *-al:* pertaining to, relating to

(Continued)

Word Element	Meaning	Word Analysis *(Continued)*
SUFFIXES		
poster/o	back (of body), behind, posterior	poster/ior (pŏs-TĒ-rē-or): pertaining to or toward the rear or caudal end *-ior:* pertaining to, relating to
proxim/o	near, nearest	proxim/al (PRŎK-sĭm-ăl): nearest the point of attachment, center of the body, or point of reference *-al:* pertaining to, relating to
ventr/o	belly, belly side	ventr/al (VĔN-trăl): pertaining to the belly side or front of the body *-al:* pertaining to, relating to
-ad	toward	medi/ad (MĒ-dē-ăd): toward the middle or center *medi-:* middle
-logist	specialist in study of	hist/o/logist (hĭs-TŎL-ō-jĭst): specialist in the study of tissue *hist/o:* tissue
-logy	study of	cyt/o/logy (sī-TŎL-ō-jē): study of cells *cyt/o:* cell
-lysis	separation; destruction; loosening	cyt/o/lysis (sī-TŎL-ĭ-sĭs): destruction or dissolution or separation of a cell *cyt/o:* cell
-toxic	poison	cyt/o/toxic (sī-tō-TŎKS-ĭk): substances that are detrimental or destructive to cells *cyt/o:* cell

SECTION REVIEW 2-1

For the following medical terms, first write the suffix and its meaning. Then translate the meaning of the remaining elements starting with the first part of the word. The first word is an example that is completed for you.

Term	Meaning
1. dist/al	-al: pertaining to, relating to; far, farthest
2. poster/ior	_____
3. hist/o/logist	_____
4. dors/al	_____
5. anter/ior	_____
6. later/al	_____
7. medi/ad	_____
8. cyt/o/toxic	_____
9. proxim/al	_____
10. ventr/al	_____

Competency Verification: Check your answers in Appendix B, Answer Key, page 508. If you are not satisfied with your level of comprehension, review the vocabulary and retake the review.

Correct Answers _____ × 10 = _____% Score

Organization of the Body

Cellular Level

2-1   Cells are the smallest living units of structure and function in the human body. Every tissue and organ in the body is composed of cells. Review the illustration depicting the cellular level in Figure 2–1.

Note the darkened area in the center, the nucleus, which is the control center of the cell and is responsible for reproduction. This spherical unit contains genetic codes for maintaining life systems of the organism and for issuing commands for growth and reproduction.

nucle/o

The combining form for nucleus is: _____ / _____.

	2-2 Any chemical substance, such as a drug that interferes with or destroys the cellular reproductive process in the nucleus, is referred to as a *nucle/o/toxic substance.* Examples of nucle/o/toxic drugs are those administered to cancer patients during chemotherapy.
	Identify the elements in this frame meaning
-toxic	poison: _____
nucle/o	nucleus: _____ / _____
cell	**2-3** Recall that **cyt/o** and -cyte are used to form words that refer to a _____.
cyt/o/logy sī-TŎL-ō-jē	**2-4** A cyt/o/logist is usually a biologist who specializes in the study of cells, especially one who uses cytologic techniques to diagnose neoplasms. Using cyt/o, build a word that means study of cells: _____ / _____ / _____.
cyt/o/logist sī-TŎL-ă-jĭst **cyt/o/lysis** sī-TŎL-ĭ-sĭs	**2-5** Use **cyt/o** to practice forming words that mean specialist in the study of cells: _____ / _____ / _____. dissolution or destruction of a cell: _____ / _____ / _____.
-logist **hist/o**	**2-6** At the tissue level, the structural organization of the human body consists of groups of cells working together to carry out a specialized activity (see Figure 2–1). The medical scientist who specializes in microscopic identification of cells and tissues is called a hist/o/logist. Identify the word elements in hist/o/logist that mean specialist in study of: _____ tissue: _____ / _____.
hist/o/logy hĭs-TŎL-ō-jē **cyt/o/logy** sī-TŎL-ō-jē	**2-7** Use -logy to form medical words meaning study of tissue: _____ / _____ / _____. study of cells: _____ / _____ / _____.

Directional Terms

The following frames introduce terms that describe regions of the body. Included are directional terms that describe a structure in relation to some defined center or reference point.

	2-8 Recall the suffixes -ac, -al, -ar, -iac, and -ior are adjective endings meaning *pertaining to, relating to.* You will find many words throughout this book that contain adjective suffixes. These suffixes help describe position, direction, body divisions, and body structures.

dors/al DŌR-săl **later/al** LĂT-ĕr-ăl **ventr/al** VĔN-trăl	Use the adjective ending -al to form words that mean pertaining to the back (of body): dors/_____. side, to one side: later/_____. belly, belly side: ventr/_____.

dors/al DŌR-săl **later/al** LĂT-ĕr-ăl **ventr/al** VĔN-trăl	**2–9** Practice building medical terms with **dors/o, later/o,** and **ventr/o.** Form medical terms that mean pertaining to or relating to the back (of body) _____ / _____. side, to one side _____ / _____. belly, belly side _____ / _____.

	2–10 The human body is capable of being in many different positions, such as standing, kneeling, and lying down. To guarantee consistency in descriptions of location, the *anatomic position* is used as a reference point to describe the location or direction of a body structure. In anatomic position, the body is erect and the eyes are looking forward. The arms hang to the sides, with palms facing forward; the legs are parallel with the toes pointing straight ahead. Review Figure 2–2 and study the terms to become acquainted with their usage in denoting positions of direction when the body is in the anatomic position. Refer to this figure to complete the following frames.

anatomic position ăn-ă-TŎM-ĭk	**2–11** When a person is standing upright facing forward, arms at the sides with palms forward, with the legs parallel and the feet slightly apart with the toes pointing forward, he or she is in the standard position called the _____ _____.

anter/ior, ventr/al ăn-TĬR-ē-or, VĔN-trăl **poster/ior, dors/al** pŏs-TĒ-rē-or, DŌR-săl	**2–12** In the anatomic position, the front (anter/ior and ventr/al) and the back (poster/ior and dors/al) consist of the largest divisions of the body. The term *anter/ior* is used to refer to the "front of the body" or the "front of any body structure." Identify the elements in this frame that refer to the front of the body: _____ / _____ and _____ / _____. back of the body: _____ / _____ and _____ / _____.

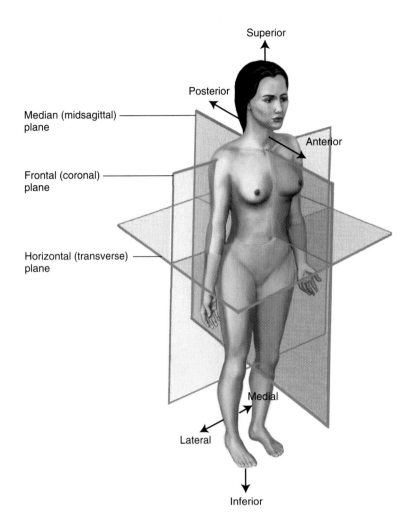

Figure 2-2   Body planes. Note the body is in the anatomic position.

front **back**	**2-13** What position of the body do the terms anter/ior and ventr/al refer to? _____ (of the body) What position of the body do the terms poster/ior and dors/al refer to? _____ (of the body)
-ior **poster/o** **anter**	**2-14** Poster/o/anter/ior refers to both the back and the front of the body. Identify the word elements in this frame that mean pertaining to, relating to: _____. back: _____ / _____. front: _____.

posterior, anterior
pŏs-TĒ-rē-or, ăn-TĬR-ē-or

2–15   Directional terms are commonly used in radiology to describe the direction of the x-ray beam from its source and its point of exit. In an anter/o/poster/ior projection, the beam enters the body anteriorly and exits posteriorly.

A poster/o/anter/ior projection indicates that the beam enters the body on the _____ side and exits on the _____ side.

anterior
ăn-TĬR-ē-or
posterior
pŏs-TĒ-rē-or

2–16   Use anterior or posterior to complete the following statements, which refer to the position of body structures.

The stomach is on the _____ side of the body.

The shoulder blades are on the _____ side of the body.

infer/ior
ĭn-FĒ-rē-or

2–17   Whereas the term *inferior* in the English language refers to something of little or less importance, when used in a medical report, it designates a position or direction meaning *lower or below.*

Combine **infer/o** *(lower, below)* + -ior *(pertaining to, relating to)* to form a directional term that literally means pertaining to lower or below.

_____ / _____.

above

2–18   In medical terms, the prefix super- designates an upper position. When you say "the head is superior to the stomach," you mean it is located above the stomach.

When you say "the eyes are superior to the mouth," you mean they are located _____ the mouth.

side

2–19   The word element **later/o** means *side, to one side.* A radiographic projection that enters through the left or right side of the body is referred to as a later/al projection.

The term later/al position refers to the _____(of the body).

!
A L E R T

Review the three basic rules for building medical words.

Rule 1: A word root links a suffix that begins with a vowel.

Rule 2: A combining form (root + **o**) links a suffix that begins with a consonant.

Rule 3: A combining form (root + **o**) links a root to another root to form a compound word. This holds true even if the next root begins with a vowel.

later/al LĂT-ĕr-ăl **anter/o/later/al** ăn-tĕr-ō-LĂT-ĕr-ăl **poster/o/later/al** pŏs-tĕr-ō-LĂT-ĕr-ăl	**2–20**　Here is a review of terms in radi/o/logy that specify direction of the x-ray beam from its source to its exit surface before striking the film. Build directional terms that mean pertaining to the side or to one side: _____ / _____ (of the body). pertaining to the anterior or front, and the side: _____ / ____ / _____ / _____ (of the body). pertaining to the posterior or back, and the side: _____ / ____ / _____ / _____ (of the body).
medi **-al**	**2–21**　Medi/al is used to describe the midline of the body or a structure. The medial portion of the face contains the nose. From the term medi/al, determine the following root meaning middle _____. suffix meaning pertaining to _____.
medi/ad MĒ-dē-ăd	**2–22**　Use -ad to form a directional medical term meaning toward the middle or center (of the body): _____ / _____.
-ad **medi** **medi/ad** MĒ-dē-ăd	**2–23**　The suffix for toward is _____, and the root for middle is _____. Combine these two elements to form a word that means toward the middle _____ / _____.
infer/ior ĭn-FĒ-rē-or **infer/ior** ĭn-FĒ-rē-or	**2–24**　Anatomists use the term infer/ior to refer to a body structure located below another body structure. They also use infer/ior to refer to the lower part of a structure. For example, your chin is situated infer/ior to your mouth (see Figure 2–2); the rectum is the infer/ior portion of the colon. To denote a structure is below another structure, use the directional term _____ / _____. To denote the lower part of a structure, use the directional term _____ / _____.
infer/ior ĭn-FĒ-rē-or **later/al** LĂT-ĕr-ăl	**2–25**　Practice using the directional terms later/al and infer/ior to describe the following positions: The legs are _____ / _____ to the trunk. The eyes are _____ / _____ to the nose.

cephal/ad SĔF-ă-lăd	**2-26** Anatomists use the term super/ior to refer to a body structure that is above another body structure or toward the head because the head is the most superior structure of the body. Cephal/ad is a term that refers to the direction toward the head. When referring to the direction going toward the head, use the term _____ / _____.
pertaining to, relating to **upper, above**	**2-27** Define the word elements in super/ior. -ior _____ _____, _____ _____. super- _____, _____.
superior soo-PĒ-rē-or **inferior** ĭn-FĒ-rē-or **superior** soo-PĒ-rē-or	**2-28** Use superior or inferior to complete the following statements that refer to the relative position of one body structure to another body structure. The chest is _____ to the stomach. The stomach is _____ to the lungs. The head is _____ to the neck.
caud/al KAWD-ăl	**2-29** The combining form **caud/o** means *tail*. In this sense, tail designates a position toward the end of the body away from the head. In humans, it also refers to an infer/ior position in the body or within a structure. Combine **caud** + -al to build a word that means relating to the tail: _____ / _____.
proxim/al PRŎK-sĭm-ăl **dist/al** DĬS-tăl	**2-30** The terms proxim/al and dist/al are used as positional and directional terms. **Proxim/al** describes a structure as being *nearest* the point of attachment to the trunk or near the beginning of a structure. **Dist/al** describes a structure as being *far from* the point of attachment to the trunk or from the beginning of a structure. Identify the terms in this frame that mean nearest the point of attachment: _____ / _____. farthest from the point of attachment: _____ / _____.
proxim/al PRŎK-sĭm-ăl	**2-31** The directional element **proxim/o** means *near or nearest* the point of attachment; **dist/o** means *far or farthest* from the point of attachment. The knee is proxim/al to the foot; the palm is dist/al to the elbow (see Figure 2–2). To describe a structure nearest the point of attachment, use the directional term _____ / _____.

dist/al DĬS-tăl	To describe a structure as being farthest from the point of attachment, use the directional term _____ / _____.

2–32   Use proxim/al or dist/al to designate the position of one structure to another structure.

proxim/al PRŎK-sĭm-ăl **proxim/al** PRŎK-sĭm-ăl **dist/al** DĬS-tăl	The wrist is _____ / _____ to the fingers. The ankle is _____ / _____ to the foot. The toes are _____ / _____ to the ankles.

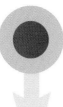

SECTION REVIEW 2-2

Using the following table, write the combining form or suffix that matches its definition in the space provided to the left of the definition. There may be more than one word element that matches a definition.

Combining Form	Suffix
caud/o	-ad
cyt/o	-al
dist/o	-ior
hist/o	-logist
infer/o	-logy
later/o	-lysis
medi/o	-toxic
proxim/o	
ventr/o	

1. _____ tissue
2. _____ pertaining to, relating to
3. _____ middle
4. _____ near, nearest
5. _____ study of
6. _____ cell
7. _____ belly, belly side
8. _____ poison

9. _____ toward
10. _____ tail
11. _____ specialist in study of
12. _____ far, farthest
13. _____ lower, below
14. _____ separation; destruction; loosening
15. _____ side, to one side

Competency Verification: Check your answers in Appendix B, Answer Key, page 508. If you are not satisfied with your level of comprehension, go back to Frame 2–1 and rework the frames.

Correct Answers _____ × 6.67 = _____% Score

Making a set of flash cards from key word elements in this chapter for each section review can help you remember the elements. Make a flash card by writing a word element on one side of a 3 × 5 or 4 × 6 index card. On the other side write the meaning of the element. Do this for all word elements in the section review. Use your flash cards to review each section. You also might use the flash cards to prepare for the chapter review at the end of this chapter.

Word Elements

This section introduces combining forms that describe a body structure. When these combining forms are attached to positional prefixes or suffixes, they form words that describe a region or position in the body. Review the following table and pronounce each word in the word analysis column aloud before you begin to work the frames.

Word Element	Meaning	Word Analysis
COMBINING FORMS		
BODY REGIONS		
abdomin/o	abdomen	abdomin/al (ăb-DŎM-ĭ-năl): pertaining to the abdomen *-al:* pertaining to, relating to
cephal/o	head	cephal/ad (SĔF-ă-lăd): toward the head *-ad:* toward
cervic/o	neck; cervix uteri (neck of uterus)	cervic/al (SĔR-vĭ-kăl): pertaining to the neck of the body or the neck of the uterus *-al:* pertaining to, relating to
crani/o	cranium (skull)	crani/al (KRĀ-nē-ăl): pertaining to the cranium or skull *-al:* pertaining to, relating to
gastr/o	stomach	gastr/ic (GĂS-trĭk): pertaining to the stomach *-ic:* pertaining to, relating to
ili/o	ilium (lateral, flaring portion of hip bone)	ili/ac (ĬL-ē-ăk): pertaining to the ilium *-ac:* pertaining to, relating to
inguin/o	groin	inguin/al (ĬNG-gwĭ-năl): pertaining to the groin *-al:* pertaining to, relating to
lumb/o	loins (lower back)	lumb/ar (LŬM-băr): pertaining to the loin area or lower back *-ar:* pertaining to, relating to
pelv/o	pelvis	pelv/ic (PĔL-vĭc): pertaining to the pelvis *-ic:* pertaining to, relating to
spin/o	spine	spin/al (SPĪ-năl): pertaining to the spine or spinal column *-al:* pertaining to, relating to
thorac/o	chest	thorac/ic (thō-RĂS-ĭk): pertaining to the chest *-ic:* pertaining to, relating to
umbilic/o	umbilicus, navel	peri/umbilic/al (pĕr-ē-ŭm-BĬL-ĭ-kăl): pertaining to the area around the umbilicus *peri-:* around *-al:* pertaining to, relating to

S E C T I O N   R E V I E W   2 – 3

For the following medical terms, first write the suffix and its meaning. Then translate the meaning of the remaining elements starting with the first part of the word. The first word is an example that is completed for you.

Term	Meaning
1. ili/ac	-ac: pertaining to, relating to; ilium (lateral, flaring portion of hip bone)
2. abdomin/al	_____
3. inguin/al	_____
4. spin/al	_____
5. peri/umbilic/al	_____
6. cephal/ad	_____
7. gastr/ic	_____
8. thorac/ic	_____
9. cervic/al	_____
10. lumb/ar	_____

Competency Verification: Check your answers in Appendix B, Answer Key, page 509. If you are not satisfied with your level of comprehenion, review the vocabulary and retake the review.

Correct Answers _____ × 10 = _____% Score

Body Planes

To visualize the structural arrangements of various organs, the body may be sectioned (cut) according to planes of reference. The three major planes are the frontal, median, and horizontal planes as shown in Figure 2–2. In addition, body cavities as shown in Figure 2–3 contain internal organs and are used as a point of reference to locate structures within body cavities.

	2-33 Review Figures 2–2 and 2–3 carefully before proceeding with the next frame. You may refer to the two figures to complete the following frames.
body plane	**2-34** A body plane is an imaginary flat surface that divides the body into two sections. Different planes divide the body into different sections, such as front and back, left side and right side, and top and bottom. These planes serve as points of reference for describing the direction from which the body is being observed. The planes are particularly useful to describe views in which radiographic images are taken.
	An imaginary flat surface that divides the body into two sections is a
	_____ _____.

median (midsagittal)
mĭd-SĂJ-ĭ-tăl
frontal (coronal)
kŏ-rō-năl
horizontal (transverse)
trăns-VĔRS

2-35 Examine Figure 2–2 and list the three major planes of the body.

_____ (_____)

_____ (_____)

_____ (_____)

When in doubt about the meaning of a word element, refer to Appendix A, page 497.

midsagittal plane
mĭd-SĂJ-ĭ-tăl plān

2-36 The _median (midsagittal)_ plane lies exactly in the middle of the body and divides the body into two equal halves (see Figure 2–2).

When the chest is divided into equal right and left sides, it is divided by the median plane, also known as the _____ _____.

median plane

2-37 When the lungs are divided into equal right and left sides, they are divided by the midsagittal plane, also known as the

_____ _____.

inferior
ĭn-FĒ-rē-or
superior
soo-PĒ-rē-or

2-38 The _horizontal (transverse) plane_ runs across the body from the right to the left side and divides the body into upper (superior) and lower (inferior) portions. Figure 2–2 shows the division of this plane.

Recall the term super/ior. It is a point of reference that refers to a structure above or oriented toward a higher place. For example, the head is superior to the heart. Infer/ior is a point of reference that refers to a structure situated below or oriented toward a lower place. For example, the feet are inferior to the legs.

Because the head is located superior to the heart, the heart is located

_____ to the head; because the feet are located inferior to ,

the legs, the legs are located _____ to the feet.

transverse plane
trăns-VĔRS plān

2-39 The plane that divides the body into superior and inferior portions is the horizontal plane. This plane is also called the

_____ _____.

cross-sectional

2-40 Many different transverse planes exist at every possible level of the body from head to foot. A trans/verse section is also called a _cross-sectional plane._ Some radiographic imaging devices produce cross-sectional images. Cross-sectioning of the body or of an organ along different planes results in different views.

The horizontal or trans/verse planes are also known as the

_____ plane.

-graph radi/o trans- -verse	**2-41** A radi/o/graph of the liver along a trans/verse plane results in a different view than a radiograph along the frontal plane. That is why a series of x-rays is often taken using different planes. Views along different planes result in a complete and comprehensive image of a body structure. Identify the elements in this frame that mean process of recording: _____. radiation, x-ray; radius (lower arm bone on thumb side): _____/____. through, across: _____. turning: _____.
coronal plane CŎR-ă-năl plān	**2-42** Locate the frontal plane in Figure 2–2. The frontal plane is also called the _____ _____.
posterior pŏs-TĒ-rē-or	**2-43** The frontal (coronal) plane is often used to take an anter/o/poster/ior (AP) chest radiograph. This indicates that the x-ray beam enters the body on the anterior side and exits the body on the _____ side. The radiograph produced shows a view from the front of the chest toward the back (of the body).

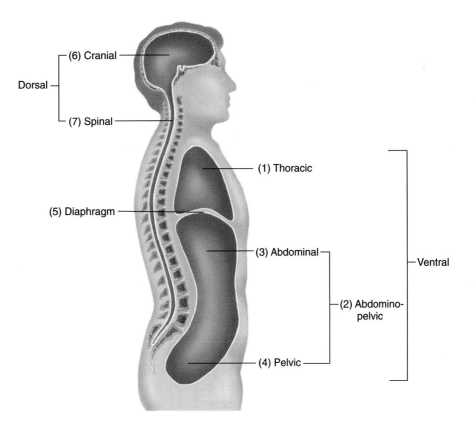

Figure 2-3   Body cavities. Ventral cavities (anterior) located in front of the body; dorsal cavities (posterior) located in the back of the body.

study of	**2-44** In the previous frame, you learned that anter/o/poster/ior is used in radi/o/logy to describe the direction or path of an x-ray beam. The combining form **radi/o** means *radiation; x-ray; radius (lower arm bone on thumb side)*. The suffix -logy means _____ _____.
radi/o/logy rā-dē-ŎL-ō-jē	**2-45** Use **radi/o** to form a word that means study of radiation or x-rays: _____ / _____ / _____.
	2-46 Identify the abbreviation in Frame 2-43 that designates the path of an x-ray beam from the anterior to the posterior part of the body: _____.

Body Cavities

cranial, spinal KRĀ-nē-ăl, SPĪ-năl **thoracic, abdominopelvic** thō-RĂS-ĭk, ăb-DŎM-ĭ-nō-PĔL-vĭk	**2-47** The body contains two major cavities, hollow spaces that contain internal organs: the dorsal and the ventral cavities. These cavities are subdivided further into two dorsal and two ventral cavities. In Figure 2-3, locate and name the dorsal cavities: _____, _____. ventral cavities: _____, _____.
	2-48 Let us continue to learn about the body cavities as you read and locate them in Figure 2-3. The (1) **thoracic cavity** contains the heart and lungs. The (2) **abdominopelvic cavity** contains organs of the reproductive and digestive systems and includes two subcavities, the (3) **abdominal** and (4) **pelvic cavities.** This subdivision is useful because of the different types of organs present in each (reproductive versus digestive). Because there is no dividing wall between them, they are actually one large cavity, the abdominopelvic cavity.
superior soo-PĒ-rē-or **inferior** ĭn-FĒ-rē-or	**2-49** Use the terms superior and inferior to describe locations, or positions, of body cavities. The thoracic cavitiy is located _____ to the abdominopelvic cavity. The spinal cavity is located _____ to the cranial cavity.
	2-50 The (5) **diaphragm**, a dome-shaped muscle, which plays an important role in breathing, separates the thorac/ic cavity from the abdomin/o/pelv/ic cavity. Locate the diaphragm in Figure 2-3.

pelv **thorac** **abdomin**	**2–51** Let us review some of the elements in the previous frame. The root that refers to the pelvis is: _____. chest is: _____. abdomen is: _____.
crani/al KRĀ-nē-ăl **spin/al** SPĪ-năl	**2–52** The *dorsal cavity* consists of the (6) **cranial** and (7) **spinal cavities**. These cavities contain the organs of the *nervous system,* the brain and spinal cord. The nervous system is one of the most complex systems of the body (see Chapter 9) and controls many vital activities of the body. Practice building words that refer to the body cavities by building a term that means pertaining to the cranium (skull): _____ / _____. pertaining to the spine: _____ / _____.
crani/al KRĀ-nē-ăl **spin/al** SPĪ-năl	**2–53** As discussed earlier, the dors/al cavity includes the crani/al cavity, which is formed by the skull and contains the brain. The spinal cavity, which is formed by the spine (backbone), contains the spinal cord. Refer to Figure 2–3 to complete the following frames. The body cavity surrounding the skull is the _____ / _____ cavity. spinal cord is the _____ / _____ cavity.

Abdominopelvic Quadrants

	2–54 Because the abdominopelvic cavity is a large area and contains many organs, it is useful to divide it into smaller sections. One method divides the abdominopelvic cavity into quadrants. A second method divides the abdominopelvic cavity into regions. Physicians and health care professionals use both of these regional divisions as a point of reference. The larger division of the abdominopelvic cavity consists of four quadrants: right upper quadrant (RUQ), left upper quadrant (LUQ), right lower quadrant (RLQ), and left lower quadrant (LLQ). Locate these quadrants in Figure 2–4A.
right upper quadrant **left upper quadrant** **right lower quadrant** **left lower quadrant**	**2–55** When you have located and reviewed the quadrants, determine the meaning of the following abbreviations RUQ: _____ _____ _____ LUQ: _____ _____ _____ RLQ: _____ _____ _____ LLQ: _____ _____ _____

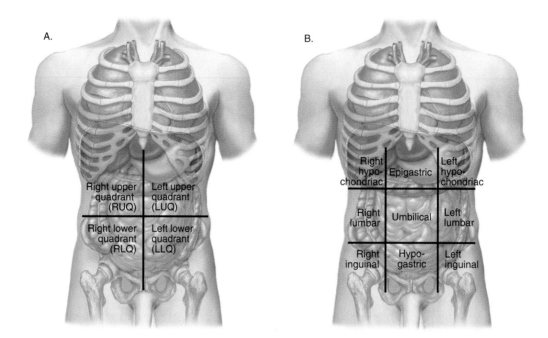

Figure 2-4   (A) Four quadrants of the abdomen. (B) Nine regions of the abdomen showing the superficial organs.

RLQ	**2–56** Quadrants are useful in describing the location in the body in which a surgical procedure will be performed. They also are useful in denoting incision sites, or the location of abnormal masses, such as tumors. A tumor located in the right lower quadrant most likely will be denoted in the medical record with the abbreviation _____.
RLQ **LLQ**	**2–57** Quadrants also may be used to describe the location of a patient's symptoms. The physician may pinpoint a patient's abdominal pain in the RLQ. This could indicate a diagnosis of appendicitis because the appendix is located in that quadrant. Pain in another quadrant, such as the LLQ, would indicate a different diagnosis. Identify the abbreviation for the: right lower quadrant: _____. left lower quadrant: _____.
left upper quadrant, **LUQ**	**2–58** Locate the quadrant that contains a major part of the stomach. This quadrant is the _____ _____ _____, and its abbreviation is _____.

Abdominopelvic Regions

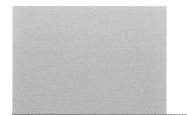	**2–59** Whereas larger sections of the abdominopelvic cavity are divided into four quadrants, the smaller sections are divided into nine regions, each of which corresponds to a region near a specific point in the body. As with quadrants, body region designation also is used to describe the location of internal organs and the origin of pain. Review Figure 2–4B to see the location of various organs within these regions.

2-60   Now that you have examined the nine regions, let us review some of the terms within each region. These terms frequently are used to describe a location of organs within the abdominal cavity.

Although the combining forms in the left-hand column below denote a body structure, when attached to directional elements, they form terms that denote specific regions of the abdomen. Study the meaning of each regional term, then divide each one in the right-hand column into its basic elements. The first term is an example that is completed for you.

Combining Form	Meaning	Regions of the Abdomen
chondr/o	cartilage	h y p o / c h o n d r / i a c
gastr/o	stomach	e p i g a s t r i c
inguin/o	groin	i n g u i n a l
lumb/o	loins (lower back)	l u m b a r
umbilic/o	umbilicus, navel	u m b i l i c a l

hypo/chondr/iac
hī-pō-KŎN-drē-ăk
epi/gastr/ic
ĕp-ĭ-GĂS-trĭk
inguin/al
ĬNG-gwĭ-năl
lumb/ar
LŬM-băr
umbilic/al
ŭm-BĬL-ĭ-kăl

2-61   Refer to Figure 2–4B to identify the terms in the regions that describe the following statements. The first one is an example that is completed for you.

The region located

near the groin: _inguin/al._

beneath the ribs: _____ / _____ / _____.

near the navel: _____ / _____.

below the stomach: _____ / _____ / _____.

hypo/chondr/iac
hī-pō-KŎN-drē-ăk
umbilic/al
ŭm-BĬL-ĭ-kăl
hypo/gastr/ic
hī-pō-GĂS-trĭk

2-62   Identify the part of speech the following suffixes.

-al, -ar, -ic, or -iac. _____

adjectives

2-63   Use **gastr/o** to develop medical words that pertain to the area under or below the stomach: _____ / _____ / _____.

above or on the stomach: _____ / _____ / _____.

hypo/gastr/ic
hī-pō-GĂS-trĭk
epi/gastr/ic
ĕp-ĭ-GĂS-trĭk

2-64   The epi/**gastr**/ic region may be the location of "heartburn" pain. Pain in this area could be symptomatic of many abnormal conditions, including indigestion or heart attack.

The area of heartburn pain may be felt in the

_____ / _____ / _____ region.

epi/gastr/ic
ĕp-ĭ-GĂS-trĭk

-iac hypo- chondr	**2–65** The right and left hypo/chondr/iac regions are located on each side of the epi/gastr/ic region and directly under the cartilage of the ribs. Identify the elements in hypo/chondr/iac that mean pertaining to, relating to: _____. under, below, deficient: _____. cartilage: _____.

 Refer to Figure 2–4B to answer the following frames. if needed, use Appendix A, Glossary of Medical Word Elements.

loins (lower back)	**2–66** The lumbar regions consist of the middle right and middle left regions located near the waistline of the body. The term lumb/ar means pertaining to the _____ (_____ _____).
lumb/o/abdomin/al lŭm-bō-ăb-DŎM-ĭ-năl	**2–67** Combine **lumb/o** + abdomin + al to form a term that means pertaining to the loins and abdomen. _____ / ____ / _____ / _____
umbilic/al region ŭm-BĬL-ĭ-kăl	**2–68** The center of the umbilic/al region marks the point where the umbilic/al cord of the mother entered the fetus. This is the navel and in layman terms is referred to as the "belly button." The region that lies between the right and left lumbar regions is designated as the _____ / _____ _____.
umbilic/al ŭm-BĬL-ĭ-kăl	**2–69** The combining form **umbilic/o** refers to *umbilicus* or *navel.* The region that literally means pertaining to the navel is: _____ / _____.
inguin/al ĬNG-gwĭ-năl	**2–70** A hernia is a protrusion or projection of an organ through the wall of the cavity that normally contains it. A common type of hernia that may occur, particularly in males, is inguin/al hernia. This hernia would be located in either the right or the left _____ / _____ region.
inguinal hernia ĬNG-gwĭ-năl HĔR-nē-ă	**2–71** Locate the right inguin/al region and the left inguin/al region in Figure 2–4B. A hernia on the right side of the groin is called an _____ / _____.

2-72   The area between the right and the left inguin/al regions is called the hypo/gastr/ic region. This region contains the large intestine (colon), which is involved with the removal of solid waste from the body. Identify the name of the region below the stomach that literally means pertaining to below the stomach:

_____ / _____ /_____.

hypo/gastr/ic
hī-pō-GĂS-trĭk

SECTION REVIEW 2 – 4

Using the following table, write the combining form, suffix, or prefix that matches its definition in the space provided to the left of the definition. There may be more than one word element that matches a definition.

Combining Forms		Suffixes	Prefixes
abdomin/o	lumb/o	-ac	epi-
chondr/o	pelv/o	-ad	hypo-
crani/o	poster/o	-al	
gastr/o	spin/o	-ic	
ili/o	thorac/o	-ior	
inguin/o			

1. _____ toward
2. _____ groin
3. _____ stomach
4. _____ pelvis
5. _____ cartilage
6. _____ above, on
7. _____ pertaining to, relating to
8. _____ loins, (lower back)
9. _____ chest
10. _____ under, below, deficient
11. _____ cranium (skull)
12. _____ spine
13. _____ ilium (lateral, flaring portion of hip bone)
14. _____ back (of body), behind, posterior
15. _____ abdomen

Competency Verification: Check your answers in Appendix B, Answer Key, page 509. If you are not satisfied with your level of comprehension, go back to Frame 2–33 and rework the frames.

Correct Answers _____ × 6.67 = _____% Score

Abbreviations

This section introduces body structure and abbreviations related to radiology and their meanings.

Abbreviation	Meaning	Abbreviation	Meaning
BODY STRUCTURE			
abd	abdomen	PA	posteroanterior
AP	anteroposterior	RLQ	right lower quadrant
Lat	lateral	RUQ	right upper quadrant
LLQ	left lower quadrant	U&L, U/L	upper and lower
LUQ	left upper quadrant		
RADIOLOGY			
CT	computed tomography	PET	positron emission tomography
CXR	chest x-ray	US	ultrasonography, ultrasound
MRI	magnetic resonance imaging	SPECT	single-photon emission computed tomography

Pathological, Diagnostic, and Therapeutic Terms

The following are additional terms related to the structure of the body. Recognizing and learning these terms will help you understand the connection between a pathological condition, its diagnosis, and the rationale behind the method of treatment selected for a particular disorder.

Pathological

adhesion (ăd-HĒ-zhŭn): band of scar tissue binding anatomical surfaces that normally are separate from each other.

Adhesions most commonly form in the abdomen, after abdominal surgery, inflammation, or injury.

inflammation (ĭn-flă-MĀ-shun): protective response of body tissues, infection, or allergy.

Signs of inflammation are redness, swelling, heat, and pain, often accompanied by loss of function.

sepsis (SĔP-sĭs): body's inflammatory response to infection, in which there is fever, elevated heart and respiratory rate, and low blood pressure.

Septicemia is a common type of sepsis.

Diagnostic

computed tomography (CT) scan (kŏm-PŪ-tĕd tō-MŎG-ră-fē): radiographic technique that uses a narrow beam of x-rays, which rotates in a full arc around the patient to image the body in cross-sectional slices. A scanner and detector send the images to a computer, which consolidates all of the data it receives from the multiple x-ray views (see Fig. 2–5A).

CT scanning is used to detect tumor masses, bone displacement, and accumulations of fluid. It may be administered with or without a contrast medium.

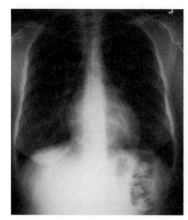

(A) Radiographic film.

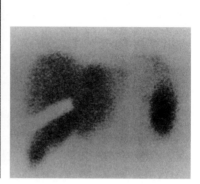

(B) Ultrasonography.

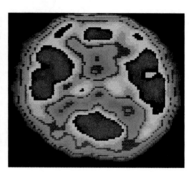

(C) Nuclear scan.

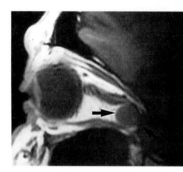

(D) CT scan.

(E) MRI scan.

(F) PET scan of brain.

Figure 2-5 Medical imaging.
A. Chest radiograph. A mediastinum suggestive of lymphatic enlargement in suspected lymphoma. From McKinnis, L: Fundamentals of Orthopedic Radiology, Page 149. FA Davis, 1997, with permission.
B. Ultrasonography. Ultrasound of blood flow, with color indicating direction. (Courtesy of Suzanne Wambold, PhD, University of Toledo.)
C. Nuclear scan. A radionucleotide scan of the liver and spleen showing a heterogeneous uptake pattern characteristic of lymphoma. From Pittiglio, DH and Sacher, RA: Clinical Hematology and Fundamentals of Hemostasis, page 302. FA Davis, 1987, with permission.
D. CT scan. A scan of eye in lateral view showing a tumor *(arrows)* below the optic nerve. From Mazziotta, JC and Gilman, S: Clinical Brain Imaging: Principles and Applications, page 27. Oxford University Press, 1992, with permission.
E. MRI scan. Midsagittal section of head. Note extreme clarity of soft tissue. From Mazziotta, JC and Gilman, S: Clinical Brain Imaging: Principles and Applications, page 298. Oxford University Press, 1992, with permission.
F. PET scan of brain. A brain scan in transverse section (frontal lobes at top). From Mazziotta, JC and Gilman, S: Clinical Brain Imaging: Principles and Applications, page 298. Oxford University Press, 1992, with permission.

endoscopy (ĕn-DŎS-kō-pē): visual examination of the interior of organs and cavities with a specialized lighted instrument called an *endoscope.*

Endoscopy also can be used to obtain tissue samples for cytological and histological examination (biopsy), to perform surgery, and to follow the course of a disease, as in the assessment of the healing of gastric and duodenal ulcers. The cavity or organ examined dictates the name of the endoscopic procedure (see Figure 2–6). A camera or video recorder frequently is used during this procedure to provide a permanent record.

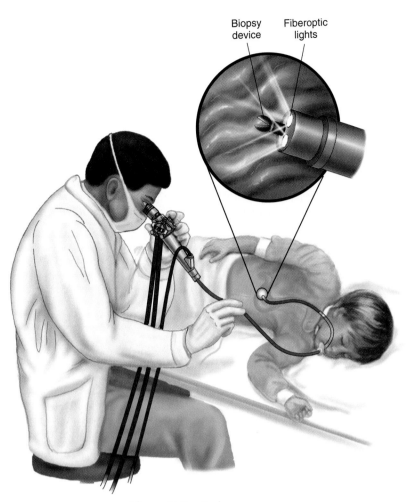

Biopsy device   Fiberoptic lights

Figure 2-6   Endoscopy.

fluoroscopy (floo-or-ŎS-kō-pē): radiographic procedure that uses a fluorescent screen instead of a photographic plate to produce a visual image from x-rays that pass through the patient. The technique offers continuous imaging of the motion of internal structures and immediate serial images.

Fluoroscopy is invaluable in diagnostic and clinical procedures. It permits the radiographer to observe organs, such as the digestive tract and heart, in motion. It also is used during biopsy surgery, nasogastric tube placement, and catheter insertion during angiography.

magnetic resonance imaging (măg-NĔT-ĭc RĔZ-ĕn-ăns ĬM-ĭj-ĭng): radiographic technique that uses electromagnetic energy to produce multiplanar cross-sectional images of the body.

Magnetic resonance imaging (MRI) does not require a contrast medium, but one may be used to enhance internal structure visualization (see Figure 2–5E). MRI is regarded as superior to CT for most central nervous system abnormalities, particularly abnormalities of the brainstem and spinal cord, and musculoskeletal and pelvic area abnormalities.

nuclear scan (NŪ-klē-ăr): diagnostic technique that produces an image by recording the concentration of a *radiopharmaceutical* (a radioactive substance known as a radionuclide combined with another chemical). The radiopharmaceutical is introduced into the body (ingested, inhaled, or injected) and specifically drawn to the area under study.

A scanning device detects the shape, size, location, and function of the organ or structure under study. It provides information about the structure and the function of an organ or system. There are a variety of nuclear scans, such as bone scans, liver scans, and brain scans (see Figure 2–5C).

positron emission tomography (PŎZ-ĭ-trŏn ē-MĬSH-ŭn tō-MŎG-ră-fē): radiographic technique that combines computed tomography with the use of radiopharmaceuticals. Positron emission tomography (PET) produces a cross-sectional (transverse) image of the dispersement of radioactivity (through emission of positrons) in a section of the body to reveal the areas where the radiopharmaceutical is being metabolized and where there is a deficiency in metabolism.

PET is a type of nuclear scan used to diagnose disorders that involve metabolic processes. It can aid in the diagnosis of neurological disorders, such as brain tumors, epilepsy, stroke, Alzheimer disease, and abdominal and pulmonary disorders (see Figure 2–5F).

radiography (rā-dē-ŎG-ră-fē): production of captured shadow images on photographic film through the action of ionizing radiation passing through the body from an external source.

Soft body tissues, such as the stomach or liver, appear black or gray on the radiograph; dense body tissues, such as bone, appear white on the radiograph, making it useful in diagnosing fractures. Figure 2–5A is a chest radiograph showing widening of the mediastinum.

radiopharmaceutical (rā-dē-ō-fărm-ă-SŪ-tĭ-kăl): drug that contains a radioactive substance that travels to an area or a specific organ that will be scanned.

Kinds of radiopharmaceuticals include diagnostic, research, and therapeutic.

scan: technique for carefully studying an area, organ, or system of the body by recording and displaying an image of the area.

A concentration of a radioactive substance that has an affinity for a specific tissue may be administered intravenously to enhance the image. The liver, brain, and thyroid can be examined; tumors can be located; and function can be evaluated by various scanning techniques.

single-photon emission computed tomography (SĬNG-gŭl FŌ-tŏn ē-MĬ-shŭn cŏm-PŪ-tĕd tō-MŎG-ră-fē): type of nuclear imaging study to scan organs after injection of a radioactive tracer. Single-photon emission computed tomography (SPECT) is similar to PET scans (See Figure 2–5F) but employs a specialized gamma camera that detects emitted radiation to produce a three-dimensional image from a composite of numerous views.

Organs commonly studied by SPECT include the brain, heart, lungs, liver, spleen, bones, and, in some cases, joints.

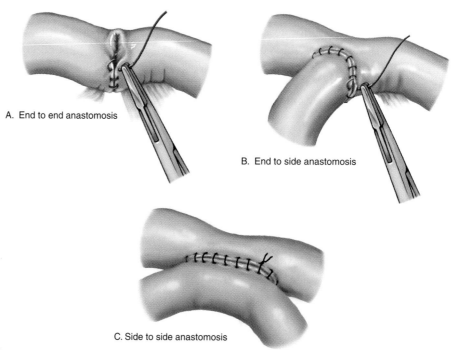

A. End to end anastomosis

B. End to side anastomosis

C. Side to side anastomosis

Figure 2-7   Anastomosis.

tomography (tō-MŎG-ră-fē): radiographic technique that produces a film representing a detailed cross-section of tissue structure at a predetermined depth.

Tomography is a valuable diagnostic tool for discovering and identifying space-occupying lesions, such as those found in the liver, brain, pancreas, and gallbladder. Various types of tomography include computed tomography (CT), positron emission tomography (PET), and single-photon emission computed tomography (SPECT).

ultrasonography (ŭl-tră-sŏn-ŎG-ră-fē): imaging technique that uses high-frequency sound waves (ultrasound) that bounce off body tissues and are recorded to produce an image of an internal organ or tissue. Ultrasonic echoes are recorded and interpreted by a computer, which produces a detailed image of the organ or tissue being evaluated.

In contrast to other imaging techniques, ultrasound (US) does not use ionizing radiation (x-ray). It is used to diagnose fetal development and internal structures of the abdomen, brain, and heart and musculoskeletal disorders. The record produced by US is called a sonogram or echogram (see Figure 2–5B.)

Therapeutic

anastomosis (ă-năs-tō-MŌ-sĭs): connection between two vessels; surgical joining of two ducts, blood vessels, or bowel segments to allow flow from one to the other (see Figure 2–7).

cauterize (KAW-tĕr-īz): process of burning tissue by thermal heat, including steam, electricity, or another agent, such as laser or dry ice.

This procedure usually is performed with the objective of destroying damaged or diseased tissues, preventing infections, or coagulating blood vessels.

PATHOLOGICAL, DIAGNOSTIC, AND THERAPEUTIC TERMS REVIEW

Match the medical term(s) with the definitions in the numbered list.

adhesion	endoscopy	radiopharmaceutical
anastomosis	fluoroscopy	sepsis
cauterize	MRI	SPECT
CT scan	PET	tomography
endoscope	radiography	US

1. _____ uses a narrow beam of x-rays, which rotates in a full arc around the patient to image the body in cross-sectional slices.

2. _____ directs x-rays through the body to a fluorescent screen to view the motion of organs, such as the digestive tract and heart.

3. _____ employs high-frequency sound waves to image internal structures of the body.

4. _____ employs magnetic energy without ionizing x-rays to produce cross-sectional images.

5. _____ is a type of nuclear scan that diagnoses disorders involving metabolic processes, such as brain tumors, epilepsy, stroke, Alzheimer disease, and abdominal and pulmonary disorders.

6. _____ is a specialized lighted instrument to view the interior of organs and cavities.

7. _____ surgically joins two ducts, blood vessels, or bowel segments to allow flow from one to the other.

8. _____ is similar to PET, but employs a specialized gamma camera that detects emitted radiation to produce a three-dimensional image based on a composite of many views.

9. _____ produces a film representing a detailed cross-section of tissue structure at a predetermined depth; three types include CT, PET, and SPECT.

10. _____ is a drug that contains a radioactive substance that travels to an area or a specific organ to be scanned.

11. _____ is a procedure to examine visually the interior of organs and cavities with a lighted instrument.

12. _____ involves burning tissue by thermal heat, including steam, electricity, or another agent, such as a laser or dry ice.

13. _____ is a band of scar tissue that binds anatomical surfaces that normally are separate from each other.

14. _____ is production of shadow images on photographic film.

15. _____ is the body's inflammatory response to infection, in which there is fever, elevated heart rate and respiratory rate, and low blood pressure.

Competency Verification: Check your answers in Appendix B, Answer Key, page 509. If you are not satisfied with your level of comprehension, review the pathological, diagnostic, and therapeutic terms and retake the review.

Correct Answers _____ × 6.67 = _____% Score

Chapter Review

Word Elements Summary

The following table summarizes combining forms, suffixes, and prefixes related to body structure.

Word Element	Meaning
COMBINING FORMS	
abdomin/o	abdomen
anter/o	anterior, front
caud/o	tail
cephal/o	head
cervic/o	neck; cervix uteri (neck of uterus)
chondr/o	cartilage
crani/o	cranium (skull)
cyt/o	cell
dist/o	far, farthest
dors/o	back (of body)
gastr/o	stomach
hist/o	tissue
ili/o	ilium (lateral, flaring portion of hip bone)
infer/o	lower, below
inguin/o	groin
later/o	side, to one side
lumb/o	loins (lower back)
medi/o	middle
nucle/o	nucleus
pelv/o	pelvis
poster/o	back (of body), behind, posterior
proxim/o	near, nearest
radi/o	radiation, x-ray; radius (lower arm bone on thumb side)
spin/o	spine
thorac/o	chest

Word Element	Meaning
umbilic/o	umbilicus, navel
ventr/o	belly, belly side
SUFFIXES	
ADJECTIVE	
-ac, -al, -ar, -iac, -ic, -ior	pertaining to, relating to
OTHER	
-ad	toward
-logist	specialist in study of
-logy	study of
-lysis	separation; destruction; loosening
-toxic	poison
-verse	turning
PREFIXES	
epi-	above, on
hypo-	under, below, deficient
medi-	middle
super-	upper, above
trans-	through, across

WORD ELEMENTS REVIEW

After you review the above Word Elements Summary, complete this activity by writing the meaning of each element or abbreviation in the space provided.

Word Element	Meaning
COMBINING FORMS	
1. abdomin/o	_____
2. anter/o	_____
3. caud/o	_____
4. cephal/o	_____
5. chondr/o	_____
6. crani/o	_____
7. cyt/o	_____
8. dist/o	_____
9. hist/o	_____
10. infer/o	_____
11. inguin/o	_____
12. later/o	_____
13. lumb/o	_____
14. medi/o	_____
15. nucle/o	_____
16. pelv/o	_____
17. proxim/o	_____
18. thorac/o	_____
19. umbilic/o	_____
20. ventr/o	_____
SUFFIXES	
21. -ac, -al, -ar, -iac, -ic, -ior	_____
22. -ad	_____
23. -logist	_____
24. -lysis	_____
25. -toxic	_____

Word Element	Meaning
PREFIXES AND ABBREVIATIONS	
26. CT	_____
27. epi-	_____
28. hypo-	_____
29. MRI	_____
30. RUQ	_____

Competency Verification: Check your answers in Appendix A, Glossary of Medical Word Elements, page 497. If you are not satisfied with your level of comprehension, review the word elements and retake the review.

Correct Answers: _____ × 3.33 = _____% Score

Chapter 2 Vocabulary Review

In figure A, label the four abdominopelvic quadrants; in figure B, label the nine abdominopelvic regions.

Right upper quadrant (RUQ)
Left upper quadrant (LUQ)
Right lower quadrant (RLQ)
Left lower quadrant (LLQ)

Right hypochondriac
Epigastric
Right lumbar
Right inguinal
Left hypochondriac
Umbilical
Left lumbar
Left inguinal
Hypogastric

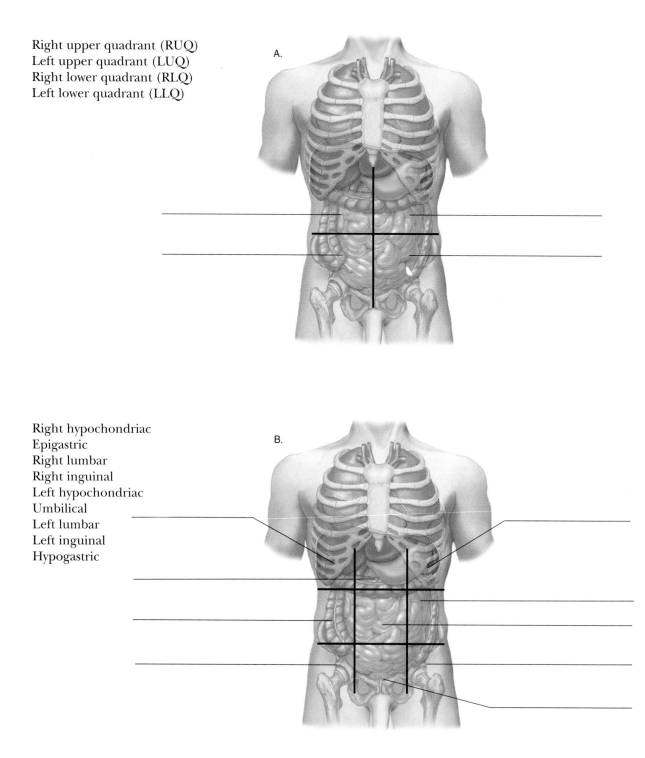

Competency Verification: Compare your answers by referring to Figure 2–4A and B, page 42.

3

Integumentary System

OBJECTIVES

Upon completion of this chapter, you will be able to:

- Describe the integumentary system and discuss its primary functions.
- Describe pathological, diagnostic, therapeutic, and other terms related to the integumentary system.
- Recognize, define, pronounce, and spell terms correctly by completing the audio CD-ROM exercises.
- Demonstrate your knowledge of this chapter by successfully completing the frames, reviews, and medical report evaluations.

The integumentary system consists of the skin and its accessory organs: the hair, nails, sebaceous glands, and sweat glands. The skin is the largest organ in the body and performs many vital functions: It shields the body against injuries, infection, dehydration, harmful ultraviolet rays, and toxic compounds. The skin is a protective interface between the body and the external environment. Beneath the skin's surface is an intricate network of sensory receptors that register sensations of temperature, pain, and pressure. The millions of sensory receptors and a vascular network aid the functions of the entire body in maintaining *homeostasis,* a stable internal environment of the body (see Figure 3–1).

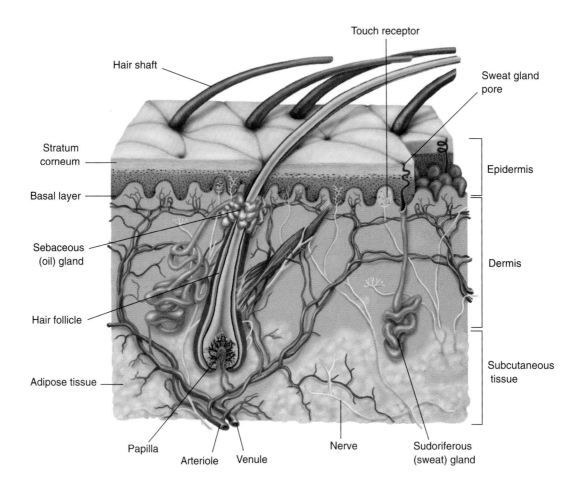

Figure 3-1   Structure of the skin and subcutaneous tissue.

Word Elements

This section introduces combining forms related to the integumentary system. Included are key suffixes; prefixes are defined in the right-hand column as needed. Review the following table, and pronounce each word in the word analysis column aloud before you begin to work the frames.

Word Element	Meaning	Word Analysis
COMBINING FORMS		
adip/o	fat	adip/o/cele (ĂD-ĭ-pō-sēl): hernia containing fat or fatty tissue *-cele:* hernia, swelling
lip/o		lip/o/cyte (LĬP-ō-sīt): fat cell *-cyte:* cell
steat/o		steat/itis (stē-ă-TĪ-tĭs): inflammation of fatty tissue *-itis:* inflammation
cutane/o	skin	cutane/ous (kū-TĀ-nē-ŭs): pertaining to the skin *-ous:* pertaining to, relating to
dermat/o		dermat/o/logist (dĕr-mă-TŎL-ō-jĭst): physician specializing in treating skin disorders *-logist:* specialist in study of

derm/o		hypo/derm/ic (hī-pō-DĔR-mĭk): under or inserted under the skin, as in a hypodermic injection
		   hypo-: under, below, deficient
		   -ic: pertaining to, relating to

hidr/o	sweat	hidr/aden/itis (hī-drăd-ĕ-NĪ-tĭs): inflammation of a sweat gland
		   aden: gland
		   -itis: inflammation
		
		Do not confuse hidr/o (sweat) with hydr/o (water).

sudor/o		sudor/esis (sū-dō-RĒ-sĭs): profuse sweating *-esis:* condition
ichthy/o	dry, scaly	ichthy/osis (ĭk-thē-Ō-sĭs): any of several dermatologic conditions characterized by noninflammatory dryness and scaling of the skin, often associated with other abnormalities of lipid metabolism *-osis:* abnormal condition; increase (used primarily with blood cells) *A mild form is called winter itch, often seen on the legs of older patients, especially during the dry winter months.*
kerat/o	horny tissue; hard; cornea	kerat/osis (kĕr-ă-TŌ-sĭs): any condition of the skin characterized by an overgrowth and thickening of skin *-osis:* abnormal condition; increase (used primarily with blood cells)
melan/o	black	melan/oma (mĕl-ă-NŌ-mă): malignant tumor of melanocytes that commonly begins in a darkly pigmented mole and can metastasize widely *-oma:* tumor *Melanomas are attributed to intense exposure to sunlight and frequently metastasize throughout the body.*

(Continued)

Word Element	Meaning	Word Analysis *(Continued)*
myc/o	fungus (plural, fungi)	dermat/o/myc/osis (dĕr-mă-tō-mī-KŌ-sĭs): fungal infection of the skin *dermat/o:* skin *-osis:* abnormal condition; increase (used primarily with blood cells)
onych/o	nail	onych/o/malacia (ŏn-ĭ-kō-mă-LĀ-shē-ă): abnormal softening of the nails *-malacia:* softening
pil/o	hair	pil/o/nid/al (pī-lō-NĪ-dăl): growth of hair in a dermoid cyst or in a sinus opening on the skin *nid:* nest *-al:* pertaining to, relating to *A pilonidal cyst commonly develops in the sacral region of the skin.*
trich/o		trich/o/pathy (trĭk-ŎP-ă-thē): any disease of the hair *-pathy:* disease
scler/o	hardening; sclera (white of eye)	scler/o/derma (sklĕr-ō-DĔR-mă): chronic disease with abnormal hardening of the skin caused by formation of new collagen *-derma:* skin
seb/o	sebum, sebaceous	seb/o/rrhea (sĕb-or-Ē-ă): increase in the amount, and often an alteration of the quality, of the fats secreted by the sebaceous glands *-rrhea:* discharge, flow
squam/o	scale	squam/ous (SKWĀ-mŭs): covered with scales; scalelike *-ous:* pertaining to, relating to
xer/o	dry	xer/o/derma (zē-rō-DĔR-mă): chronic skin condition characterized by excessive roughness and dryness *-derma:* skin *Xeroderma is a mild form of ichthyosis.*

SUFFIXES		
-derma	skin	py/o/derma (pī-ō-DĔR-mă): any pyogenic infection of the skin *py/o:* pus
-phoresis	carrying, transmission	dia/phoresis (dī-ă-fō-RĒ-sĭs): condition of profuse sweating; sudoresis; hyperhidrosis *dia-:* through, across
-plasty	surgical repair	dermat/o/plasty (DĔR-mă-tō-plăs-tē): surgical repair of the skin *dermat/o:* skin
-therapy	treatment	cry/o/therapy (krī-ō-THĔR-ă-pē): treatment using cold as a destructive medium *cry/o:* cold *Warts and actinic keratosis are some of the common skin disorders responsive to cryotherapy.*

Listen and Learn, the audio CD-ROM that accompanies this book, will help you master the pronunciation of selected medical words. Use it to practice pronunciations of the above-listed medical terms and for instructions to complete the *Listen and Learn* exercise on the CD-ROM for this section.

For the following medical terms, first write the suffix and its meaning. Then translate the meaning of the remaining elements starting with the first part of the word. The first word is an example that is completed for you.

Term	Meaning
1. hypo/derm/ic	-ic: pertaining to, relating to; under, below, deficient; skin
2. melan/oma	
3. kerat/osis	
4. cutane/ous	
5. lip/o/cyte	
6. onych/o/malacia	
7. scler/o/derma	
8. dia/phoresis	
9. dermat/o/myc/osis	
10. cry/o/therapy	

Competency Verification: Check your answers in Appendix B, Answer Key, page 510. If you are not satisfied with your level of comprehension, review the vocabulary and retake the review.

Correct Answers _____ × 10 = _____% Score

Throughout the frames in this book, prefixes that stand alone are pink; word roots and combining forms that stand alone are **bold;** and suffixes that stand alone are blue.

ALERT

Skin

	3-1 The skin is considered an organ and is composed of two layers of tissue: the outer epidermis, which is visible to the naked eye, and the inner layer, the dermis. Identify and label the (1) **epidermis** and the (2) **dermis** in Figure 3–2.
epi/derm/is ĕp-ĭ-DĔR-mĭs **derm/is** DĔR-mĭs	**3-2** The epi/derm/is forms the protective covering of the body and does not have a blood or nerve supply. It is dependent on the dermis for its network of capillaries for nourishment. As oxygen and nutrients flow out of the capillaries in the dermis, they pass through tissue fluid supplying nourishment to the deeper layers of the epidermis. When you talk about the outer layer of skin, you are referring to the _____ / _____ / _____. When you talk about the deeper layer of skin, consisting of nerve and blood vessels, you are talking about the _____ / _____.
epi- **-is**	**3-3** The epi/derm/is is thick on the palms of the hands and the soles of the feet but relatively thin over most other areas. Identify the element in epi/derm/is that denotes: above or upon: _____. a part of speech (noun): _____.
skin	**3-4** The combining form **derm/o** refers to the *skin*. Derm/o/pathy is a disease of the _____.
-pathy **derm/o**	**3-5** Identify the elements in derm/o/pathy that mean disease: _____. skin: _____ / ____.
	3-6 Although the epidermis is composed of several layers, the (3) **stratum corneum** and the (4) **basal layer** are of greatest importance. The stratum corneum is composed of dead flat cells that lack a blood supply and sensory receptors. Its thickness is correlated with normal wear of the area it covers. Only the stratum germivatum is composed of living cells and includes a basal layer where new cells are formed. Label the two structures in Figure 3–2.
	3-7 As new cells form in basal layer, they move toward the stratum corneum to replace the cells that have been sloughed off, they die and become filled with a hard protein material called *keratin*. The relatively waterproof characteristic of keratin prevents body fluids from evaporating and moisture from entering the body. The entire process by which a cell forms in the basal layers, rises to the surface, becomes keratinized, and sloughs off takes about 1 month. Check the basal layer in Figure 3–1 to see the single row of newly formed cells in the deepest layer of the epi/derm/is.

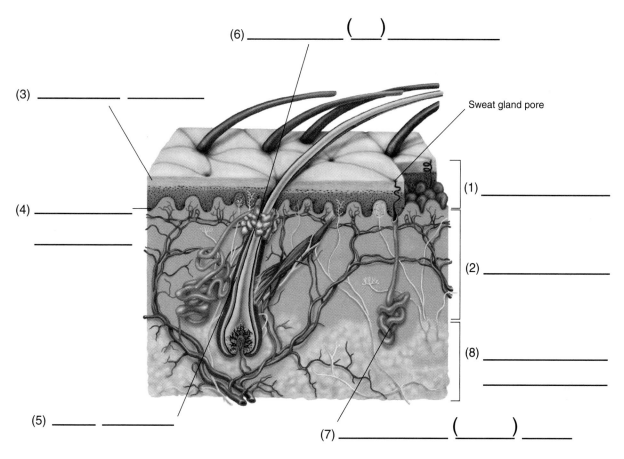

(6) _____ ( ) _____

(3) _____ _____

Sweat gland pore

(1) _____

(4) _____

(2) _____

(8) _____

_____

(5) ___ ___ ___

(7) _____ ( ) ___

Figure 3-2   Identifying integumentary structures.

skin **study, skin**	**3-8** Besides **derm/o,** two other combining forms for *skin* are **cutane/o** and **dermat/o.** Cutane/ous means pertaining to the _____; dermat/o/logy is the _____ of the _____.
dermat/o/logist dĕr-mă-TŎL-ō-jĭst	**3-9** A physician who specializes in treating skin diseases is called a _____ /o/_____.
dermat/itis dĕr-mă-TĪ-tĭs	**3-10** Use **dermat** to build a word meaning inflammation of the skin. _____ / _____.
skin **skin**	**3-11** The prefix sub- means *under* or *below;* the prefix hypo- means *under, below, deficient.* A sub/cutane/ous injection occurs beneath the _____. A hypo/derm/ic needle is inserted under the _____.

skin	**3-12** Sub/cutane/ous literally means pertaining to under the _____.
skin	**3-13** When you see the terms *derm/a, derm/is,* and *derm/oid,* you will know the roots refer to the _____.
skin	**3-14** The suffixes -ic, -is, and -oid designate a part of speech. It is not necessary for you always to be able to identify the part of speech, but it is important for you to remember that derm/a, derm/is, and derm/ic all refer to the _____.
melan/o/cyte MĔL-ăn-ō-sīt **melan/oma** mĕl-ă-NŌ-mă	**3-15** In the basal layer, specialized cells, called *melan/o/cytes,* produce a black pigment called *melanin.* The production of melanin increases with exposure to strong ultraviolet light. This exposure creates a suntan that provides a protective barrier from the damaging effects of the sun. The number of melan/o/cytes is about the same in all races. Differences in skin color are attributed to production of melanin. In people with dark skin, melanocytes continuously produce large amounts of melanin. In people with light skin, melanocytes produce less melanin. The combining form **melan/o** refers to the color *black.* Build a word that literally means black cell: _____ / _____ / _____. black tumor: _____ / _____.
adjective **adjective**	**3-16** The term *derm/is* is a noun. Identify the part of speech in derm/ic: _____ derm/al: _____
	3-17 Label Figure 3–2 as you learn about the parts of the dermis. The second layer of skin, the derm/is, contains the (5) **hair follicle**, (6) **sebaceous (oil) gland**, and (7) **sudoriferous (sweat) gland**.
inflammation, skin	**3-18** Dermat/itis is an _____ of the _____.
disease, skin	**3-19** Derm/o/pathy is a disease of the skin; dermat/o/pathy is also a _____ of the _____.
epi/derm/is, derm/is ĕp-ĭ-DĔR-mĭs, DĔR-mĭs	**3-20** The two layers of the skin are the _____ / _____ / _____ and _____ / _____.
hidr/osis hī-DRŌ-sĭs	**3-21** The combining form for sweat is **hidr/o.** Use -osis to form a word meaning an abnormal condition of sweat: _____ / _____.

sweat; gland **inflammation** **excessive, above normal** **sweat** **abnormal condition**	**3-22** The term *diaphoresis* denotes a condition of profuse or excessive sweating. The following two terms also refer to sweating. hidr/aden/itis means hidr: _____; aden: _____ -itis: _____. hyper/hidr/osis means hyper-: _____, _____ _____ hidr/o: _____ -osis: _____ _____.
sweat **water**	**3-23** Although **hidr/o** and **hydr/o** sound alike, they have different meanings. **Hidr/o** refers to _____; **hydr/o** refers to _____.
an/hidr/osis ăn-hī-DRŌ-sĭs	**3-24** An/hidr/osis is an abnormal condition characterized by inadequate perspiration. When a person suffers from an absence of sweating, you would say they have a condition called _____ / _____ / _____.
aden/oma ăd-ĕ-NŌ-mă	**3-25** An aden/oma is a benign (not malignant) epithelial neoplasm in which the tumor cells form glands or glandlike structures. The tumor usually is well circumscribed, tending to compress rather than infiltrate or invade adjacent tissue. When you want to build a word that means tumor composed of glandular tissue, you use the term _____ / _____.
adip/ectomy ăd-ĭ-PĔK-tō-mē	**3-26** **Lip/o** and **adip/o** are combining forms meaning *fat*. A lip/ecto-my is the excision of fat or adipose tissue. Use **adip/o** to form another surgical term meaning excision of fat: _____ / _____.
adip/o, lip/o **steat/o**	**3-27** Adip/oma and lip/oma refer to a fatty tumor. Both are benign tumors consisting of fat cells. Two combining forms in this frame that mean fat are _____ / ____ and _____ / ____. A third combining form that refers to fat is _____ / ____.
	3-28 The dermis is attached to the underlying structures of the skin by (8) **subcutaneous tissue.** Identify and label the layer of subcutaneous tissue in Figure 3–2.

sub/cutane/ous sŭb-kū-TĀ-nē-ŭs **lip/o/cytes** LĬP-ō-sītz	**3-29** Sub/cutane/ous tissue forms lip/o/cytes, also known as fat cells. Determine the words in this frame that mean pertaining to under, below the skin: _____ / _____ / _____. fat cells: _____ / _____ / _____.
cell **tumor**	**3-30** Whereas a lip/o/cyte is a fat _____, an adip/oma is a fatty _____.

Competency Verification: Check your labeling of Figure 3–2 in Appendix B, Answer Key, page 510.

	3-31 Suction lip/ectomy, also called *lip/o/suction,* is the removal of sub/cutane/ous fat tissue using a blunt-tipped cannula (tube) introduced into the fatty area through a small incision. Suction is applied, and fat tissue is removed. Locate the sub/cutane/ous tissue in Figure 3–1.
sub/cutane/ous sŭb-kū-TĀ-nē-ŭs **lip/ectomy** or lĭ-PĔK-tō-mē **liposuction** LĬP-ō-sŭk-shŭn	**3-32** Identify the terms in Frame 3–31 that mean under the skin: _____ / _____ / _____. excision of fat: _____ / _____.
fat	**3-33** Lip/o/suction is used primarily to remove or reduce localized areas of fat around the abdomen, breasts, legs, face, and upper arms, where skin is contractile enough to redrape in a normal manner, and is performed for cosmetic reasons. Lip/o/suction literally means suction of _____.
derm/o, dermat/o, **cutane/o**	**3-34** List the three combining forms that refer to the skin: _____ / _____, _____ / _____, and _____ / _____.
dermat/o/plasty DĔR-mă-tō-plăs-tē	**3-35** Use **dermat/o** to form a word meaning surgical repair (of the) skin: _____ / _____ / _____.
log **-ist**	**3-36** The following noun suffixes include the same root and are easier to remember if you analyze their components. The -y and -ist denote a noun ending. **-log**y means study of **-log**ist means specialist in study of The root in each suffix that means study of is _____. The element in the suffix -logist that means specialist is _____.

dermat/o/logy dĕr-mă-TŎL-ō-jē **dermat/o/logist** dĕr-mă-TŎL-ō-jĭst	**3-37** Refer to Frame 3–36 and use **dermat/o** to develop words meaning study of the skin: _____ / ____ / _____. specialist who treats skin disorders: _____ / ____ / _____.
dermat/oma dĕr-mă-TŌ-mă **dermat/o/pathy** dĕr-mă-TŌ-pă-thē **dermat/o/logy** dĕr-mă-TŎL-ō-jē	**3-38** Use **dermat/o** to practice forming words meaning tumor of the skin: _____ / _____. disease of the skin: _____ / ____ / _____. study of the skin: _____ / ____ / _____.
dermat/o/logist dĕr-mă-TŎL-ō-jĭst	**3-39** A physician specializing in treating diseases of the stomach is a gastr/o/logist. A physician specializing in treating diseases of the skin is a _____ / ____ / _____.
dermat/o/logy dĕr-mă-TŎL-ō-jē	**3-40** The medical specialty concerned with the treatment of stomach diseases is gastr/o/logy. The medical specialty concerned with the treatment of skin diseases is _____ / ____ / _____.
hardening	**3-41** Scler/osis is an abnormal condition of _____.
skin	**3-42** Scler/o/derma, a chronic hardening and thickening of the skin, is caused by new collagen formation. It is characterized by inflammation that ultimately develops into fibrosis (scarring), then sclerosis (hardening) of tissues. Systemic scler/o/derma can be defined as hardening of the _____.
system/ic sĭs-TĔM-ĭk **scler/osis** sklĕ-RŌ-sĭs **hardening**	**3-43** System/ic scler/osis, a form of scler/o/derma, is characterized by formation of thickened collagenous fibrous tissue, thickening of the skin, and adhesion to underlying tissues. The disease progresses to involve the tissues of the heart, lungs, muscles, genitourinary tract, and kidneys. A form of scler/o/derma that causes fibrosis and sclerosis of multiple body systems is known as _____ / _____ _____ / _____. If you check **scler/o** in Appendix A, Glossary of Medical Word Elements, you will see that **scler/o** means *hardening; sclera (white of eye)*. In the integumentary system, however, it specifically refers to _____.

horny tissue *or* **hard** **cornea**	**3-44** The combining form **kerat/o** means *horny tissue, hard,* and *cornea.* The cornea of the eye is covered in Chapter 11. When **kerat/o** is used in discussions of the skin, it refers to: _____ _____ or _____. of the eye, it refers to the: _____.
kerat/osis kĕr-ă-TŌ-sĭs	**3-45** Kerat/osis, a skin condition, is characterized by hard, horny tissue. A person with a skin lesion in which there is overgrowth and thickening of the epidermis most likely would be diagnosed with _____ / _____.
tumor	**3-46** A kerat/oma is a horny _____; also called kerat/osis.
sub/cutane/ous sŭb-kū-TĀ-nē-ŭs	**3-47** Sub/cutane/ous surgery is performed through a small opening in the skin. The word that means pertaining to under, below the skin is _____ / _____ / _____ (adjective ending).

Accessory Organs of the Skin

sebaceous sē-BĀ-shŭs **sudoriferous** sū-dŏr-ĬF-ĕr-ŭs	**3-48** The accessory organs of the skin include the integumentary glands, hair, and nails. Refer to Figure 3–1 to complete this frame. The oil-secreting glands of the skin are called _____ glands. The sweat glands are called _____ glands.
cutane/ous kū-TĀ-nē-ŭs	**3-49** Combine **cutane** + -ous to build a medical word meaning pertaining to the skin: _____ / _____.
derm/o/pathy dĕr-MŎP-ă-thē	**3-50** Use **derm/o** to form a medical term that means disease of the skin: _____ / ____ / _____.
myc/osis mī-KŌ-sĭs	**3-51** The combining form **myc/o** refers to a *fungus* (plural, fungi). Combine **myc/o** + -osis to form a word meaning an abnormal condition caused by fungi: _____ / _____.
skin	**3-52** Dermat/o/myc/osis, a fungal infection of the skin, is caused by dermatophytes, yeasts, and other fungi. When you see this term in a medical report, you will know it means a fungal infection of the _____.

dermat/itis děr-mă-TĪ-tĭs	**3-53** Form a medical word that means an inflammation of the skin: _____ / _____.
fungus FŬN-gŭs	**3-54** Myc/o/dermat/itis, an inflammation of the skin, is caused by a _____.
trich/o/pathy trĭk-ŎP-ă-thē **trich/osis** trĭ-KŌ-sĭs	**3-55** The combining form **trich/o** refers to the *hair*. Construct medical terms meaning disease of the hair: _____ / ____ / _____. abnormal condition of the hair: _____ / _____.
trich/o/myc/osis trĭk-ō-mī-KŌ-sĭs	**3-56** Combine **trich/o** + **myc** + -osis to form a medical term that means an abnormal condition of the hair caused by a fungus: _____ / ____ / _____ / _____.
hair	**3-57** Another combining form for the hair is **pil/o**. Whenever you see **pil/o** or **trich/o** in a word, you will know it refers to the _____.
pil/o **-oid**	**3-58** Pil/o/cyst/ic refers to a derm/oid cyst containing hair. The element in this frame that refers to hair is _____ / ____; the element in this frame that means resembling is _____.
	3-59 Label the structures of the fingernail in Figure 3–3 as you read the following material. Each nail is formed in the (1) **nail root** and is composed of keratin, a hard fibrous protein, which is also the main component of hair. As the nail grows from a (2) **matrix** of active cells beneath the (3) **cuticle,** it stays attached and slides forward over the epithelial layer called the (4) **nail bed.** Most of the (5) **nail body** appears pink because of the underlying blood vessels. The (6) **lunula** is the crescent-shaped area at the base of the nail. It has a whitish appearance because the vascular tissue underneath does not show through.

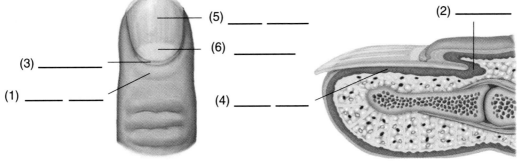

Figure 3-3 Structure of a fingernail.

ALERT

Here is a review of the three basic rules of word building.

Rule 1: A word root links a suffix that begins with a vowel.

Rule 2: A combining form (root + **o**) links a suffix that begins with a consonant.

Rule 3: A combining form (root + **o**) links a root to another root to form a compound word. This holds true even if the next root begins with a vowel.

---

onych/oma ŏn-ĭ-KŌ-mă **onych/o/pathy** ŏn-ĭ-KŎP-ăth-ē	**3-60** The combining form **onych/o** refers to the *nail*(s). Form medical words meaning tumor of the nail (or nailbed): _____ / _____. disease of the nails: _____ / ___ / _____.
onych/o/malacia ŏn-ĭ-kō-mă-LĀ-shē-ă	**3-61** The term **malacia** refers to an abnormal softening of tissue. This term also is used in words as a suffix. Build a word with the suffix -malacia that means softening of the nail(s): _____ / ___ / _____.
onych/o **myc** **-osis**	**3-62** The nails become white, opaque, thickened, and brittle when a person has a disease called *onych/o/myc/osis*. Identify the word elements in onych/o/myc/osis that mean nail: _____ / ___. fungus: _____. abnormal condition: _____.
nail(s)	**3-63** When you see the term onych/o/myc/osis in a medical chart, you will know it means a fungus infection of the _____.
xer/o	**3-64** The noun suffix -derma also is used to denote *skin*. A person with excessive dryness of skin has a condition called xer/o/derma. From xer/o/derma, identify the combining form that means dry: _____ / ___.
hernia **swelling**	**3-65** The suffix -cele refers to a _____ or _____.

lip/o/cele LĬP-ō-sēl	**3-66** A hernia containing fat or fatty tissue is called an adip/o/cele or _____ /_____ /_____.

Competency Verification: Check your labeling of Figure 3–3 in Appendix B, Answer Key, page 510.

Listen and Learn, the audio CD-ROM that accompanies this book, will help you master the pronunciation of selected medical words. Use it to practice pronunciations *of selected terms from frames 3–1 to 3–66* for instructions to complete the *Listen and Learn* exercise on the CD-ROM for this section.

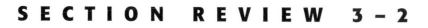

SECTION REVIEW 3 – 2

Using the following table, write the combining form, suffix, or prefix that matches its definition in the space provided to the left of the definition. There may be more than one word element that matches a definition.

Combining Forms	Suffixes	Prefixes
adip/o	-cele	epi-
cutane/o	-derma	hypo-
derm/o	-logist	
dermat/o	-malacia	
hidr/o	-osis	
lip/o	-pathy	
onych/o	-rrhea	
pil/o		
scler/o		
steat/o		
trich/o		
xer/o		

1. _____ disease
2. _____ dry
3. _____ fat
4. _____ discharge, flow
5. _____ hair
6. _____ hardening; sclera (white of eye)
7. _____ hernia, swelling
8. _____ nail

9. _____ skin
10. _____ softening
11. _____ specialist in study of
12. _____ above, upon
13. _____ abnormal condition; increase (used primarily with blood cells)
14. _____ sweat
15. _____ under, below, deficient

Competency Verification: Check your answers in Appendix B, Answer Key, page 510. If you are not satisfied with your level of comprehension, go back to Frame 3–1 and rework the frames.

Correct Answers _____ × 6.67 = _____% Score

Making a set of flash cards from key word elements in this chapter for each section review can help you remember the elements. Make a flash card by writing a word element on one side of a 3 × 5 or 4 × 6 index card. On the other side, write the meaning of the element. Do this for all word elements in the section review. Use your flash cards to review each section. You also might use the flash cards to prepare for the chapter review at the end of this chapter.

Combining Forms Denoting Colors

3-67 Examine the combining forms and their meanings that denote color in the left-hand column below. Examples of medical terms with their definitions are provided in the middle column. In the far right-hand column of this frame, use a slash to break down each word into its basic elements.

Combining Form	Medical Term	Word Breakdown
albin/o: white	albinism: *white condition*	a l b i n i s m
cyan/o: blue	cyanoderma: *blue skin*	c y a n o d e r m a
erythr/o: red	erythroderma: *red skin*	e r y t h r o d e r m a
leuk/o: white	leukoderma: *white skin*	l e u k o d e r m a
melan/o: black	melanoderma: *black skin*	m e l a n o d e r m a
xanth/o: yellow	xanthoma: *yellow tumor*	x a n t h o m a

albin/ism
ĂL-bĭn-ĭzm
cyan/o/derma
sī-ă-nō-DĔR-mă
erythr/o/derma
ĕ-rĭth-rō-DĔR-mă
leuk/o/derma
loo-kō-DĔR-mă
melan/o/derma
mĕl-ăn-ō-DĔR-mă
xanth/oma
zăn-THŌ-mă

3-68 The -a ending in cyanoderma, erythroderma, leukoderma, and melanoderma designates that these words are (adjectives, nouns) _____.

nouns

3-69 Use **-derma** to build medical words meaning

skin that is red: _____ / ____ / _____.

skin that is black: _____ / ____ / _____.

skin that is yellow: _____ / ____ / _____.

skin that is dry: _____ / ____ / _____.

erythr/o/derma
ĕ-rĭth-rō-DĔR-mă
melan/o/derma
mĕl-ăn-ō-DĔR-mă
xanth/o/derma
zăn-thō-DĔR-mă
xer/o/derma
zē-rō-DĔR-mă

Cells

3-70 You have already learned that a cell is the smallest basic unit of the human organism and that every tissue and organ in your body is made up of cells. Cyt/o/logy is the study of _____.

cyt/o and -cyte are used to build words that designate a _____.

cells
cell

3-71 Cyt/o/logy is the study of _____.

cells

erythr/o/cyte ĕ-RĬTH-rō-sīt **leuk/o/cyte** LOO-kō-sīt **melan/o/cyte** MĔL-ăn-ō-sīt **xanth/o/cyte** ZĂN-thō-sīt	**3-72** Use -cyte (cell) to form words meaning cell that is red: _____ / ____ / _____. cell that is white: _____ / ____ / _____. cell that is black: _____ / ____ / _____. cell that is yellow: _____ / ____ / _____.
-penia **leuk/o** **cyt/o**	**3-73** Leuk/o/cyt/o/penia, an abnormal decrease in white blood cells (WBCs), may be caused by an adverse drug reaction, radiation poisoning, or a pathological condition. One or all kinds of WBCs may be affected. The word leuk/o/cyt/o/penia is formed from the following word elements: The suffix meaning decrease or deficiency is _____. The combining form for white is _____ / ____. The combining form for cell is _____ / ____.
leuk/o/cyt/o/penia loo-kō-sī-tō-PĒ-nē-ă	**3-74** A person with a decrease or deficiency in white blood cell production may be diagnosed with a condition known as leuk/o/penia or _____ / ____ / _____ / ____ / _____.
WBC	**3-75** The abbreviation for white blood count or white blood cell(s) is _____.
blood	**3-76** The suffix -emia is used in words to mean *blood condition*. Xanth/emia, an occurrence of yellow pigment in the blood, literally means yellow _____.
xanth/omas zăn-THŌ-măs	**3-77** High cholesterol levels may cause small yellow tumors called _____ / _____.
blood **white**	**3-78** Leuk/emia is a progressive malignant disease of the blood-forming organs characterized by proliferation and development of immature leuk/o/cytes in the blood and bone marrow. Leuk/emia literally means white _____. Leuk/o/cytes are _____ blood cells.
leuk/emia loo-KĒ-mē-ă	**3-79** A disease of unrestrained growth of immature white blood cells is called _____ / _____.

3-80   The activity of melan/o/cytes, which produce melanin, is geneti-
cally regulated and inherited. Local accumulations of melanin are seen in
pigmented moles and freckles. Environmental and physiological factors
also play a role in skin color. Locate the basal layer (stratum germinativum)
in Figure 3–1.

3-81   The absence of pigment in the skin, eyes, and hair is most likely
due to an inherited inability to produce melanin. This lack of melanin
results in the condition called *albin/ism*. A person with this condition is
called an *albino*.

When a person has a deficiency or absence of pigment in the skin, hair,
and eyes due to an abnormality in production of melanin, the condition

is known as _____ / _____.

albin/ism
ĂL-bĭn-ĭzm

3-82   The number of melan/o/cytes is about the same in all races.
Differences in skin color are attributed to production of melanin. In
people with dark skin, melan/o/cytes continuously produce large
amounts of melanin. In people with light skin, melan/o/cytes produce less

_____ .

melanin
MĔL-ă-nĭn

3-83   Melan/oma is a malignant neoplasm that originates in the skin
and is composed of melan/o/cytes.

Form medical words that literally mean

black cell: _____ / ____ / _____.

black tumor: _____ / _____.

melan/o/cyte
mĕl-ĂN-ō-sīt
melan/oma
mĕl-ă-NŌ-mă

3-84   The lesion of melan/oma is characterized by its asymmetry,
irregular border, and lack of uniform color. Malignant melan/oma is the
most dangerous form of skin cancer because of its tendency to metastasize
rapidly .

The medical term that literally means black tumor is

_____ / _____.

melan/oma
mĕl-ă-NŌ-mă

3-85   Cyan/osis, also called *cyan/o/derma*, is caused by a deficiency of
oxygen and an excess of carbon dioxide in the blood. A person who is
rescued from drowning exhibits a dark bluish or purplish discoloration
of the skin. This condition is known as cyan/osis or

_____ / ____ / _____ .

cyan/o/derma
sī-ă-nō-DĔR-mă

cyan/osis sī-ă-NŌ-sĭs	**3–86** Use -osis to develop medical words meaning abnormal condition of blue (skin): _____ / _____.
erythr/osis ĕr-ĭ-THRŌ-sĭs	abnormal condition of red (skin): _____ / _____.
melan/osis mĕl-ăn-Ō-sĭs	abnormal condition of black (pigmentation): _____ / _____.
xanth/osis zăn-THŌ-sĭs	abnormal condition of yellow (skin): _____ / _____.

increase **leuk/o/cyt/osis** loo-kō-sī-TŌ-sĭs	**3–87** As you already know, the suffix -osis is used in words to mean abnormal condition. When -osis is used in a word related to blood, however, it means increase. The complete meaning of -osis is *abnormal condition; increase (used primarily with blood cells).* Erythr/o/cyt/osis is defined as an _____ in red blood cells. Use leuk/o *(white)* to build a term meaning increase in white blood cells: _____ / _____ / _____ / _____.

melan/oma mĕl-ă-NŌ-mă	**3–88** Skin cancer is the most common type of cancer. There has been an increase in the rate of skin cancer, mainly caused by exposure to ultraviolet rays in sunlight. Sun exposure, especially excessive tanning of the skin, can cause the lethal black tumor called _____ / _____.

Other Related Terms

carcin/oma kăr-sĭ-NŌ-mă	**3–89** Basal cell carcin/oma is a type of skin cancer that affects the basal cell layer of the epidermis (see Figure 3–4). Metastasis is rare, but local invasion destroys underlying and adjacent tissue. This condition occurs most frequently on areas of the skin exposed to the sun. A type of skin cancer that affects the basal layer is called basal cell _____ / _____.

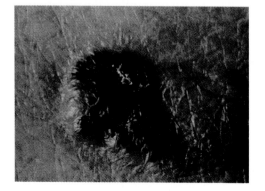
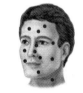

Figure 3-4 Basal cell carcinoma (late stage). From Goldsmith, LA, Lazarus, GS, and Tharp, MD: Adult and Pediatric Dermatology: A Color Guide to Diagnosis and Treatment, page 144. FA Davis, 1997, with permission.

AIDS **Kaposi sarcoma** KĂP-ō-sē săr-KŌ-mă	**3-90** Kaposi sarcoma, a malignant skin tumor frequently associated with patients who have acquired immunodeficiency syndrome (AIDS), is often fatal. Initially the tumor appears as a purplish brown lesion. The abbreviation for acquired immunodeficiency syndrome is _____. A type of skin cancer associated with the AIDS virus is _____ _____.
death	**3-91** The combining form **necr/o** is used in words to denote *death* or *necr/osis*. Necr/o/tic is a word that means pertaining to necr/osis or _____.
dead	**3-92** The term necr/osis is used to denote the death of areas of tissue or bone surrounded by healthy tissue. Cellular necr/osis means that the cells are _____.
dead	**3-93** Necr/o/cyt/osis also means that the cells are _____.
necr/osis nĕ-KRŌ-sĭs	**3-94** Bony necr/osis occurs when dead bone tissue results from the loss of blood supply (for example, after a fracture). The term that means abnormal condition of death is _____ / _____.
gangrene GĂNG-grēn	**3-95** Gangrene is a form of necr/osis associated with loss of blood supply. Before healing can take place, the dead matter must be removed. When there is an injury to blood flow, a form of necr/osis may develop that is known as _____.
self **self** **self**	**3-96** In the English language, an auto/graph is a signature written by oneself. In medical words, auto- is used as a prefix and means *self, own*. Auto/hypnosis is hypnosis of one's _____. Auto/examination is an examination of one's _____. An auto/graft is skin transplanted from one's _____.
auto/grafts AW-tō-grăfts	**3-97** A graft is tissue that is transplanted or implanted in a part of the body to repair a defect. Grafts done with tissue transplanted from the patient's own skin are called _____ / _____.

derm/a/tome
DĔR-mă-tōm

3-98   A derm/a/tome* is an instrument used to incise or cut. When the physician wants to graft a thin slice of skin, the physician asks for an instrument called a _____ / _____ / _____.

auto/graft
AW-tō-grăft

3-99   Skin transplanted from another person will not survive long, so a graft is performed using tissue transplanted from the patient's own skin. This surgical procedure is called an _____ / _____.

Listen and Learn, the audio CD-ROM that accompanies this book, will help you master the pronunciation of selected medical words. Use it to practice pronunciations *of selected terms from frames 3–67 to 3–99* for instructions to complete the *Listen and Learn* exercise on the CD-ROM for this section.

*The use of *a* as the connecting vowel is an exception to the rule of using an *o.*

SECTION REVIEW 3 – 3

Using the following table, write the combining form, suffix, or prefix that matches its definition in the space provided to the left of the definition. There may be more than one word element that matches a definition.

Combining Forms	Suffixes	Prefixes
cyan/o	-cyte	auto-
cyt/o	-derma	
erythr/o	-emia	
leuk/o	-oma	
melan/o	-osis	
necr/o	-pathy	
xanth/o	-penia	
	-rrhea	

1. _____ black
2. _____ blue
3. _____ blood condition
4. _____ cell
5. _____ decrease, deficiency
6. _____ disease
7. _____ discharge, flow
8. _____ red
9. _____ self, own
10. _____ skin
11. _____ tumor
12. _____ white
13. _____ yellow
14. _____ death, necrosis
15. _____ abnormal condition; increase (used primarily with blood cells)

Competency Verification: Check your answers in Appendix B, Answer Key, page 511. If you are not satisfied with your level of comprehension, go back to Frame 3–67 and rework the frames.

Correct Answers _____ × 6.67 = _____% Score

Abbreviations

This section introduces integumentary system–related abbreviations and their meanings. Included are abbreviations contained in the medical record activities that follow.

Abbreviation	Meaning	Abbreviation	Meaning
AIDS	acquired immunodeficiency syndrome	ID	intradermal
BCC	basal cell carcinoma	I&D	incision and drainage
Bx	biopsy	IM	intramuscular
decub	decubitus	oint, ung	ointment
derm	dermatology	PE	physical examination
FH	family history	WBC	white blood cell(s), white blood count
FS	frozen section		

Pathological, Diagnostic, and Therapeutic Terms

The following are additional pathological, diagnostic, and therapeutic terms related to the integumentary system. Recognizing and learning these terms will help you understand the connection between a pathological condition, its diagnosis, and the types of treatment used to treat integumentary disorders.

Pathological

abrasion (ă-BRĀ-zhŭn): scraping away of a portion of skin or of a mucous membrane as a result of injury or by mechanical means, as in dermabrasion for cosmetic purposes.

acne (ĂK-nē): inflammatory disease of the sebaceous follicles of the skin, marked by comedones (blackheads), papules, and pustules.

Acne is especially common in puberty and adolescence. It usually affects the face, chest, back, and shoulders.

alopecia (ăl-ō-PĒ-shē-ă): absence or loss of hair, especially of the head; also known as *baldness*.

carbuncle (KĂR-bŭng-kĕl): deep-seated pyogenic infection of the skin usually involving subcutaneous tissues (see Figure 3–5).

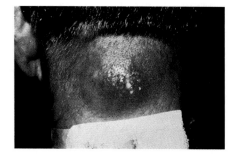

Figure 3-5 Carbuncle-furuncle. From Goldsmith, LA, Lazarus, GS, and Tharp, MD: Adult and Pediatric Dermatology: A Color Guide to Diagnosis and Treatment, page 364. FA Davis, 1997, with permission.

comedo (KŎM-ē-dō): blackhead; discolored dried sebum plugging an excretory duct of the skin.

contusion (kŏn-TOO-zhŭn): injury in which the skin is not broken; also known as a *bruise*.

cyst (SĬST): closed sac or pouch in or under the skin, with a definite wall, that contains fluid, semifluid, or solid material.

decubitus ulcer (dē-KŪ-bĭ-tŭs ŬL-sĕr): skin ulceration caused by prolonged pressure, usually in a person who is bedridden; also known as a *bedsore*.

ecchymosis (ĕk-ĭ-MŌ-sĭs): skin discoloration consisting of a large, irregularly formed hemorrhagic area with colors changing from blue-black to greenish brown or yellow; commonly called a *bruise* (see Figure 3–6).

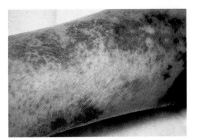

Figure 3-6   Ecchymosis. From Harmening, DM: Clinical Hematology and Fundamentals of Hemostasis, 4th edition, page 489. FA Davis, 2001, with permission.

eczema (ĔK-zĕ-mă): general term for an itchy red rash that initially weeps or oozes serum and may become crusted, thickened, or scaly.

Eczematous rash may result from various causes, including allergies, irritating chemicals, drugs, scratching or rubbing the skin, or sun exposure. It may be acute or chronic.

furuncle (FŪ-rŭng-k'l): tender, dome-shaped lesion, typically caused by infection around a hair follicle. As furuncles mature, they form localized abscesses with pus; commonly called a *boil* (see Figure 3–5).

Lesions drain a creamy pus when incised and may heal with scarring.

hirsutism (HŬR-sūt-ĭzm): condition characterized by excessive growth of hair, or presence of hair, in unusual places, especially in women.

impetigo (ĭm-pĕ-TĪ-gō): inflammatory skin disease characterized by isolated pustules that become crusted and rupture.

petechia (pē-TĒ-kē-ă): minute, pinpoint hemorrhagic spot of the skin.

A petechia is a smaller version of an ecchymosis.

psoriasis (sō-RĪ-ă-sĭs): chronic skin disease characterized by itchy red patches covered with silvery scales (see Figure 3–7). The condition runs in families and may be brought on by anxiety.

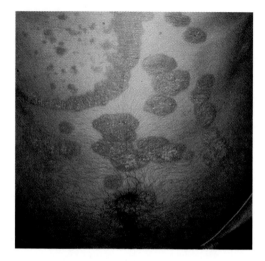

Figure 3-7   Psoriasis. From Goldsmith, LA, Lazarus, GS, and Tharp, MD: Adult and Pediatric Dermatology: A Color Guide to Diagnosis and Treatment, page 258. FA Davis, 1997, with permission.

scabies (SKĀ-bēz): contagious skin disease transmitted by the itch mite.

skin lesions (LĒ-zhŭn): areas of pathologically altered tissue caused by disease, injury, or a wound due to external factors or internal disease.

Evaluation of skin lesions, injuries, or changes to tissue helps establish the diagnosis of skin disorders. Lesions are described as primary or secondary.

primary lesions: initial reaction to pathologically altered tissue; may be flat or elevated.

secondary lesions: result from the changes that take place in the primary lesion due to infection, scratching, trauma, or various stages of a disease.

Lesions also are described by their appearance, color, location, and size as measured in centimeters. Review the primary and secondary lesions illustrated in Figure 3–8.

tinea (TĬN-ē-ă): any fungal skin disease occurring on various parts of the body. Its name indicates the body part affected; commonly called *ringworm.*

Examples of tinea include tinea barbae (beard), tinea corporis (body), tinea pedis (athlete's foot), and tinea versicolor (skin).

urticaria (ŭr-tĭ-KĀ-rē-ă): allergic reaction of the skin characterized by eruption of pale-red elevated patches that are intensely itchy; also called *wheals (hives).*

vitiligo (vĭt-ĭl-Ī-gō): localized loss of skin pigmentation characterized by milk-white patches.

wart (wort): rounded epidermal growths caused by a virus.

Types of warts include plantar warts, juvenile warts, and venereal warts; removable by cryosurgery, electrocautery, or acids; able to regrow if virus remains in the skin.

PRIMARY LESIONS

FLAT LESIONS
Flat, discolored, circumscribed lesions of any size

Macule
Flat, pigmented, circumscribed area less than 1 cm in diameter.
Examples: freckle, flat mole, or rash that occurs in rubella.

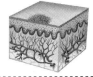

ELEVATED LESIONS

Solid   *Fluid-filled*

Papule
Solid, elevated lesion less than 1 cm in diameter that may be the same color as the skin or pigmented.
Examples: nevus, wart, pimple, ringworm, psoriasis, eczema.

Vesicle
Elevated, circumscribed, fluid-filled lesion less than 0.5 cm in diameter.
Examples: poison ivy, shingles, chickenpox.

Nodule
Palpable, circumscribed lesion; larger and deeper than a papule (0.6 to 2 cm in diameter); extends into the dermal area.
Examples: intradermal nevus, benign or malignant tumor.

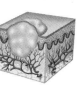

Pustule
Small, raised, circumscribed lesion that contains pus; usually less than 1 cm in diameter.
Examples: acne, furuncle, pustular psoriasis, scabies.

Tumor
Solid, elevated lesion larger than 2 cm in diameter that extends into the dermal and subcutaneous layers.
Examples: lipoma, steatoma, dermatofibroma, hemangioma.

Bulla
A vesicle or blister larger than 1 cm in diameter.
Examples: second degree burns, severe poison oak, poison ivy.

Wheal
Elevated, firm, rounded lesion with localized skin edema (swelling) that varies in size, shape, and color; paler in the center than its surrounding edges; accompanied by itching.
Examples: hives, insect bites, urticaria.

SECONDARY LESIONS

DEPRESSED LESIONS
Depressed lesions caused by loss of skin surface

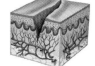
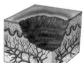

Excoriations
Linear scratch marks or traumatized abrasions of the epidermis.
Examples: scratches, abrasions, chemical or thermal burns.

Fissure
Small slit or cracklike sore that extends into the dermal layer; could be caused by continuous inflammation and drying.

Ulcer
An open sore or lesion that extends to the dermis and usually heals with scarring.
Examples: pressure sore, basal cell carcinoma.

Figure 3-8 Primary and secondary lesions.

Diagnostic

biopsy (BĪ-ŏp-sē): removal of a small piece of living tissue from an organ or other part of the body for microscopic examination to confirm or establish a diagnosis, estimate prognosis, or follow the course of a disease.

Types of biopsy include aspiration biopsy, needle biopsy, punch biopsy, and shave biopsy.

skin test: method for determining induced sensitivity (allergy) by applying or inoculating a suspected allergen or sensitizer into the skin. Sensitivity (allergy) to the specific antigen is indicated by an inflammatory skin reaction to it.

The most commonly used tests are the intradermal, patch, and scratch tests.

Therapeutic

chemical peel: chemical removal of the outer layers of skin to treat acne scaring and general keratoses; also used for cosmetic purposes to remove fine wrinkles on the face; also called *chemabrasion.*

cryosurgery (krī-ō-SĔR-jĕr-ē): use of subfreezing temperature (commonly with liquid nitrogen) to destroy abnormal tissue cells, such as unwanted, cancerous, or infected tissue.

debridement (dā-brēd-MŎNT): removal of foreign material and dead or damaged tissue, especially in a wound; used to promote healing and prevent infection.

dermabrasion (DĔRM-ă-brā-zhŭn): removal of acne scars, nevi, tattoos, or fine wrinkles on the skin through the use of sandpaper, wire brushes, or other abrasive materials on the epidermal layer.

electrodessication (ē-lĕk-trō-dĕs-ĭ-KĀ-shŭn): process in which high-frequency electrical sparks are used to dehydrate and destroy diseased tissue.

incision and drainage (I&D): incision of a lesion, such as an abscess, followed by the drainage of its contents.

Listen and Learn, the audio CD-ROM that accompanies this book, will help you master the pronunciation of selected medical words. Use it to practice pronunciations of the above-listed medical terms and for instructions to complete the *Listen and Learn* exercise on the CD-ROM for this section.

PATHOLOGICAL, DIAGNOSTIC, AND THERAPEUTIC TERMS REVIEW

Match the medical term(s) below with the definitions in the numbered list.

alopecia
biopsy
comedo
cryosurgery
debridement

decubitus ulcer
dermabrasion
eczema
electrodesiccation
petechia

scabies
tinea
urticaria
vitiligo
wart

1. _____ is a rounded epidermal growth caused by a virus.

2. _____ is localized loss of skin pigmentation characterized by appearance of milk-white patches.

3. _____ is a fungal skin disease, commonly called ringworm, whose name indicates the body part affected.

4. _____ is ulceration caused by prolonged pressure; also called bedsore.

5. _____ is a general term for an itchy red rash that may become crusted, thickened, or scaly.

6. _____ is an allergic reaction of the skin characterized by eruption of pale red elevated patches that are intensely itchy; also called hives.

7. _____ refers to excision of a small piece of living tissue from an organ or other part of the body for microscopic examination.

8. _____ refers to use of revolving wire brushes or sandpaper to remove superficial scars on the skin.

9. _____ refers to the procedure in which diseased tissue is dehydrated and destroyed by high-frequency electrical sparks.

10. _____ refers to use of liquid nitrogen to destroy or eliminate abnormal tissue cells.

11. _____ refers to removal of foreign material and dead or damaged tissue, especially in a wound.

12. _____ is a contagious skin disease transmitted by the itch mite.

13. _____ is absence or loss of hair, especially of the head; baldness.

14. _____ is a blackhead.

15. _____ is a minute hemorrhagic spot on the skin that is a smaller version of ecchymosis.

Competency Verification: Check your answers in Appendix B, Answer Key, page 511. If you are not satisfied with your level of comprehension, review the pathological, diagnostic, and therapeutic terms and retake the review.

Correct Answers _____ × 6.67 = _____% Score

PRIMARY AND SECONDARY LESIONS REVIEW

Identify and label the following skin lesions using the terms listed below.

bulla	excoriations	vesicle	nodule
wheal	macule	tumor	ulcer
pustule	fissure	papule	

PRIMARY LESIONS

FLAT LESIONS
Flat, discolored, circumscribed lesions of any size

Flat, pigmented, circumscribed area less than 1 cm in diameter.
Examples: freckle, flat mole, or rash that occurs in rubella.

- **ELEVATED LESIONS** -

Solid · *Fluid-filled*

Solid, elevated lesion less than 1 cm in diameter that may be the same color as the skin or pigmented.
Examples: nevus, wart, pimple, ringworm, psoriasis, eczema.

Elevated, circumscribed, fluid-filled lesion less than 0.5 cm in diameter.
Examples: poison ivy, shingles, chickenpox.

Palpable, circumscribed lesion; larger and deeper than a papule (0.6 to 2 cm in diameter); extends into the dermal area.
Examples: intradermal nevus, benign or malignant tumor.

Small, raised, circumscribed lesion that contains pus; usually less than 1 cm in diameter.
Examples: acne, furuncle, pustular psoriasis, scabies.

Solid, elevated lesion larger than 2 cm in diameter that extends into the dermal and subcutaneous layers.
Examples: lipoma, steatoma, dermatofibroma, hemangioma.

A vesicle or blister larger than 1 cm in diameter.
Examples: second degree burns, severe poison oak, poison ivy.

Elevated, firm, rounded lesion with localized skin edema (swelling) that varies in size, shape, and color; paler in the center than its surrounding edges; accompanied by itching.
Examples: hives, insect bites, urticaria.

- -

SECONDARY LESIONS

DEPRESSED LESIONS
Depressed lesions caused by loss of skin surface

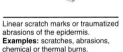

Linear scratch marks or traumatized abrasions of the epidermis.
Examples: scratches, abrasions, chemical or thermal burns.

Small slit or cracklike sore that extends into the dermal layer; could be caused by continuous inflammation and drying.

An open sore or lesion that extends to the dermis and usually heals with scarring.
Examples: pressure sore, basal cell carcinoma.

Competency Verification: Check your answers by referring to Figure 3–8, page 85. Review material that you did not answer correctly.

Medical Record Activities

The two medical records included in the following activities reflect common real-life clinical scenarios to show how medical terminology is used in documenting patient care. The physician who specializes in the treatment of skin disorders is called a *dermatologist;* the medical specialty concerned in the diagnoses and treatment of skin disorders is called *dermatology.*

✓ MEDICAL RECORD ACTIVITY 3–1. Compound Nevus

Terminology

The terms listed in the chart come from the medical record *Compound Nevus* that follows. Use a medical dictionary such as *Taber's Cyclopedic Medical Dictionary,* the appendices of this book, or other resources to define each term. Then practice the pronunciations aloud for each term.

Term	Definition
circumscribed SĔR-kŭm-skrībd	
crusting KRUST-ĭng	
lesion LĒ-zhŭn	
melanoma mĕl-ă-NŌ-mă	
nevus NĒ-vŭs	
trauma TRAW-mă	
vermilion border vĕr-mĭl-yŏn	

Listen and Learn Online! will help you master the pronunciation of selected medical words from this medical record activity. Visit www.fadavis.com/gylys/simplified for instructions in completing the *Listen and Learn Online!* exercise for this section and then to practice pronunciations.

COMPOUND NEVUS

Reading

Practice pronunciation of medical terms by reading the following medical report aloud.

A 29-year-old married white woman was referred for surgical treatment of a nevus of the right lower lip. The patient has had a small nevus located at the vermilion border of her lower lip all of her life, but recently it has enlarged and has become irritated with crusting and bleeding, through local trauma.

The lesion was evaluated initially about 1 month ago during a period of trauma, but it could not be removed at that time because the patient had a prominent upper respiratory infection. Subsequently, there has been healing of the local inflammatory component, and the nevus is clear at this time.

Examination reveals a brownish lesion with a flat, irregular border that is fairly circumscribed, measuring 0.5 cm in the greatest diameter and located just at the edge of the vermilion border on the right side of the lower lip.

IMPRESSION: Compound nevus, lower lip, rule out melanoma.

Evaluation

Review the medical record above to answer the following questions.

1. What is a nevus?

   _____

   _____

2. Locate the vermilion border on your lip. Where is it located?

   _____

   _____

3. Was the lesion limited to a certain area?

   _____

   _____

4. In the impression, the pathologist has ruled out melanoma. What does this mean?

   _____

   _____

5. Is a melanoma a dangerous condition? If so, explain why.

   _____

   _____

Terminology

The terms listed in the chart come from the medical record *Psoriasis* that follows. Use a medical dictionary such as *Taber's Cyclopedic Medical Dictionary,* the appendices of this book, or other resources to define each term. Then practice the pronunciations aloud for each term.

Term	Definition
Bartholin gland BĂR-tō-lĭn	
colitis kō-LĪ-tĭs	
diabetes mellitus dī-ă-BĒ-tēz MĔ-lĭ-tŭs	
diaphoresis dī-ă-fō-RĒ-sĭs	
Dx	
enteritis ĕn-tĕr-Ī-tĭs	
erythematous ĕr-ĭ-THĔM-ă-tŭs	
FH	
histiocytoma hĭs-tē-ō-sī-TŌ-mă	
macules MĂK-ūls	
papules PĂP-ūls	
pruritus proo-RĪ-tŭs	
psoriasis sō-RĪ-ă-sĭs (see Figure 3–7)	
sclerosed sklă-RŌST	
sinusitis sī-nŭs-Ī-tĭs	
syncope SĬN-kō-pē	
vulgaris vŭl-GĀ-rĭs	

Listen and Learn Online! will help you master the pronunciation of selected medical words from this medical record activity. Visit www.fadavis.com/gylys/simplified for instructions in completing the *Listen and Learn Online!* exercise for this section and then to practice pronunciations.

PSORIASIS

Reading

Practice pronunciation of medical terms by reading the following medical report aloud.

Patient is a 24-year-old white woman who has experienced intermittent psoriasis since her early teens in various stages of severity. Since May, her condition has become more troublesome because of an increase of symptoms after being exposed to the sun. Her past history indicates she had chronic sinusitis of 3 years' duration. Her Bartholin gland was excised in 20XX. She has had pruritus of the scalp and abdominal regions. There is no FH of psoriasis. An uncle has had diabetes mellitus since age 43. Patient has occasional abdominal pains accompanied by diaphoresis and/or syncope. PE showed the patient to have psoriatic involvement of the scalp, external ears, trunk, and, to a lesser degree, legs. There are many scattered erythematous (light ruby), thickened plaques covered by thick, yellowish white scales. A few areas on the legs and arms show multiple, sclerosed, brown macules and papules.

DIAGNOSIS: 1. Psoriasis vulgaris.
2. Multiple histiocytomas.
3. Abdominal pain, by history.
4. Rule out colitis, regional enteritis.

Evaluation

Review the medical record above to answer the following questions.

1. What causes psoriasis?

   _____

   _____

2. On what parts of the body does psoriasis typically occur?

   _____

   _____

3. How is psoriasis treated?

   _____

   _____

4. What is a histiocytoma?

   _____

   _____

Chapter Review

Word Elements Summary

The following table summarizes combining forms, suffixes, and prefixes related to the integumentary system.

Word Element	Meaning
COMBINING FORMS	
adip/o, lip/o, steat/o	fat
cutane/o, derm/o, dermat/o	skin
cyt/o	cell
hidr/o, sudor/o	sweat
hydr/o	water
ichthy/o	dry, scaly
kerat/o	horny tissue; hard; cornea
myc/o	fungus
necr/o	death, necrosis
pil/o, trich/o	hair
onych/o	nail
scler/o	hardening; sclera (white of eye)
squam/o	scale
xer/o	dry
COMBINING FORMS OF COLOR	
cyan/o	blue
erythr/o, erythemat/o	red
leuk/o	white
melan/o	black
xanth/o	yellow
SUFFIXES	
SURGICAL	
-plasty	surgical repair
-tome	instrument to cut

Word Element	Meaning
DIAGNOSTIC, SYMPTOMATIC, AND RELATED	
-cele	hernia, swelling
-cyte	cell
-derma	skin
-emia	blood condition
-esis	condition
-itis	inflammation
-logist	specialist in study of
-logy	study of
-malacia	softening
-oma	tumor
-osis	abnormal condition; increase (used primarily with blood cells)
-pathy	disease
-penia	decrease, deficiency
-phagia	swallowing, eating
-phoresis	carrying, transmission
-rrhea	discharge, flow
-therapy	treatment
ADJECTIVE	
-al, -ous	pertaining to, relating to
PREFIXES	
auto-	self, own
epi-	above, on
hypo-	under, below, deficient
sub-	under, below

After you review the Word Elements Summary, complete this activity by writing the meaning of each element in the space provided.

Word Element	Meaning
COMBINING FORMS	
1. adip/o, lip/o, steat/o	
2. cutane/o, derm/o, dermat/o	
3. cyt/o	
4. hidr/o, sudor/o	
5. hydr/o	
6. ichthy/o	
7. kerat/o	
8. myc/o	
9. necr/o	
10. onych/o	
11. pil/o, trich/o	
12. scler/o	
13. squam/o	
14. xer/o	
COMBINING FORMS OF COLOR	
15. cyan/o	
16. erythr/o	
17. leuk/o	
18. melan/o	
19. xanth/o	
SUFFIXES	
SURGICAL	
20. -plasty	
21. -tome	

Word Element	Meaning
DIAGNOSTIC, SYMPTOMATIC, AND RELATED	
22. -cele	
23. -cyte	
24. -emia	
25. -esis	
26. -itis	
27. -logist	
28. -logy	
29. -malacia	
30. -oma	
31. -osis	
32. -pathy	
33. -penia	
34. -phagia	
35. -phoresis	
36. -rrhea	
37. -therapy	
PREFIXES	
38. auto-	
39. epi-	
40. sub-	

Competency Verification: Check your answers in Appendix A, Glossary of Medical Word Elements, page 497. If you are not satisfied with your level of comprehension, review the word elements and retake the review.

Correct Answers: _____ × 2.5 = _____% Score

Chapter 3 Vocabulary Review

Match the medical term(s) below with the definitions in the numbered list.

autograft	hirsutism	onychoma	subcutaneous
decubitus ulcer	Kaposi sarcoma	onychomalacia	suction lipectomy
diaphoresis	leukemia	onychomycosis	trichopathy
ecchymosis	lipocele	papules	xanthoma
erythrocyte	melanoma	pustule	xeroderma

1. _____ means beneath the skin.

2. _____ is a condition in which a person sweats excessively; profuse perspiration.

3. _____ refers to any disease of the hair.

4. _____ refers to a graft transferred from one part to another part of a patient's body.

5. _____ is a type of malignant skin tumor associated with AIDS.

6. _____ refers to excision of subcutaneous fat tissue by use of a blunt-tipped cannula (tube), done for cosmetic reasons.

7. _____ is a fungal infection of the nails.

8. _____ is caused by prolonged pressure against an area of skin from a bed or chair.

9. _____ refers to excessive production of white blood cells; literally means white blood.

10. _____ is a black-and-blue mark on the skin; a bruise.

11. _____ is a benign tumor of the nail bed.

12. _____ means excessive body hair, especially in women.

13. _____ is an elevated lesion containing pus, as seen in acne, furuncles, and psoriasis.

14. _____ is a medical term for warts, moles, and pimples.

15. _____ is a red blood cell.

16. _____ means excessive dryness of skin.

17. _____ is a black tumor.

18. _____ refers to a hernia that contains fat or fatty cells.

19. _____ refers to a tumor containing yellow material.

20. _____ is an abnormal softening of the nail or nailbed.

Competency Verification: Check your answers in Appendix B, Answer Key, page 512. If you are not satisfied with your level of comprehension, review the chapter vocabulary and retake the review.

Correct Answers: _____ × 5 = _____% Score

chapter

4

Respiratory System

OBJECTIVES

Upon completion of this chapter, you will be able to:

■ Describe the respiratory system and discuss its primary functions.

■ Describe pathological, diagnostic, therapeutic, and other terms related to the respiratory system.

■ Recognize, define, pronounce, and spell terms correctly by completing the audio CD-ROM exercises.

■ Demonstrate your knowledge of this chapter by successfully completing the frames, reviews, and medical report evaluations.

The respiratory system consists of the upper respiratory tract—the nose, pharynx, larynx, and trachea—and the lower respiratory tract—the left and the right primary bronchi, bronchioles, alveoli, and the lungs (see Figure 4–1). The main function of the respiratory system is to perform the pulmonary ventilation of the body. These structures, along with the cardiovascular system, transport oxygen and remove carbon dioxide (a waste product) from the cells of the body. This is accomplished by the events of respiration, exchanging oxygen and carbon dioxide between the environmental air and the blood circulating through the lungs. Secondary functions of the respiratory system include warming the air as it passes into the body and assisting in the speech function (providing air for the larynx and the vocal cords).

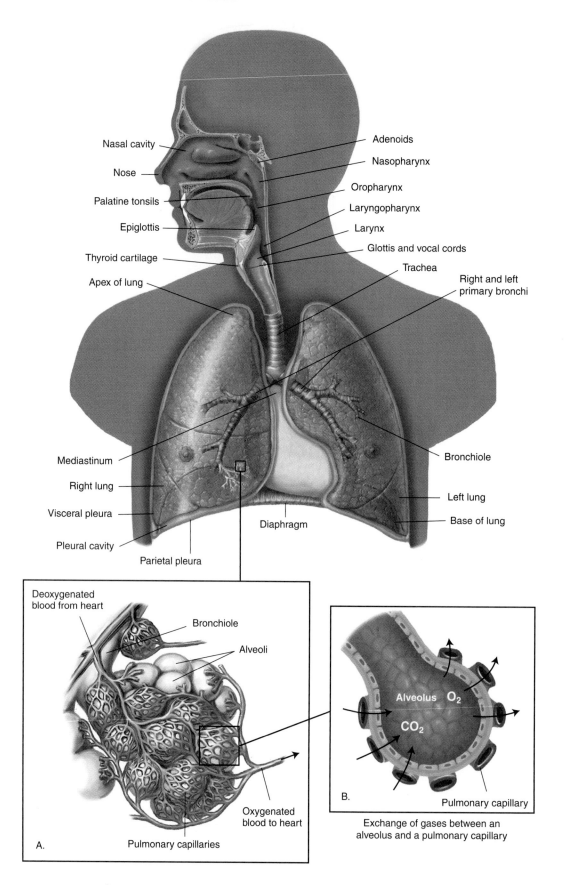

Figure 4-1 Anterior view of the upper and lower respiratory tracts.

Word Elements

This section introduces combining forms related to the respiratory system. Included are key suffixes; prefixes are defined in the right-hand column as needed. Review the following table and pronounce each word in the word analysis column aloud before you begin to work the frames.

Word Element	Meaning	Word Analysis
COMBINING FORMS		
UPPER RESPIRATORY TRACT		
adenoid/o	adenoids	adenoid/ectomy (ăd-ĕ-noyd-ĔK-tō-mē): excision of the adenoids *-ectomy:* excision, removal
laryng/o	larynx (voice box)	laryng/o/scope (lăr-ĬN-gō-skōp): instrument for examining the larynx *-scope:* instrument for examining
nas/o	nose	nas/al (NĀ-zl): pertaining to the nose *-al:* pertaining to, relating to
rhin/o		rhin/o/rrhea (rī-nō-RĒ-ă): thin watery discharge from the nose *Rhinorrhea also can be caused by the flow of cerebrospinal fluid from the nose after an injury to the head.* *-rrhea:* discharge, flow
pharyng/o	pharynx (throat)	pharyng/itis (făr-ĭn-JĪ-tĭs): inflammation of the pharynx, usually due to infection *-itis:* inflammation

tonsill/o	tonsils	peri/tonsill/ar (pĕr-ĭ-TŎN-sĭ-lăr): pertaining to the area surrounding the tonsils
		   peri-: around
		   -ar: pertaining to, relating to

trache/o	trachea (windpipe)	trache/o/stomy (trā-kē-ŎS-tō-mē): surgical opening through the neck into the trachea to provide and secure an open airway *-stomy:* forming an opening (mouth) *When performed as an emergency, the tracheostomy is closed after normal breathing is restored. If the procedure is permanent, such as with a laryngectomy, the patient is taught self-care*
LOWER RESPIRATORY TRACT		
alveol/o	alveolus (plural, alveoli)	alveol/ar (ăl-VĒ-ō-lăr): pertaining to the alveoli *-ar:* pertaining to, relating to

(Continued)

Word Element	Meaning	Word Analysis (Continued)
bronchi/o	bronchus (plural, bronchi)	bronchi/ectasis (brŏng-kē-ĔK-tă-sĭs): chronic dilation of a bronchus or bronchi, usually in the lower portions of the lung -ectasis: dilation, expansion *Bronchiectasis can be caused by the damaging effects of a long-standing infection.*
bronch/o		bronch/o/scope (BRŎNG-kō-skōp): curved, flexible tube with a light for visual examination of the bronchi -scope: instrument for examining *A bronchoscope is used to examine the bronchi, secure a specimen for biopsy or culture, or aspirate secretions of a foreign body from the respiratory tract.*
bronchiol/o	bronchiole	bronchiol/itis (brŏng-kē-ō-LĪ-tĭs): inflammation of the bronchioles -itis: inflammation
pneum/o	air; lung	pneum/ectomy (nū-MĔK-tō-mē): excision of all or part of a lung -ectomy: excision, removal
pneumon/o		pneumon/ia (nū-MŌ-nē-ă): acute inflammation and infection of alveoli, which fill with pus or products of the inflammatory reaction -ia: condition *Pneumonia is caused most often by inhaled pneumonococci and less frequently by staphylococci, fungi, or viruses.*
pulmon/o	lung	pulmon/o/logist (pool-mă-NŎL-ă-jĭst): physician who specializes in treating pathological conditions of the lungs -logist: specialist in study of
pleur/o	pleura	pleur/itic (ploo-RĬT-ĭk): pertaining to a condition of pleurisy -itic: pertaining to, relating to
thorac/o	chest	thorac/o/pathy (thō-răk-ŎP-ă-thē): any disease involving the thorax or the organs it contains -pathy: disease

SUFFIXES		
-algia	pain	pleur/algia (ploo-RĂL-jē-ă): pain in the pleura *pleur:* pleura
-dynia		thorac/o/dynia (thō-răk-ō-DĬN-ē-ă): pain in the chest *thorac:* chest
-ectasis	dilation, expansion	atel/ectasis (ăt-ĕ-LĔK-tă-sĭs): abnormal condition characterized by the collapse of alveoli *atel:* incomplete; imperfect *Atelectasis is characterized by the collapse of alveoli, preventing the respiratory exchange of carbon dioxide and oxygen in a part of the lungs.*

Word Element	Meaning	Word Analysis
-osmia	smell	an/osmia (ăn-ŎZ-mē-ă): loss or impairment of the sense of smell; usually occurs as a temporary condition *an-:* without, not
-osis	abnormal condition; increase (used primarily with blood cells)	cyan/osis (sī-ă-NŌ-sĭs): bluish discoloration of the skin and mucous membranes caused by a deficiency of oxygen in the blood *cyan:* blue
-oxia	oxygen	hyp/oxia (hī-PŎKS-ē-ă): inadequate oxygen at the cellular level characterized by tachycardia, hypertension, and dizziness *hyp-:* under, below, deficient
-phagia	swallowing, eating	aer/o/phagia (ĕr-ō-FĀ-jē-ă): swallowing of air *aer/o:* air
-pnea	breathing	a/pnea (ăp-NĒ-ă): temporary cessation of breathing *a-:* without, not *Apnea may be a serious symptom, especially in patients with other potentially life-threatening conditions. Some types of apnea include newborn, cardiac, and sleep.*
-spasm	involuntary contraction, twitching	pharyng/o/spasm (făr-ĬN-gō-spăzm): spasm of the muscles in the pharynx *pharyng/o:* pharynx (throat)
-thorax	chest	py/o/thorax (pī-ō-THŌ-răks): accumulation of pus in the thorax *py/o:* pus

Listen and Learn, the audio CD-ROM that accompanies this book, will help you master the pronunciation of selected medical words. Use it to practice pronunciations of the above-listed medical terms and for instructions to complete the *Listen and Learn* exercise on the CD-ROM for this section.

S E C T I O N   R E V I E W   4 – 1

For the following medical terms, first write the suffix and its meaning. Then translate the meaning of the remaining elements starting with the first part of the word. The first word is an example that is completed for you.

Term	Meaning
1. laryng/o/scope	-scope: instrument for examining; larynx (voice box)
2. py/o/thorax	_____
3. hyp/oxia	_____
4. trache/o/stomy	_____
5. a/pnea	_____
6. pulmon/o/logist	_____
7. pneumon/ia	_____
8. rhin/o/rrhea	_____
9. an/osmia	_____
10. pneum/ectomy	_____

Competency Verification: Check your answers in Appendix B, Answer Key, page 512. If you are not satisfied with your level of comprehension, review the vocabulary and retake the review.

Correct Answers _____ × 10 = _____% Score

Respiratory System

Upper Respiratory Tract

nose, stomach	**4-1** The external openings of the nose are referred to as the *nostrils* or *nares* (singular, naris). *Nas/o/gastr/ic* refers to the nose and stomach. This term is used to describe procedures and devices associated with the nose and the stomach, such as nas/o/gastr/ic feeding and nas/o/gastr/ic suction. When you see the term nas/o/gastr/ic tube, you will know it refers to a device inserted into the _____ and into the _____.
pharynx (throat) FĂR-ĭnks	**4-2** When the term tube is used in association with a procedure, it usually refers to a catheter. A catheter, a hollow flexible tube, can be inserted into a vessel or cavity of the body to withdraw or instill fluids into a body cavity or vessel. A pharyng/eal suction catheter is used to suction the pharynx during direct visualization. The combining form **pharyng/o** means _____ (_____).

nas/o

rhin/o

4-3   Two combining forms for the nose are _____ / _____ and _____ / _____.

4-4   The prefix para- is a directional element meaning *near, beside; beyond.* The para/nas/al sinuses are hollow spaces within the skull that open into the nasal cavities and are lined with *ciliated epithelium*, which is continuous with the mucosa of the nasal cavities.

The term in this frame that means around the nose is

_____ / _____ / _____.

para/nas/al
păr-ă-NĀ-săl

4-5   Both **rhin/o** and **nas/o** refer to the *nose.* As a general rule, **nas/o** is not used to build surgical terms, but if you are in doubt about which element to use, consult a medical dictionary.

Form operative terms meaning

surgical repair of the nose: _____ / _____ / _____.

incision of the nose: _____ / _____ / _____.

rhin/o/plasty
RĪ-nō-plăs-tē
rhin/o/tomy
rī-NŎT-ō-mē

4-6   *Rhin/o/rrhea* is a discharge from the nose—a runny nose. Sneezing, tearing, and a runny nose are common symptoms of a cold.

Build a term that means discharge from the nose:

_____ / _____ / _____.

rhin/o/rrhea
rī-nō-RĒ-ă

4-7   *Rhin/o/rrhea* refers to a runny nose, whereas *rhin/o/rrhagia* is a nosebleed. When profuse bleeding from the nose occurs, the diagnosis is

_____ / _____ / _____;

when a runny discharge from the nose occurs, the diagnosis is

_____ / _____ / _____.

rhin/o/rrhagia
rī-nō-RĂ-jē-ă

rhin/o/rrhea
rī-nō-RĒ-ă

4-8   Practice building some more medical terms with **rhin/o.**

An inflammation of the nose is called _____ / _____.

A physician who specializes in diseases of the nose is a

_____ / _____ / _____.

rhin/itis
rī-NĪ-tĭs

rhin/o/logist
rī-NŎL-ă-jĭst

When in doubt about the meaning of a word element, refer to Appendix A, Glossary of Medical Word Elements.

aer/o	**4-9** Air enters the nose and passes through the (1) **nasal cavity,** where fine hairs catch many of the dust particles that we inhale. Label the nasal cavity in Figure 4–2. **Pneum/o, pneumon/o,** and _____ /_____ are combining forms for air.
aer/o/phagia ĕr-ō-FĀ-jē-ă	**4-10** Swallowing air is not unusual for infants. It can occur as they suck on a nipple to obtain milk, water, or any liquid substance. Many times it causes gaseous discomfort, which is relieved when the infant is burped. Combine **aer/o** + -phagia to form a medical term meaning swallowing air: _____ /_____ /_____.
air	**4-11** The suffix -therapy is used in words to mean treatment. Aer/o/therapy is the treatment of diseases by the use of _____.
water	**4-12** Hydr/o/therapy is treatment of diseases by means of _____.
air **water**	**4-13** Using air and water to treat a disease or injury is also a form of therapy. *Aer/o/hydr/o/therapy* is treatment by application of _____ and _____.
aer/o/therapy ĕr-ō-THĔR-ă-pē **hydr/o/therapy** hī-drō-THĔR-ă-pē **aer/o/hydr/o/therapy** ĕr-ō-hī-drō-THĔR-ă-pē	**4-14** Use -therapy to develop words meaning treatment by air: _____ /_____ /_____. treatment by water: _____ /_____ /_____. treatment by air and water: _____ /_____ /_____ /_____ /_____.
	4-15 After passing through the nasal cavity, air reaches the (2) **pharynx (throat).** Label the pharynx in Figure 4–2.
pharyng/o **myc** **-osis**	**4-16** From pharyng/o/myc/osis, determine the elements meaning: pharynx (throat): _____ /_____. fungus: _____. abnormal condition: _____.
pharynx FĂR-ĭnks	**4-17** Pharyng/o/myc/osis is a fungal disease of the _____.
pharynx FĂR-ĭnks	**4-18** The suffix -plegia means *paralysis.* Pharyng/o/plegia and pharyng/o/paralysis are used to describe muscle paralysis of the _____.

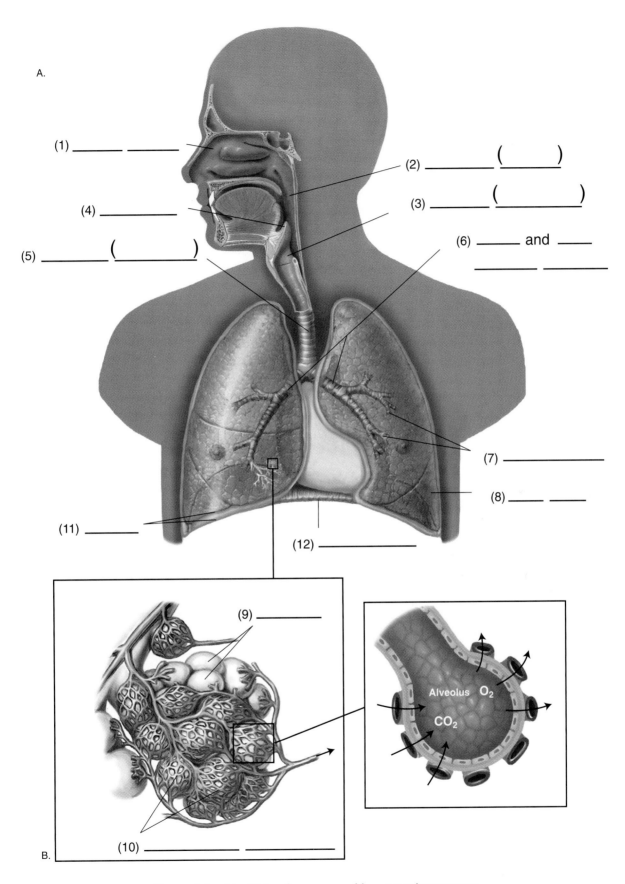

A.

(1) _____ _____

(2) _____ (_____)

(3) _____ (_____)

(4) _____ _____

(6) _____ and _____

(5) _____ (_____)

_____ _____

(7) _____

(8) _____ _____

(11) _____

(12) _____

(9) _____

Alveolus O$_2$

CO$_2$

(10) _____ _____

B.

Figure 4-2   Identifying the upper and lower respiratory tracts.

cancer
KĂN-sĕr

4-19 Smoking, drinking alcohol, and chewing tobacco can cause cancer (CA) of the pharynx. Patients with CA of the pharynx may require some type of plastic surgery.

When you see CA in a medical chart, you will know it is an abbreviation for _____.

---

pharyng/itis
făr-ĭn-JĪ-tĭs

pharyng/o/plasty
făr-ĬN-gō-plăs-tē
pharyng/o/tomy
făr-ĭn-GŎT-ō-mē

pharyng/o/tome
făr-ĬN-gō-tōm

pharyng/o/spasm
făr-ĬN-gō-spăzm

4-20 Use **pharyng/o** to form medical words meaning

inflammation of the pharynx (throat): _____ / _____.

surgical repair of the pharynx (throat):
_____ / _____ / _____.

incision of the pharynx (throat): _____ / _____ / _____.

instrument to incise the pharynx (throat):
_____ / _____ / _____.

involuntary contraction or twitching of the pharynx (throat):
_____ / _____ / _____.

---

pharyng/o/cele
făr-ĬN-gō-sēl

4-21 Use -cele to build a word that literally means *hernia or swelling* of the pharynx: _____ / _____ / _____.

---

stricture
STRĬK-chūr
pharynx
FĂR-ĭnks

4-22 Pharyng/o/stenosis is a narrowing, or _____,
of the _____.

4-23 The (3) **larynx (voice box)** is responsible for sound production and makes speech possible. Label the larynx in Figure 4–2.

---

laryng/o
lăr-ĬN-gō

4-24 From laryng/itis (inflammation of the larynx), construct the combining form of the larynx: _____ / _____.

---

laryng/o/scope
lăr-ĬN-gō-skōp

4-25 Combine **laryng/o** + -scope to form a word meaning instrument to view the larynx: _____ / _____ / _____.

---

laryng/ectomy
lăr-ĭn-JĔK-tō-mē

4-26 When laryng/eal CA is detected in its early stages, a partial laryng/ectomy may be recommended. For extensive CA of the larynx, the entire larynx is removed. In either case, when excision of the larynx is performed, the surgery is called a

_____ / _____.

laryng/o/spasm
lăr-ĬN-gō-spazm

4-27   Spasms of the larynx impede breathing.

The medical word meaning spasm of the larynx is

_____ / _____ / _____.

-stenosis
stĕ-NŌ-sĭs
laryng/o

4-28   Laryng/o/stenosis is a stricture of the larynx.

Determine the elements that mean:

narrowing, stricture: _____.

larynx: _____ / _____.

---

laryng/itis
lăr-ĭn-JĪ-tĭs

laryng/o/scope
lăr-ĬN-gō-skōp

laryng/o/scopy
lăr-ĭn-GŎS-kō-pē

laryng/o/stenosis
lăr-ĭn-gō-stĕ-NŌ-sĭs

4-29   Form medical words meaning:

inflammation of the larynx: _____ / _____.

instrument to view or examine the larynx:

_____ / _____ / _____.

visual examination of the larynx:

_____ / _____ / _____.

narrowing or stricture of the larynx:

_____ / _____ / _____.

4-30   Label the structures in Figure 4–2 as you continue to read the material in this frame. A small leaf-shaped cartilage called the (4) **epiglottis** is located in the super/ior portion of the larynx. During swallowing, it closes off the larynx so that food and liquid are directed into the esophagus. If anything but air passes into the larynx, a cough reflex attempts to expel the material to avoid a serious blockage of breathing.

SECTION REVIEW 4 – 2

Using the following table, write the combining form, suffix, or prefix that matches its definition in the space provided to the left of the definition. There may be more than one word element that matches a definition.

Combining Forms	Suffixes	Prefixes
aer/o	-cele	a-
hydr/o	-ectasis	an-
laryng/o	-phagia	neo-
myc/o	-plegia	para-
nas/o	-scopy	
pharyng/o	-stenosis	
rhin/o	-stomy	
trache/o	-therapy	
	-tome	
	-tomy	

1. _____ air
2. _____ near, beside; beyond
3. _____ fungus
4. _____ dilation, expansion
5. _____ forming an opening (mouth)
6. _____ incision
7. _____ instrument to cut
8. _____ larynx (voice box)
9. _____ hernia, swelling
10. _____ new

11. _____ nose
12. _____ paralysis
13. _____ pharynx (throat)
14. _____ narrowing, stricture
15. _____ swallowing, eating
16. _____ trachea (windpipe)
17. _____ treatment
18. _____ without, not
19. _____ visual examination
20. _____ water

Competency Verification: Check your answers in Appendix B, Answer Key, page 512. If you are not satisfied with your level of comprehension, go back to Frame 4–1 and rework the frames.

Correct Answers _____ × 5 = _____% Score

 Making a set of flash cards from key word elements in this chapter for each section review can help you remember the elements. Make a flash card by writing a word element on one side of a 3 × 5 or 4 × 6 index card. On the other side, write the meaning of the element. Do this for all word elements in the section reviews. Use your flash cards to review each section. You might also use the flash cards to prepare for the chapter review at the end of this chapter.

Lower Respiratory Tract

bronchus
BRŎNG-kŭs

bronchi/oles
BRŎNG-kē-ōlz

4-31 Continue to label the structures in Figure 4–2, page 107, as you read the material in this frame.

The (5) **trachea (windpipe)** is a cylindrical tube composed of smooth muscle embedded with a series of 16 to 20 C-shaped rings of cartilage. The trachea extends downward into the thoracic cavity, where it divides to form the (6) **right** and **left primary bronchi** (singular, bronchus). Each bronchus enters a lung and continues to subdivide into increasingly finer, smaller branches known as the (7) **bronchioles**.

The singular form of bronchi is _____.

The smaller segments of the bronchus are called

_____ / _____.

4-32 The intricate network of air passages that supply the lungs looks like an inverted tree, with the trachea resembling the trunk. The term *bronch/ial tree* is often used to describe the series of respiratory tubes that branch into progressively narrower tubes as they extend into the lungs. Because each segment of the bronchial tree is an air passage that distributes the air throughout the lungs, surgical removal of any single segment is possible. Refer to Figure 4–1 to examine these structures.

cartilage
KĂR-tĭ-lĭj

4-33 The trachea's cartilaginous rings provide the necessary rigidity to keep the air passage open at all times. The combining form **chondr/o** refers to *cartilage*. Chondr/itis is an inflammation of _____.

chondr/o/plasty
KŎN-drō-plăs-tē
chondr/o/pathy
kŏn-DRŎP-ă-thē
chondr/oma
kŏn-DRŌ-mă

4-34 Form medical words meaning

surgical repair of cartilage: _____ / ____ / _____.

any disease of cartilage: _____ / ____ / _____.

tumor (or tumor-like growth) of cartilage: _____ / _____.

trache/o/stomy
trā-kē-ŎS-tō-mē

trache/o/stomy
trā-kē-ŎS-tō-mē

4-35 On its way to the lungs, air passes from the larynx to the trachea, the airway commonly known as the *windpipe*. In a life-threatening situation, when trache/al obstruction causes cessation of breathing, a trache/o/stomy is performed through the neck into the trachea to gain access to an airway below a blockage (see Figure 4–3).

When an emergency situation warrants the creation of an opening into the

trachea, the procedure performed is

_____ / ____ / _____.

The surgical procedure meaning forming an opening (mouth) into the

trachea is _____ / ____ / _____.

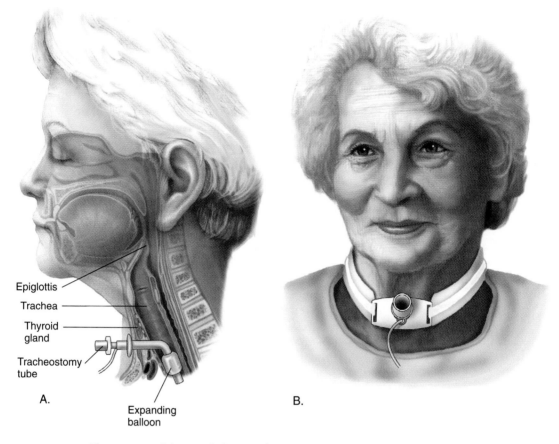

Epiglottis

Trachea

Thyroid gland

Tracheostomy tube

A.

Expanding balloon

B.

Figure 4-3 (A) Lateral view, tracheostomy tube in place. (B) Frontal view.

---

trache/o/malacia
trā-kē-ō-mă-LĀ-shē-ă

4–36 Softening of trache/al cartilage may be caused by pressure of the left pulmonary artery on the trachea. Use -malacia to form a word that literally means *softening of the trachea:*

_____ / ____ / _____.

---

trache/o/pathy
trā-kē-ŎP-ă-thē
trache/o/plasty
TRĀ-kē-ō-plăs-tē
trache/o/stenosis
trā-kē-ō-stĕn-Ō-sĭs
trache/o/tomy
trā-kē-ŎT-ō-mē

4–37 Use trache/o to develop medical terms that mean

disease of the trachea: _____ / ____ / _____.

surgical repair of the trachea: _____ / ____ / _____.

narrowing or stricture of the trachea:

_____ / ____ / _____.

incision of the trachea: _____ / ____ / _____.

---

trachea, larynx
TRĀ-kē-ă, LĂR-inks

4–38 Trache/o/laryng/o/tomy is an incision of the

_____ and _____.

4-39   Label the left lung in Figure 4–2 as you continue to read the material in this frame. Then review the position of the trachea to see how it branches into a right and left primary bronchus. Each primary *bronchus (plural, bronchi)* leads to a separate lung, the right and the (8) **left lung.** The structures of the bronchi and the alveoli are part of the lungs, which are the organs of *respiration* (act of breathing).

---

bronchi
BRŎNG-kē

4-40   Change the singular form of bronchus to a plural form:

_____ .

---

bronch/itis
brŏng-KĪ-tĭs

bronch/o/spasm
BRŎNG-kō-spăzm

bronch/o/stenosis
brŏng-kō-stĕn-Ō-sĭs

4-41   Use **bronch/o** to build medical words meaning

inflammation of the bronchi: _____ / _____ .

involuntary contraction or twitching of the bronchus:
_____ / _____ / _____ .

narrowing or stricture of the bronchi:
_____ / _____ / _____ .

---

bronch/o/spasm
BRŎNG-kō-spăzm

4-42   Patients with asthma (see Figure 4–4.) experience wheezing caused by bronch/ial spasms. The medical term for this condition is bronchi/o/spasm or _____ / _____ / _____ .

---

bronchi/ectasis
brŏng-kē-ĔK-tă-sĭs

4-43   A chronic dilation of the bronchi is called bronchi/ectasis. Chronic pneumon/ia or flu may result in a chronic dilation of the bronchi. The medical term for this condition is

_____ / _____ .

4-44   Structurally, each primary bronchus is similar to that of the trachea, but as they subdivide into finer branches, the amount of cartilage in the walls decreases and finally disappears in the bronchi/oles. As the cartilage diminishes, a layer of smooth muscle surrounding the tube becomes more prominent. The smooth muscles in the walls of the bronchioles can constrict or dilate these airways to maintain unobstructed air passages. The bronchi/oles eventually distribute air to the (9) **alveoli** (singular, alveolus), the small clusters of grapelike air sacs of the lungs. Each alveolus is surrounded by a network of microscopic (10) **pulmonary capillaries.** It is through these walls that an exchange of carbon dioxide (CO_2) and oxygen (O_2) takes place. Label the alveoli and pulmonary capillaries in Figure 4–2.

---

micro/scope
MĪ-krō-skōp

4-45   Macro/scopic structures are visible to the naked eye. Micro/scopic structures, such as the alveoli, are visible only by the use of a micro/scope. Micro/scopic capillaries are visible to the naked eye by use of a magnifying instrument called a _____ / _____ .

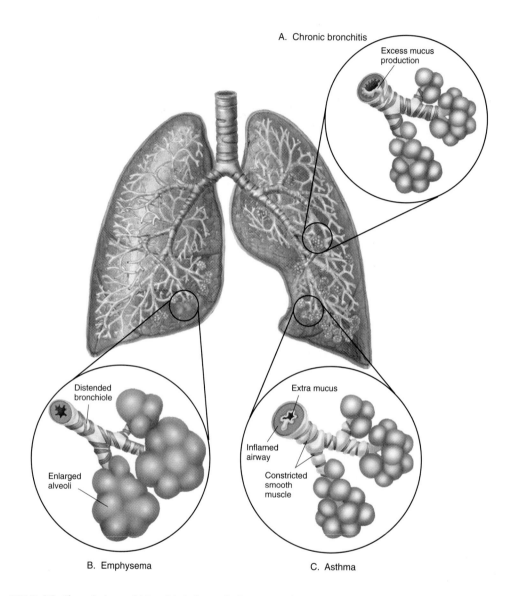

Figure 4-4   COLD (A) Chronic bronchitis with inflamed airways and excessive mucous. (B) Emphysema with distended bronchioles and alveoli. (C) Asthma with narrowed bronchial tubes and swollen mucous membranes.

alveoli ăl-VĒ-ō-lī	**4–46** If a lung disorder destroys or damages enough alveol/ar sacs, there is less surface area for gas exchange, and breathlessness results. The clusters of air sacs at the end of the bronchial tree are called _____ (plural).
external respiration **internal respiration**	**4–47** The entire process of gas exchange between the atmosphere and body cells is called _respiration,_ which occurs in two processes. _External respiration_ occurs each time we _inhale_ (breathe in) air. This process results in a gas exchange (oxygen loading and carbon dioxide unloading) between the air-filled chambers of the lungs and the blood in the pulmonary capillaries (see Figure 4–2, structure 10). _Internal (cellular) respiration_ is the exchange of gases (oxygen unloading and carbon dioxide loading) between the blood and body tissue cells. This occurs in body tissues when oxygen (carried in blood from the lungs to nourish the body's cells) is exchanged for carbon dioxide. The carbon dioxide travels in the bloodstream to the lungs and is _exhaled_ through the mouth or nose. You may have to read this frame a few times to understand the process of respiration. Nevertheless, see if you can differentiate between the two types of respiration. Gas exchange between the body and the outside environment is called _____ _____. Gas exchange at the cellular level between the blood and body tissue cells is called _____ _____.
O₂ **CO₂**	**4–48** You may see symbols O_2 and CO_2 in laboratory reports. If you forget what they mean, use Appendix E, which is a reference of abbreviations and symbols. The symbol for oxygen is _____. The symbol for carbon dioxide is _____.
inflammation, lung(s) ĭn-flă-MĀ-shŭn	**4–49** **Pneum/o** and **pneumon/o** are the combining forms that refer to the _lung(s)_ or _air._ Pneumon/itis is an _____ of the _____.
air, lung **condition**	**4–50** Pneumon/ia, an acute inflammation and infection of the lungs in which the alveoli fill with secretions, is the fifth leading cause of death in the United States. Analyze pneumon/ia by defining the word elements: **pneumon/o** means _____ or _____. -ia means _____ (noun ending).
pneumon/ectomy nū-mōn-ĔK-tō-mē	**4–51** In patients with lung cancer, it may be necessary to remove part or all of the lung. Use **pneumon/o** to form a word meaning herniation of a lung: _____ / _____.

pneumon/o/cele nū-MŌN-ō-sēl	**4–52** A hernial protrusion of lung tissue may be caused by a partial airway obstruction Use **pneumon/o** to form a word meaning herniation of the lung: _____ / ____ / _____.
pneumon/osis nū-mōn-Ō-sĭs **pneumon/o/pathy** nū-mō-NŎP-ăth-ē **pneumon/ectomy** nū-mōn-ĔK-tō-mē	**4–53** Use **pneumon/o** to build medical words meaning: abnormal condition of the lungs: _____ / _____. disease of the lung: _____ / ____ / _____. excision of a lung: _____ / _____.
lung(s)	**4–54** The suffix -centesis is used in words to denote a *surgical puncture*. Pneum/o/centesis is a surgical puncture to aspirate the _____.
	4–55 If you are not sure what *aspirate* means in the previous frame, take a few minutes to use your medical dictionary to define the term. _____ _____
pneumon/o/centesis nū-mō-nō-sĕn-TĒ-sis	**4–56** Lung abscess, an abnormal localized collection of fluid, may be caused by pneumonia. Therapeutic treatment of pneum/o/centesis may be required. Construct another word that means surgical puncture of a lung: _____ / ____ / _____.
lung(s), air **black** **abnormal condition**	**4–57** Pneumon/o/melan/osis is an abnormal condition of black lung caused by inhalation of black dust, which is a disease common among coal miners; also called *pneumomelanosis* and *pneumoconiosis*. Analyze pneumon/o/melan/osis by defining the word elements: **pneumon/o** means: _____ or _____. **melan/o** means: _____. -osis means: _____ _____.
oxygen **carbon dioxide**	**4–58** The lungs are divided into five lobes: three lobes in the right lung and two lobes in the left lung. Both lungs supply the blood with O_2 inhaled from outside the body and dispose of waste CO_2 in the exhaled air. O_2 refers to _____; CO_2 refers to _____ _____.
excision *or* removal ĕk-SĬ-zhŭn	**4–59** A person with lung cancer may undergo a lob/ectomy, which is a(n) _____ of a lobe.

lob/o	**4-60** From lob/ar (pertaining to the lobe), construct the combining form for lobe: _____ / _____.
lob/itis lō-BĪ-tĭs **lob/o/tomy** lō-BŎT-ō-mē **lob/ectomy** lō-BĔK-tō-mē	**4-61** Develop medical words meaning inflammation of a lobe: _____ / _____. incision of the lobe: _____ / _____ / _____. excision of a lobe: _____ / _____.
	4-62 Each lung is enclosed in a double-folded membrane called the (11) **pleura.** Label the pleura in Figure 4–2.
inflammation	**4-63** Pleur/itis is an _____ of the pleura.
pleur/o	**4-64** From pleur/o/dynia, identify the combining form for pleura: _____ / _____.
pleur/o/dynia ploo-rō-DĬN-ē-ă **pleur/algia** ploo-RĂL-jē-ă	**4-65** A pain in the pleura is known as _____ / _____ / _____ or _____ / _____.
pneumon/o *or* **pneum/o**	**4-66** Pleur/o/pneumon/ia is pleurisy complicated with pneumonia. The combining form for air or lung is _____ / _____.
pleur/itis ploo-RĪ-tĭs **pleur/o/cele** PLOO-rō-sēl	**4-67** Form medical words meaning inflammation of the pleura: _____ / _____. hernia or swelling of the pleura: _____ / _____ / _____.
inflammation, pleura PLOO-ră	**4-68** Pleurisy is an inflammation of the pleura. Pleur/itis is also an _____ of the _____.
inflammation, pleura PLOO-ră	**4-69** Whenever you see pleur/isy or pleur/itis, you will know it means _____ of the _____.
pleur/o/dynia ploo-rō-DĬN-ē-ă	**4-70** The suffixes -algia and -dynia refer to pain. The *pleura* often becomes inflamed when a person has *pneumonia.* This condition may cause pleur/algia, also called _____ / _____ / _____.

without, not slow bad, painful, difficult good, normal rapid breathing	**4–71** The prefixes a-, brady-, dys-, eu-, and tachy- are commonly attached to -pnea to describe an abnormality of the breathing process. Write the meanings of each element before continuing with subsequent frames. a-: _____, _____. brady-: _____. dys-: _____, _____, _____. eu-: _____, _____. tachy-: _____. -pnea: _____.
a/pnea ăp-NĒ-ă	**4–72** A/pnea is a temporary cessation of breathing that affects the body's intake of oxygen and the release of carbon dioxide. It is a serious symptom, especially in patients with other potentially life-threatening conditions. A term that literally means without breathing is _____ / _____
a/pnea ăp-NĒ-ă	**4–73** An infant whose mother used cocaine during pregnancy is more likely to develop life-threatening a/pnea. In this frame, the word meaning temporary cessation of breathing is _____ / _____.
dys/pnea dĭsp-NĒ-ă	**4–74** Use dys- to form a word meaning painful or difficult breathing: _____ / _____
dys/pnea dĭsp-NĒ-ă	**4–75** Dys/pnea is normal when it is due to vigorous work or athletic activity. Dys/pnea also can occur as a result of various disorders of the respiratory system, such as pleurisy. A person with pleurisy may experience _____ / _____.
dys/pnea dĭsp-NĒ-ă	**4–76** Asthma is a respiratory condition marked by recurrent attacks of labored breathing accompanied by wheezing (see Figure 4–4A). Generally the person has difficulty breathing. The medical term for bad, painful, or difficult breathing is _____ / _____.
eu- **-pnea**	**4–77** Eu/pnea is normal breathing, as distinguished from dys/pnea and a/pnea. From eu/pnea, determine the word elements meaning good, normal: _____. breathing: _____.

4-78   Here is a review of forming words with -pnea.

Construct medical words meaning

without breathing: _____ / _____.

a/pnea
ăp-NĒ-ă

dys/pnea   difficult or labored breathing: _____ / _____.
dĭsp-NĒ-ă

eu/pnea   normal breathing: _____ / _____.
ūp-NĒ-ă

tachy/pnea   rapid breathing: _____ / _____.
tăk-ĭp-NĒ-ă

4-79   Orth/o/pnea is a condition in which there is labored breathing in any posture except in the erect sitting or standing position.

Identify the word element that means

-pnea   breathing: _____.

orth/o   straight: _____ / ____.

4-80   The combining form thorac/o means chest. Form a word

thorac/o/tomy   meaning an incision of the chest: _____ / ____ / _____.
thō-răk-ŎT-ō-mē

4-81   To remove fluid from the thorac/ic (pertaining to the chest) cavity, a surgical puncture of the chest is performed. This procedure is

thorac/o/centesis   called thor/a/centesis, or _____ / ____ / _____
thō-răk-ō-sĕn-TĒ-sĭs   (see Figure 4–5).

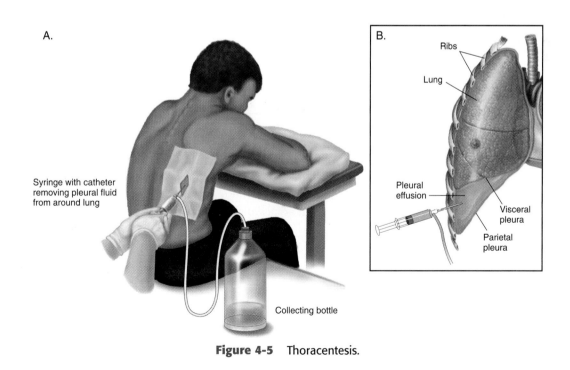

A.

Syringe with catheter
removing pleural fluid
from around lung

Collecting bottle

B.

Ribs

Lung

Pleural
effusion

Visceral
pleura

Parietal
pleura

Figure 4-5   Thoracentesis.

thorac/o/centesis thō-răk-ō-sĕn-TĒ-sĭs	**4-82** Fluid often builds up around the lung(s) in patients with CA or pneumonia. To remove fluid from the thorac/ic cavity, the physician performs the surgical procedure called thor/a/centesis, also known as _____ / _____ / _____.
	4-83 The (12) **diaphragm** is a muscular partition that separates the lungs from the abdominal cavity and aids in the process of breathing. The combining form **phren/o** refers to the *diaphragm*. Label the diaphragm in Figure 4–2.
phren/o	**4-84** The combining form **phren/o** also refers to the *mind*. When you want to build words that refer to the diaphragm or mind, use the combining form _____ / _____.
diaphragm DĪ-ă-frăm	**4-85** Phren/o/logy is the study of the mind, whereas phren/o/ptosis refers to a prolapse or downward displacement of the _____.
phren/o/spasm FRĔN-ō-spăzm	**4-86** Build a medical word that means involuntary contraction or twitching of the diaphragm: _____ / _____ / _____.

Competency Verification: Check your labeling of Figure 4–2 with Appendix B, Answer Key, page 512.

inspiration or **inhalation** ĭn-spĭ-RĀ-shŭn, ĭn-hă-LĀ-shŭn **expiration** or **exhalation** ĕks-pĭ-RĀ-shŭn, ĕks-hă-LĀ-shŭn	**4-87** Identify the words in Figure 4–6 that mean the process of breathing air into the lungs: _____. out of the lungs: _____.
inter/cost/al ĭn-tĕr-KŎS-tăl	**4-88** During normal, relaxed inspiration, the important muscles are the diaphragm and the inter/cost/al muscles. As its name implies, the muscles between adjacent ribs are known as the _____ / _____ / _____ muscles.
descends **ascends**	**4-89** Examine Figure 4–6A and B and use the words "ascends" or "descends" to complete this frame. During inspiration (or inhalation), the diaphragm _____. During expiration (or exhalation), the diaphragm _____.

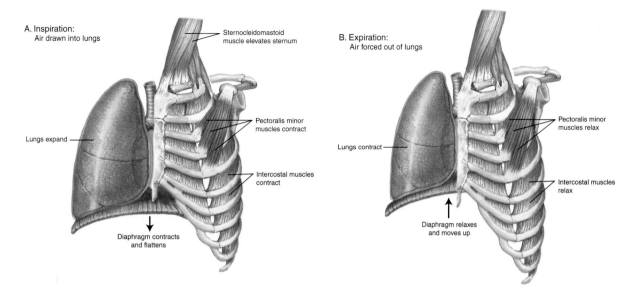

A. Inspiration:
Air drawn into lungs

Sternocleidomastoid
muscle elevates sternum

Lungs expand

Pectoralis minor
muscles contract

Intercostal muscles
contract

Diaphragm contracts
and flattens

B. Expiration:
Air forced out of lungs

Lungs contract

Pectoralis minor
muscles relax

Intercostal muscles
relax

Diaphragm relaxes
and moves up

Figure 4-6   The position of the diaphragm during (A) inspiration and (B) expiration.

my/o/rrhaphy mī-OR-ă-fē	**4–90** The combining form *my/o* means muscle. Some muscle injuries may necessitate the surgical procedure my/o/rrhaphy. When a torn muscle needs repair, the surgeon sutures the muscle using a surgical procedure known as _____ / _____ / _____.
my/o/plasty MĪ-ō-plăs-tē	**4–91** Another surgical procedure, my/o/plasty, requires the use of muscular tissue to correct a muscular injury or defect. My/o/rrhaphy and my/o/plasty are involved in the treatment of muscular disorders. Nevertheless, when the surgeon uses muscular tissue to correct a defect, you will know the surgical procedure is called _____ / _____ / _____.
my/oma mī-Ō-mă **my/o/pathy** mī-ŎP-ă-thē **my/o/rrhaphy** mī-OR-ă-fē	**4–92** Develop medical words meaning tumor of muscle: _____ / _____. any disease of the muscle: _____ / _____ / _____. suture of muscle: _____ / _____ / _____.
air	**4–93** Recall that **aer/o** is the combining form for _____.
aer/o/phobia ĕr-ō-FŌ-bē-ă	**4–94** Aer/o/phobia is a fear of air, drafts of air, airborne influences, or "bad air" (body odor). The medical word meaning fear of air is _____ / _____ / _____.

hem/o/phobia hē-mō-FŌ-bē-ă	**4-95** Combine **hem/o** and -phobia to form a word meaning fear of blood: _____ / _____ / _____ .
muc/o **myc/o**	**4-96** Although the combining forms **muc/o** and **myc/o** look similar, they have different meanings. Determine the combining form that means mucus: _____ / _____ . fungus: _____ / _____ .
air, lung **fungus** **abnormal condition**	**4-97** Analyze pneumon/o/myc/osis by defining the word elements: **pneumon/o** refers to _____ or _____ . **myc** refers to a _____ . -osis refers to an _____ _____ .
chronic bronch/itis brŏng-KĪ-tĭs	**4-98** Bronch/itis sometimes leads to chronic bronch/itis, an inflammation of the bronchi that persists for a long time (see Figure 4–4B). This pulmon/ary disease is often caused by cigarette smoking and is characterized by increased production of mucus from the bronchi/al mucosa and obstruction of the respiratory passages. It results in the ejection of mucus, sputum, or fluids from the trachea and lungs by coughing or spitting. Bronch/itis may be of short duration, but when it persists for a long time, it may be a more serious pulmon/ary disease called _____ _____ / _____ .
bronchi/al BRŎNG-kē-ăl **bronch/itis** brŏng-KĪ-tĭs	**4-99** Use **bronchi/o** to build a term meaning pertaining to the bronchi: _____ / _____ . Use **bronch/o** to build a term meaning inflammation of the bronchi: _____ / _____ .
laryng/itis lăr-ĭn-JĪ-tĭs	**4-100** The larynx contains the organ of sound called the vocal cords. When the vocal cords become inflamed from overuse or infection, laryng/itis occurs, causing hoarseness and difficulty speaking. The medical term for an inflamed larynx is _____ / _____ .

bronch/o **pneumon** **-ia**	**4-101** Pneumon/ia is a lung inflammation caused by bacteria, a virus, or chemical irritants. Some pneumon/ias affect only one lobe of the lung (lobar pneumon/ia). Others, such as bronch/o/pneumon/ia, involve the lungs and bronchioles. Identify the elements in bronch/o/pneumon/ia that mean bronchus: _____ /____. air; lung: _____. condition: _____.
bronch/o/pneumon/ia brong-kō-nū-MŌ-nē-ă	**4-102** A type of pneumon/ia that involves the lungs and bronchi/oles is called _____ /____ /_____ /_____.
-oles	**4-103** In Frame 4-102 the element that means small or minute is _____.
compromised, **immunocompromised** ĭm-ū-nō-KŎM-pră-mīzd	**4-104** Another type of pneumon/ia called *Pneumocystis carinii* pneumonia (PCP) is closely associated with persons whose immune systems are *compromised*, particularly patients with *acquired immunodeficiency syndrome* (AIDS). Studies indicate PCP is caused by a fungus that resides in or on the *normal flora* (potentially pathogenic organisms that reside in, but are harmless to healthy individuals). The fungus becomes an aggressive pathogen in *immunocompromised* persons. Identify two terms in this frame that mean a person's immune system is incapable of resisting pathogenic organisms. In other words, their immune system is _____ or _____.
PCP **AIDS**	**4-105** The abbreviation for *Pneumocystis carinii* pneumon/ia is _____; the abbreviation for acquired immunodeficiency syndrome is _____.
Pneumocystis carinii **pneumonia** nū-mō-SĬS-tĭs kă-RĪ-nē-ī nū-MŌ-nē-ă	**4-106** A type of pneumonia seen in patients with AIDS is _____ _____ _____.
emphysema ĕm-fĭ-SĒ-mă	**4-107** Emphysema, a chronic disease characterized by overexpansion and destruction of the alveoli, is often associated with cigarette smoking. Destruction of alveoli occurs in the respiratory disease called _____.

COLD

asthma
ĂZ-mă
emphysema
ĕm-fĭ-SĒ-mă

4-108   Chronic obstructive lung disease (COLD), a group of respiratory disorders, is characterized by a chronic, partial obstruction of the bronchi and lungs. The three major disorders included in COLD are asthma, chronic bronch/itis, and emphysema (see Figure 4–4).

The abbreviation for chronic obstructive lung disease is _____.

As described previously, three major pathological conditions associated with COLD are chronic bronch/itis, _____, and

_____ (see Figure 4–4B).

bronch/itis
brong-KĪ-tĭs

4-109   Chronic bronch/itis, an inflammation of the mucous membranes lining the bronchial airways, is characterized by increased mucus production resulting in a chronic productive cough (see Figure 4–4A). Cigarette smoking, environmental irritants, allergic response, and infectious agents are causative factors of this condition.

The medical term for inflammation of the bronchi is

_____ / _____.

metastasize or **metastasis**
mĕ-TĂS-tă-sīz,
mĕ-TĂS-tă-sĭs

4-110   Lung cancer, associated with smoking, is the leading cause of cancer-related deaths in men and women in the United States. It usually spreads rapidly and metastasizes to other parts of the body, making it difficult to diagnose and treat in its early stages.

When cancer spreads to other parts of the body, the medical term used to describe that condition is _____.

tuberculosis
tū-bĕr-kū-LŌ-sĭs

tubercles
TŪ-bĕr-klz

4-111   Tuberculosis (TB), an infectious disease, produces small lesions or tubercles in the lungs. If left untreated, it infects the bones and organs of the entire body. An increase in tuberculosis is attributed to the increasing prevalence of AIDS.

The abbreviation TB refers to _____.

The name tuberculosis is derived from small lesions that appear in the lungs called _____.

Listen and Learn, the audio CD-ROM that accompanies this book, will help you master the pronunciation of selected medical words. Use it to practice pronunciations *of selected terms from frames 4–1 to 4–111* for instructions to complete the *Listen and Learn* exercise on the CD-ROM for this section.

SECTION REVIEW 4 – 3

Using the following table, write the combining form, suffix, or prefix that matches its definition in the space provided to the left of the definition. There may be more than one word element that matches a definition.

Combining Forms	Suffixes	Prefixes
bronch/o	-cele	a-
bronchi/o	-centesis	brady-
chondr/o	-ectasis	dys-
hem/o	-osis	eu-
melan/o	-phobia	macro-
myc/o	-pnea	micro-
orth/o	-scope	tachy-
pleur/o	-spasm	
pneum/o	-stenosis	
pneumon/o		
thorac/o		

1. _____ abnormal condition; increase (used primarily with blood cells)
2. _____ slow
3. _____ bad; painful; difficult
4. _____ black
5. _____ breathing
6. _____ bronchus (plural, bronchi)
7. _____ blood
8. _____ chest
9. _____ dilation, expansion
10. _____ fear
11. _____ fungus
12. _____ good, normal
13. _____ hernia, swelling
14. _____ instrument for examining
15. _____ involuntary contraction, twitching
16. _____ large
17. _____ rapid
18. _____ air; lung
19. _____ pleura
20. _____ small
21. _____ straight
22. _____ narrowing, stricture
23. _____ surgical puncture
24. _____ without, not
25. _____ cartilage

Competency Verification: Check your answers in Appendix B, Answer Key, page 513. If you are not satisfied with your level of comprehension, go back to Frame 4–31 and rework the frames.

Correct Answers _____ × 4 = _____% Score

Abbreviations

This section introduces respiratory system–related abbreviations and their meanings. Included are abbreviations contained in the medical record activities that follow.

Abbreviation	Meaning	Abbreviation	Meaning
ARDS	adult respiratory distress syndrome, acute respiratory distress syndrome	MRI	magnetic resonance imaging
CF	cystic fibrosis	NMT	nebulized mist treatment
COLD	chronic obstructive lung disease	PFT	pulmonary function test
COPD	chronic obstructive pulmonary disease	PND	paroxysmal nocturnal dyspnea
CPR	cardiopulmonary resuscitation	RD	respiratory disease
CT scan	computed tomography scan	SIDS	sudden infant death syndrome
DPT	diphtheria pertussis, tetanus	SOB	shortness of breath
HMD	hyaline membrane disease	TB	tuberculosis
IPPB	intermittent positive-pressure breathing	URI	upper respiratory infection
IRDS	infant respiratory distress syndrome	VC	vital capacity

Pathological, Diagnostic, and Therapeutic Terms

The following are additional terms related to the respiratory system. Recognizing and learning these terms will help you understand the connection between a pathological condition, its diagnosis, and the rationale behind the method of treatment selected for a particular disorder.

Pathological

acidosis (ăs-i-DŌ-sĭs): excessive acidity of blood due to an accumulation of acids or an excessive loss of bicarbonate.

Respiratory acidosis is caused by abnormally high levels of carbon dioxide (CO_2) in the body.

acute respiratory distress syndrome (ă-KŪT rĕs-PĪR-ă-tō-rē dĭs-TRĔS SĬN-drŏm): respiratory insufficiency marked by progressive hypoxia. This syndrome is due to severe inflammatory damage causing abnormal permeability of the alveolar-capillary membrane; also called *adult respiratory distress syndrome (ARDS).*

The alveoli fill with fluid, which interferes with gas exchange.

atelectasis (ăt-ĕ-LĔK-tă-sĭs): collapse of lung tissue, preventing the respiratory exchange of oxygen and carbon dioxide.

Atelectasis can be caused by a variety of conditions, including obstruction of foreign bodies, excessive secretions, or pressure on the lung from a tumor.

coryza (kō-RĪ-ză): acute inflammation of the nasal passages accompanied by profuse nasal discharge; also called a *cold*.

crackle (KRĂK-ăl): adventitious lung sound heard on auscultation of the chest, produced by air passing over retained airway secretions or the sudden opening of collapsed airways.

A crackle may be heard on inspiration or expiration and is a discontinuous adventitious lung sound as opposed to a wheeze, which is continuous; formerly called rale.

croup (croop): acute respiratory syndrome that occurs primarily in children and infants and is characterized by laryngeal obstruction and spasm, barking cough, and stridor.

cystic fibrosis (SĬS-tĭk fī-BRŌ-sĭs): inherited disease of the exocrine glands with production of thick mucus that causes severe congestion within the lungs and digestive systems.

The average life expectancy of a person with cystic fibrosis (CF) is approximately 20 years.

empyema (ĕm-pī-Ē-mă): pus in a body cavity, especially in the pleural cavity (pyothorax).

Empyema is usually the result of a primary infection in the lungs.

epiglottitis (ĕp-ĭ-glŏt-Ī-tĭs): in the acute form, epiglottitis is a severe, life-threatening infection of the epiglottis and surrounding area; occurs most often in children between ages 2 and 12.

In the classic form, a sudden onset of fever, dysphagia, inspiratory stridor, and severe respiratory distress occurs that often requires intubation or tracheotomy to open the obstructed airway.

epistaxis (ĕp-ĭ-STĂK-sĭs): hemorrhage from the nose; also called *nosebleed*.

hypoxemia (hī-pŏks-Ē-mē-ă): deficiency of oxygen in the blood; usually a sign of respiratory impairment; also called *anoxemia*.

hypoxia (hī-PŎKS-ē-ă): deficiency of oxygen in the tissues; usually a sign of respiratory impairment; also called *anoxia*.

influenza (ĭn-floo-ĔN-ză): acute, contagious respiratory infection characterized by sudden onset of fever, chills, headache, and muscle pain.

lung cancer (LŬNG KĂN-sĕr): pulmonary malignancy commonly attributable to cigarette smoking. Survival rates are low due to rapid metastasis and late detection.

pertussis (pĕr-TŬS-ĭs): acute infectious disease characterized by a "whoop"-sounding cough. Immunization of infants as part of the diphtheria and tetanus (DPT) vaccine prevents contraction; also called *whooping cough*.

pleural effusion (PLOO-răl ĕ-FŪ-zhŭn): abnormal presence of fluid in the pleural cavity. The fluid may contain blood (hemothorax), serum (hydrothorax), or pus (pyothorax).

pneumothorax (nū-mō-THŌ-răks): collection of air in the pleural cavity, causing the complete or partial collapse of a lung

Pneumothorax can occur with pulmonary disease (emphysema, lung cancer, or tuberculosis) when pulmonary lesions rupture near the pleural surface allowing communication between an alveolus or bronchus and the pleural cavity. It may also be the result of an open chest wound, or a perforation of the chest wall that permits the entrance of air (see Figure 4–7).

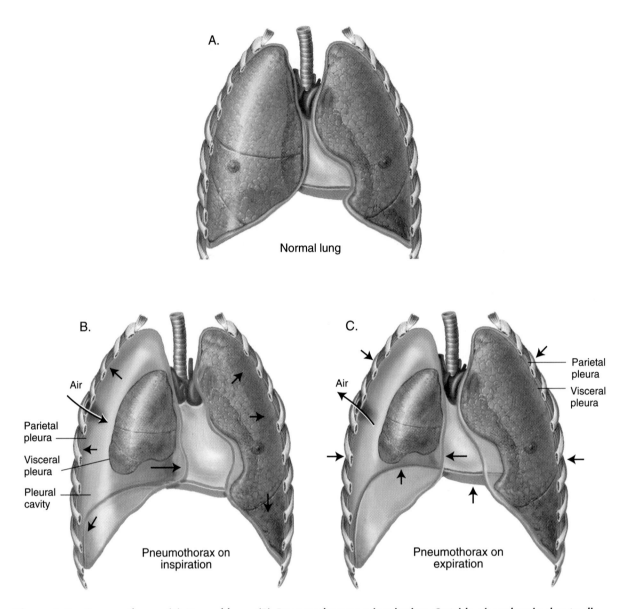

Figure 4-7 Pneumothorax. (A) Normal lung. (B) Pneumothorax on inspiration. Outside air rushes in due to disruption of chest wall and parietal pleura; the mediastinal contents shift to the side opposite the injury compressing the uninjured lung. (C) Pneumothorax on expiration. Lung air rushes out due to disruption of visceral pleura; the mediastinal contents move toward the center.

rhonchi (RONG-kē): abnormal chest sounds resembling snoring, produced in airways with accumulated fluids.

stridor (STRĪ-dor): abnormal high-pitched musical sound made on inspiration caused by an obstruction in the trachea or larynx.
Stridor is one of the characteristics of the upper respiratory disorder called croup.

sudden infant death syndrome (SIDS): completely unexpected and unexplained death of an apparently well, or virtually well, infant. The most common cause of death between the second week and first year of life; also known as *crib death.*

wheezes (HWĒZ-ĕz): whistling or sighing sounds resulting from narrowing of the lumen of a respiratory passageway that is noted by use of a stethoscope.

Wheezing occurs in conditions such as asthma, croup, hay fever, obstructive emphysema, and many other obstructive respiratory conditions.

Diagnostic

arterial blood gases (ăr-TĒ-rē-ăl): group of tests that measure the oxygen and carbon dioxide concentration in an arterial blood sample.

bronchoscopy (brŏng-KŎS-kō-pē): direct visual examination of the interior bronchi using a bronchoscope (curved, flexible tube with a light).

A bronchoscopy may be performed to remove obstructions, obtain a biopsy specimen, or observe directly for pathological changes.

chest x-ray: radiograph of the chest taken from anteroposterior (AP), posteroanterior (PA), or lateral projections (see Figure 2–5A).

Chest x-ray is used to diagnose atelectasis, tumors, pneumonia, emphysema, and many other lung diseases.

computed tomography (CT) scan (cŏm-PŪ-tĕd tō-MŎG-ră-fē SKĂN): radiographic technique that uses a narrow beam of x-rays, which rotates in a full arc around the patient to image the body in cross-sectional slices. A scanner and detector send the images to a computer, which consolidates all of the data it receives from the multiple x-ray views (see Figure 2–5D).

CT scanning is used to detect lesions in the lungs and thorax, blood clots, and pulmonary embolism (PE). CT scan may be performed with or without a contrast medium.

magnetic resonance imaging (măg-NĔT-ĭc RĔZ-ĕn-ăns ĬM-ĭj-ĭng): radiographic technique that uses electromagnetic energy to produce multiplanar cross-sectional images of the body (see Figure 2–5E).

In the respiratory system, magnetic resonance imaging (MRI) is used to produce an MRI scan of the chest and lungs. MRI does not require a contrast medium, but it may be used to enhance internal structure visualization.

pulmonary function tests (PŬL-mō-nĕ-rē): include any of several tests to evaluate the condition of the respiratory system. Measures of expiratory flow and lung volume capacity are obtained.

spirometry (spī-RŎM-ĕ-trē): measures the breathing capacity of the lungs.

Therapeutic

bronchodilators (brŏng-kō-DĪ-lā-tŏrz): drugs used to dilate the walls of the bronchi of the lungs to increase airflow.

Bronchodilators are used to treat asthma, emphysema, chronic obstructive pulmonary lung disease (COLD), and exercise-induced bronchospasm. (See figure 4–4)

corticosteroids (kor-tĭ-kō-STĒR-oydz): hormonal agents that reduce tissue edema and inflammation associated with chronic lung disease.

nebulized mist treatment (NMT): use of a device for producing a fine spray (nebulizer) to deliver medication directly into the lungs (see Figure 4–8.).

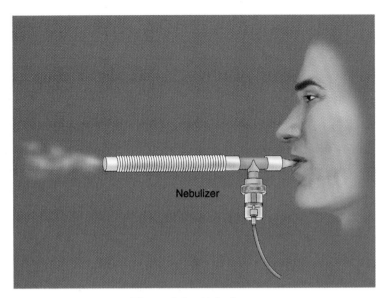

Figure 4-8 Nebulizer.

postural drainage (PŎS-chur-ăl DRĀN-ăj): use of body positioning to assist in the removal of secretions from specific lobes of the lung, bronchi, or lung cavities.

Listen and Learn, the audio CD-ROM that accompanies this book, will help you master the pronunciation of selected medical words. Use it to practice pronunciations of the above medical terms and for instructions to complete the *Listen and Learn* exercise on the CD-ROM for this section.

PATHOLOGICAL, DIAGNOSTIC, AND THERAPEUTIC TERMS REVIEW

Match the medical term(s) below with the definitions in the numbered list.

acidosis	coryza	hypoxia	pleural effusion
ARDS	crackle	influenza	pneumothorax
atelectasis	cystic fibrosis	lung cancer	rhonchi
bronchodilators	epiglottitis	MRI	stridor
CT scan	epistaxis	pertussis	SIDS

1. _____ is a high-pitched breathing sound resembling the blowing of wind caused by obstruction of air passages.

2. _____ refers to nosebleed.

3. _____ is a contagious respiratory infection characterized by onset of fever, chills, headache, and muscle pain.

4. _____ is excessive acidity of blood due to an accumulation of acids or an excessive loss of bicarbonate.

5. _____ is acute inflammation of the nasal passages accompanied by profuse nasal discharge; a cold.

6. _____ is a genetic disease of the exocrine glands with production of excessive mucus, causing severe congestion within the lungs and digestive systems.

7. _____ refers to pulmonary malignancy commonly attributable to cigarette smoking.

8. _____ is an abnormal presence of fluid in the pleural cavity.

9. _____ refers to accumulation of air in the pleural cavity.

10. _____ is an adventitious lung sound heard on auscultation of the chest, produced by air passing over retained airway secretions; formerly called *rale*.

11. _____ is used to dilate the walls of the bronchi of the lungs to increase airflow.

12. _____ is a form of restrictive lung disease that follows severe infection or trauma in young and previously healthy individuals.

13. _____ is a radiographic technique that uses electromagnetic energy to produce multiplanar cross-sectional images of the body; used to produce scan of the chest and a radioactive lung scan.

14. _____ refers to a collapsed lung,

15. _____ is a severe life-threatening infection of the epiglottis that occurs most often in children.

16. _____ is an acute infectious disease characterized by an explosive cough; also called *whooping cough.*

17. _____ is a radiographic technique that uses a narrow beam of x-rays, which rotates in a full arc around the patient to image the body in cross-sectional slices, then a scanner and detector send the images to a computer to consolidate all of the data.

18. _____ refers to the unexpected and unexplained death of an apparently well, or virtually well, infant.

19. _____ is a deficiency of oxygen in the tissues; usually a sign of respiratory impairment.

20. _____ refers to abnormal chest sounds resembling snoring, produced in obstructed airways.

Competency Verification: Check your answers in Appendix B, Answer Key, page 513. If you are not satisfied with your level of comprehension, review the pathological, diagnostic, and therapeutic terms and retake the review.

Correct Answers: _____ × 5 = _____% Score

Medical Record Activities

The medical records included in the following activities reflect common real-life clinical scenarios using medical terminology to document patient care. The physician who specializes in the treatment of respiratory disorders is called a *pulmonologist;* the medical specialty concerned in the diagnoses and treatment of respiratory disorders is called *pulmonology.*

✓ MEDICAL RECORD ACTIVITY 4–1. Papillary Carcinoma

Terminology

The terms listed in the chart come from the medical record *Papillary Carcinoma* that follows. Use a medical dictionary such as *Taber's Cyclopedic Medical Dictionary,* the appendices of this book, or other resources to define each term. Then practice reading the pronunciations aloud for each term.

Term	Definition
anesthesia ăn-ĕs-THĒ-zē-ă	
biopsy BĪ-ŏp-sē	
carcinoma kăr-sĭ-NŌ-mă	
diagnosis dī-ăg-NŌ-sĭs	
expire	
hemorrhage HĔM-ĕ-rĭj	
lymph node lĭmf nōd	
meatus mē-Ā-tŭs	
metastatic mĕt-ă-STĂT-ĭk	
necropsy NĔK-rŏp-sē	
needle biopsy BĪ-ŏp-sē	
nodular NŎD-ū-lăr	

(Continued)

Term	Definition *(Continued)*
papillary PĂP-ĭ-lăr-ē	
pneumonia nū-MŌ-nē-ă	
polyp PŎL-ĭp	
polypectomy pŏl-ĭ-PĔK-tō-mē	
pulmonary PŬL-mō-nĕ-rē	
snare snār	

Listen and Learn Online! will help you master the pronunciation of selected medical words from this medical record activity. Visit www.fadavis.com/gylys/simplified for instructions in completing the *Listen and Learn Online!* exercise for this section and then to practice pronunciations.

PAPILLARY CARCINOMA

Reading

Practice pronunciation of medical terms by reading the following medical report aloud.

A 55-year-old white man was seen 2 years ago because of upper airway obstruction due to large polyps in the right nasal cavity. On examination, a large polypoid mass was observed to fill most of the right nasal cavity. The mass originated in the middle meatus. With the use of a nasal snare, polypectomy was performed to remove several sections. There was a slight hemorrhage. On the next day, a 4 × 3 cm oval soft mass was excised from beneath the left submaxillary region, with the patient under local anesthesia. The mass was just beneath the superficial fascia and appeared to be an enlarged lymph node unconnected with the nasal disease.

The pathological diagnosis of the nasal growth was low-grade papillary carcinoma. The diagnosis of the lymph node was metastatic carcinoma. A chest film was taken that indicated the presence of pulmonary densities attributed to unresolved pneumonia. Also, a needle biopsy of the enlarged liver nodes yielded no results.

After discharge from the hospital, the patient expired at home, and no necropsy was obtained.

Evaluation

Review the medical record above to answer the following questions.

1. What types of patients are at risk for nasal polyps?

_____

_____

2. When is a polypectomy indicated?

_____

_____

3. Were the patient's nasal polyps cancerous?

_____

_____

4. What contributed to the patient's expiration?

_____

_____

5. Why was a biopsy of the liver performed?

_____

_____

✓ MEDICAL RECORD ACTIVITY 4–2. Lobar Pneumonia

Terminology

The terms listed in the chart come from the medical record *Lobar Pneumonia* that follows. Use a medical dictionary such as *Taber's Cyclopedic Medical Dictionary,* the appendices of this book, or other resources to define each term. Then practice reading the pronunciations aloud for each term.

Term	Definition
asthma ĂZ-mă (see Figure 4–4C)	
excursion ĕks-KŬR-zhŭn	
lobe lōb	
nasal polyps NĀ-zl pŏl-ĭps	

(Continued)

Term	Definition (Continued)
percussion pĕr-KŬSH-ŭn	
phlegm flĕm	
resonance RĔZ-ō-năns	
tactile fremitus TĂK-tĭl FRĔM-ĭ-tŭs	

Listen and Learn Online! will help you master the pronunciation of selected medical words from this medical record activity. Visit www.fadavis.com/gylys/simplified for instructions in completing the *Listen and Learn Online!* exercise for this section and then to practice pronunciations.

LOBAR PNEUMONIA

Reading

Practice pronunciation of medical terms by reading the following medical report aloud.

EMERGENCY ROOM NUMBER: 543985720

CHIEF COMPLAINT: Cough and fever.

HISTORY OF PRESENT ILLNESS: Patient reports with 7 days' history of sinus drainage, cough, and yellow phlegm.

REVIEW OF SYSTEMS: She denies ear pain, sore throat, abdominal pain, dysuria, frequency or infrequency of urination.

PAST MEDICAL HISTORY OF ASTHMA. History of nasal polyps with nasal polypectomy performed at the beginning of this year.

SOCIAL/FAMILY HISTORY: Noncontributory.

PHYSICAL EXAMINATION: Temperature 39°C, pulse 128 beats/min, respiratory rate 28/minute, blood pressure 112/68 mm Hg. Ears are clear, all pharynx unremarkable, some sinus tenderness to percussion. Neck is supple. Chest shows diminished excursion on the right side with each inspiratory effort; diminished resonance to percussion and increased tactile fremitus noted over right middle lobe anteriorly. Lungs have clear breath sounds over all left lung fields and right upper lobe; bronchial breath sounds noted over right middle lobe.

DIAGNOSIS: Right middle lobe pneumonia.

Evaluation

Review the medical record to answer the following questions.

1. What physical examination techniques are useful in this case?

2. What explains the unilateral chest expansion?

3. What explains the decrease in resonance and increase in tactile fremitus?

4. What is the significance of bronchial breath sounds in this case?

5. What laboratory data are useful to confirm the diagnosis?

Chapter Review

Word Elements Summary

The following table summarizes combining forms, suffixes, and prefixes related to the respiratory system.

Word Element	Meaning
COMBINING FORMS	
adenoid/o	adenoids
alveol/o	alveolus (plural, alveoli)
bronch/o, bronchi/o	bronchus (plural, bronchi)
chondr/o	cartilage
epiglott/o	epiglottis
laryng/o	larynx (voice box)
nas/o, rhin/o	nose
or/o	mouth

(Continued)

Word Element	Meaning *(Continued)*
pharyng/o	pharynx (throat)
pleur/o	pleura
pneum/o, pneumon/o	air; lung
pulmon/o	lung
sinus/o	sinus, cavity
thorac/o	chest
tonsill/o	tonsils
trache/o	trachea (windpipe)

OTHER COMBINING FORMS

aer/o	air
carcin/o	cancer
gastr/o	stomach
hem/o	blood
hepat/o	liver
hydr/o	water
melan/o	black
muc/o	mucus
my/o	muscle
myc/o	fungus
orth/o	straight

SUFFIXES

SURGICAL

-centesis	surgical puncture
-ectomy	excision, removal
-plasty	surgical repair
-rrhaphy	suture
-tome	instrument to cut
-tomy	incision

DIAGNOSTIC, SYMPTOMATIC, AND RELATED

-algia, -dynia	pain
-cele	hernia, swelling

Word Element	Meaning
-ectasis	dilation, expansion
-itis	inflammation
-logist	specialist in study of
-malacia	softening
-oma	tumor
-osis	abnormal condition, increase (used primarily with blood cells)
-pathy	disease
-phagia	swallowing, eating
-phobia	fear
-plasm	formation, growth
-plegia	paralysis
-pnea	breathing
-rrhagia	bursting forth (of)
-scope	instrument for examining
-scopy	visual examination
-spasm	involuntary contraction, twitching
-stenosis	narrowing, stricture
-therapy	treatment
ADJECTIVE	
-ous	pertaining to, relating to
NOUN	
-ia	condition
-ist	specialist
PREFIXES	
epi-	above, upon
eu-	good, normal
macro-	large
micro-	small
neo-	new
peri-	around

WORD ELEMENTS REVIEW

After you review the Word Elements Summary, complete this activity by writing the meaning of each element in the space provided.

Word Element	Meaning
COMBINING FORMS	
1. bronch/o, bronchi/o	
2. chondr/o	
3. nas/o, rhin/o	
4. or/o	
5. pharyng/o	
6. pleur/o	
7. pneum/o, pneumon/o	
8. pulmon/o	
9. thorac/o	
10. tonsill/o	
11. trache/o	
OTHER COMBINING FORMS	
12. aer/o	
13. carcin/o	
14. hem/o	
15. hydr/o	
16. melan/o	
17. muc/o	
18. myc/o	
19. my/o	
SUFFIXES	
SURGICAL	
20. -centesis	
21. -plasty	
22. -rrhaphy	
23. -tome	
24. -tomy	

Word Element	Meaning
DIAGNOSTIC, SYMPTOMATIC, AND RELATED	
25. -algia, -dynia	
26. -cele	
27. -ectasis	
28. -itis	
29. -logist	
30. -malacia	
31. -oma	
32. -osis	
33. -pathy	
34. -phagia	
35. -phobia	
36. -plasm	
37. -plegia	
38. -pnea	
39. -rrhagia	
40. -scope	
41. -scopy	
42. -spasm	
43. -stenosis	
44. -therapy	
PREFIXES	
45. epi-	
46. eu-	
47. macro-	
48. micro-	
49. neo-	
50. peri-	

Competency Verification: Check your answers in Appendix A, Glossary of Medical Word Elements, page 497. If you are not satisfied with your level of comprehension, review the word elements and retake the review.

Correct Answers: _____ × 2 = _____% Score

Chapter 4 Vocabulary Review

Match the medical terms(s) with the definitions in the numbered list.

aerophagia	atelectasis	diagnosis	pyothorax
anosmia	catheter	pharyngoplegia	rhinoplasty
apnea	chondroma	pleurisy	thoracentesis
aspirate	COLD	*Pneumocystis carinii*	tracheostomy
asthma	croup	pneumothorax	TB

1. _____ refers to presence of pus in the chest.

2. _____ is surgical puncture of the chest to remove fluid.

3. _____ is a respiratory condition marked by recurrent attacks of difficult or labored breathing accompanied by wheezing.

4. _____ is an acute respiratory syndrome of childhood characterized by laryngeal obstruction and spasm, barking cough, and stridor.

5. _____ refers to creating an opening through the neck into the trachea.

6. _____ refers to use of scientific methods and medical skill to establish the cause and nature of a person's illness.

7. _____ is temporary cessation of breathing.

8. _____ refers to swallowing air.

9. _____ refers to using suction to remove fluids from a body cavity.

10. _____ is a cartilaginous tumor.

11. _____ is an abnormal condition characterized by the collapse of alveoli.

12. _____ is loss or impairment of the sense of smell.

13. _____ is paralysis of muscles of the pharynx.

14. _____ is inflammation of the pleura.

15. _____ is a type of pneumonia seen in patients with AIDS and in debilitated children.

16. _____ is a hollow flexible tube that can be inserted into a vessel or cavity of the body; used to withdraw or instill fluids.

17. _____ refers to surgical repair or plastic surgery of the nose.

18. _____ is an infectious disease that produces small lesions or tubercles in the lungs.

19. _____ refers to a group of respiratory disorders characterized by chronic bronchitis, asthma, and emphysema.

20. _____ is presence of air in the pleural cavity.

Competency Verification: Check your answers in Appendix B, Answer Key, page 514. If you are not satisfied with your level of comprehension, review the chapter vocabulary and retake the review.

Correct Answers: _____ × 5 _____% Score

Cardiovascular and Lymphatic Systems

OBJECTIVES

Upon completion of this chapter, you will be able to:

- Describe the cardiovascular system and discuss its primary functions.
- Describe the lymphatic system and discuss its primary functions.
- Describe pathological, diagnostic, therapeutic, and other terms related to the cardiovascular and lymphatic systems.
- Recognize, define, pronounce, and spell terms correctly by completing the audio CD-ROM exercises.
- Demonstrate your knowledge of this chapter by successfully completing the frames, reviews, and medical report evaluations.

The *cardiovascular (CV) system* is composed of the heart, which is essentially a muscular pump, and an extensive network of tubes called blood vessels. The main purpose of the CV system, also called circulatory system, is to deliver oxygen, nutrients, and other essential substances to the cells of the body and to remove the waste products of cellular metabolism. Delivery and removal of these substances are achieved by a complex network of blood vessels: the arteries, capillaries, and veins—all of which are connected to the heart. Without a healthy CV system that provides adequate circulation, tissues are deprived of oxygen and nutrients. In addition, waste removal ceases. When this happens, an irreversible change in the cells takes place that may result in a person's death. The CV system is vital for survival.

Because the lymphatic system does not have a pump, it depends on the pumping action of the heart to circulate its substances (see Figure 5–1). The lymphatic system is composed of lymph nodes, lymph vessels, and lymph fluid. It is responsible for draining fluid from the tissues and returning it to the bloodstream.

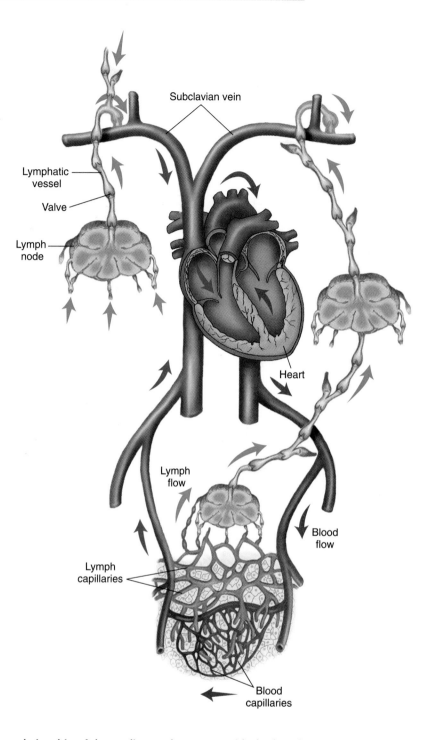

Figure 5-1   Interrelationship of the cardiovascular system with the lymphatic system. Blood flows from the heart to blood capillaries and back to the heart. Lymph capillaries collect tissue fluid, which is returned to the blood. The arrows indicate direction of flow of the blood and lymph.

Word Elements

This section introduces combining forms related to the cardiovascular system. Included are key suffixes; prefixes are defined in the right-hand column as needed. Review the following table and pronounce each word in the word analysis column aloud before you begin to work the frames.

Word Element	Meaning	Word Analysis
COMBINING FORMS		
angi/o	vessel (usually blood or lymph)	angi/o/graphy (ăn-jē-ŎG-ră-fē): x-ray visualization of internal anatomy of the heart and blood vessels after the intravascular introduction of a contrast medium *-graphy:* process of recording *Angiography is used as a diagnostic aid to visualize blood vessel and heart abnormalities.*
aort/o	aorta	aort/o/stenosis (ā-ōr-tō-stĕn-Ō-sĭs): narrowing of the aorta *-stenosis:* narrowing, stricture
arteri/o	artery	arteri/o/scler/osis (ăr-tē-rē-ō-sklĕ-RŌ-sĭs): disorder characterized by thickening, loss of elasticity, and calcification of arterial walls *scler:* hardening; sclera (white of eye) *-osis:* abnormal condition; increase (used primarily with blood cells) *Arteriosclerosis results in a decreased blood supply, especially to the cerebrum and lower extremities.*
ather/o	fatty plaque	ather/oma (ăth-ĕr-Ō-mă): fatty degeneration or thickening of the larger arterial walls, as occurs in atherosclerosis *-oma:* tumor
atri/o	atrium	atri/o/ventricul/ar (ā-trē-ō-vĕn-TRĬK-ū-lăr): pertaining to the atrium and the ventricle *ventricul:* ventricle (of heart or brain) *-ar:* pertaining to, relating to
cardi/o	heart	cardi/o/megaly (kăr-dē-ō-MĔG-ă-lē): enlargement of the heart *-megaly:* enlargement
phleb/o	vein	phleb/itis (flĕb-Ī-tĭs): inflammation of a vein *-itis:* inflammation
thromb/o	blood clot	thromb/o/lysis (thrŏm-BŎL-ĭ-sĭs): breaking up of a thrombus *-lysis:* separation; destruction; loosening
vas/o	vessel; vas deferens; duct	vas/o/spasm (VĂS-ō-spăzm): spasm of a blood vessel *-spasm:* involuntary contraction, twitching
vascul/o	vessel	vascul/ar (VĂS-kū-lăr): pertaining to or composed of blood vessels *-ar:* pertaining to, relating to
ven/o	vein	ven/ous (VĒ-nŭs): pertaining to the veins or blood passing through them *-ous:* pertaining to, relating to

(Continued)

Word Element	Meaning	Word Analysis *(Continued)*
ventricul/o	ventricle (of heart or brain)	inter/ventricul/ar (ĭn-tĕr-vĕn-TRĬK-ū-lăr): within a ventricle *ventricul:* ventricle (of heart or brain) *-ar:* pertaining to, relating to

SUFFIXES

Word Element	Meaning	Word Analysis *(Continued)*
-cardia	heart condition	tachy/cardia (tăk-ē-KĂR-dē-ă): rapid heart rate *tachy-:* rapid
-gram	record, writing	electr/o/cardi/o/gram (ē-lĕk-trō-KĂR-dē-ō-grăm): record of electrical activity of the heart *electr/o:* electricity *cardi/o:* heart
-graph	instrument for recording	electr/o/cardi/o/graph (ē-lĕk-trō-KĂR-dē-ŏ-grăf): instrument for recording electrical activity of the heart *electr/o:* electricity *cardi/o:* heart
-graphy	process of recording	electr/o/cardi/o/graphy (ē-lĕk-trō-kăr-dē-Ŏ-grăf-ē): process of recording electrical activity of the heart *electr/o:* electricity *cardi/o:* heart *Electrocardiography is a noninvasive test that records the electrical activity of the heart. It is used to diagnose abnormal cardiac rhythm and the presence of myocardial damage.*
-ic	pertaining to, relating to	trans/aort/ic (trăns-ā-OR-tĭk): surgical procedure performed through the aorta *trans-:* through, across *aort:* aorta *Transaortic is a term used especially in reference to surgical procedures on the aortic valve, performed through an incision in the wall of the aorta.*
-stenosis	narrowing, stricture	arteri/o/stenosis (ăr-tē-rē-ō-stĕ-NŌ-sĭs): narrowing of an artery *arteri/o:* artery *The narrowing of an artery may be caused by fatty plaque buildup, scar tissue, or a blood clot.*
-um	structure, thing	endo/cardi/um (ĕn-dō-KĂR-dē-ŭm): structure within the heart *endo-:* in, within *cardi:* heart

Listen and Learn, the audio CD-ROM that accompanies this book, will help you master the pronunciation of selected medical words. Use it to practice pronunciations of the above-listed medical terms and for instructions to complete the *Listen and Learn* exercise on the CD-ROM for this section.

For the following medical terms, first write the suffix and its meaning. Then translate the meaning of the remaining elements starting with the first part of the word. The first word is an example that is completed for you.

Term	Meaning
1. endo/cardi/um	-um: structure, thing; in, within; heart
2. cardi/o/megaly	_____
3. aort/o/stenosis	_____
4. tachy/cardia	_____
5. phleb/itis	_____
6. thromb/o/lysis	_____
7. vas/o/spasm	_____
8. ather/oma	_____
9. electr/o/cardi/o/graphy	_____
10. atri/o/ventricul/ar	_____

Competency Verification: Check your answers in Appendix B, Answer Key, page 514. If you are not satisfied with your level of comprehension, review the vocabulary and retake the review.

Correct Answers _____ × 10 = _____% Score

Cardiovascular System

Walls of the Heart

	5-1 The heart is a four-chambered muscular organ located in the *mediastinum,* the area of the chest between the lungs. Its primary purpose is to pump blood through the arteries, veins, and capillaries. The walls of the heart are composed of the: (1) **endocardium,** the (2) **myocardium,** and the (3) **pericardium.** Review the structures of the heart and label its three layers in Figure 5–2.
my/o/cardi/um mī-ō-KĂR-dē-ŭ m **peri/cardi/um** pĕr-ĭ-KĂR-dē-ŭm	**5-2** The *endo/cardi/um,* the inner membranous layer, lines the interior of the heart and the heart valves. The *myocardium,* the middle muscular layer, is composed of a special type of muscle arranged in such a way that the contraction of muscle bundles results in squeezing or wringing of the heart chambers to eject blood from the particular chambers. The *peri/cardi/um,* a fibrous sac, surrounds and encloses the entire heart. When we talk about the muscular layer of the heart, we are referring to the _____ / ____ / _____ / ____; when we talk about the fibrous sac, that encloses the entire heart, we are referring to the _____ / _____ / _____.
peri/card/itis pĕr-ĭ-kăr-DĪ-tĭs	**5-3** The prefix peri- means *around.* Peri/card/itis is an inflammation of the peri/cardi/um. This condition causes an accumulation of fluid around the heart and decreases the heart's ability to pump blood. A term that means inflammation around the heart is _____ / _____ / _____.
peri/cardi/ectomy pĕr-ĭ-kăr-dē-ĔK-tō-mē	**5-4** The surgical procedure meaning excision of all or part of the peri/cardi/um is _____ / _____ / _____.
peri/cardi/o/rrhaphy pĕr-ĭ-kăr-dē-OR-ă-fē	**5-5** Suturing a wound in the peri/cardi/um is called _____ / _____ / ____ / _____.
my/o/cardi/um mī-ō-KĂR-dē-ŭm	**5-6** The cross-striations of cardi/ac muscle provide the mechanics of squeezing blood out of the heart chambers to maintain the flow of blood in one direction. Identify the muscul/ar layer of the heart responsible for this function. _____ / ____ / _____ / ____.

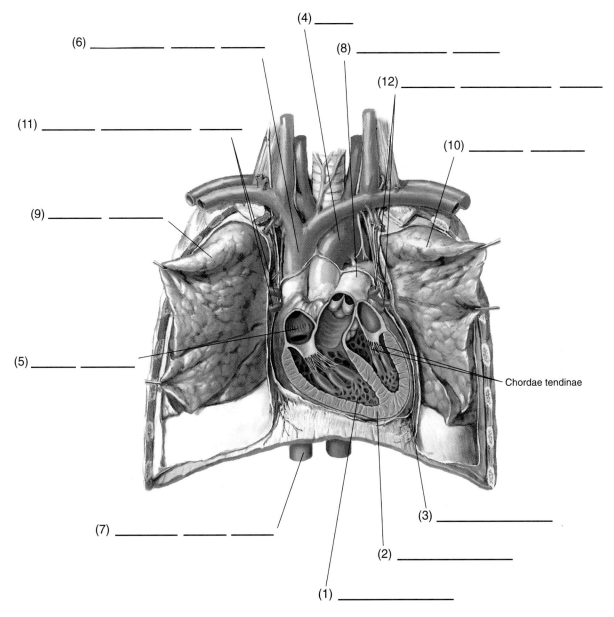

(4) _____

(6) _____ _____ _____

(8) _____ _____

(12) _____ _____ _____

(11) _____ _____ _____

(10) _____ _____

(9) _____ _____ _____

(5) _____ _____

Chordae tendinae

(3) _____

(7) _____ _____ _____

(2) _____

(1) _____

Figure 5-2   Heart structures.

5-7   Review the three layers of the heart by completing the following statements:

The layer that lines the heart and the heart valves is known as the

_____ / _____ / _____.

The fibrous sac surrounding the entire heart, which is composed of two membranes separated by fluid, is called the

_____ / _____ / _____.

The middle specialized muscular layer is called the

_____ / _____ / _____ / _____.

endo/cardi/um
ĕn-dō-KĂR-dē-ŭm

peri/cardi/um
pĕr-ĭ-KĂR-dē-ŭm

my/o/cardi/um
mī-ō-KĂR-dē-ŭm

Circulation and Heart Structures

	5–8 The circulatory system is frequently divided into the *cardiovascular system,* which consists of the heart and blood vessels, and the *lymphatic system,* which consists of lymph vessels, lymph nodes, and lymphoid organs (spleen, thymus, and tonsils). Review Figure 5–1 to see the interrelationship of the cardiovascular system with the lymphatic system.
	5–9 Some of the main vessels associated with circulation are illustrated in Figure 5–2. Observe the locations and label the structures as you read the following material. The (4) **aorta,** the largest blood vessel in the body, is the main trunk of systemic circulation. It starts and arches out at the left ventricle. Deoxygenated blood enters the (5) **right atrium** via two large veins, the *vena cavae* (singular, vena cava). The (6) **superior vena cava** conveys blood from the upper portion of the body (head and arms); the (7) **inferior vena cava** conveys blood from the lower portion of the body (legs).
deoxygenated dē-ŏk-sĭ-jĕn-Ā-tĕd	**5–10** Blood in the veins except for pulmonary veins has a low oxygen content (deoxygenated) and a relatively high concentration of carbon dioxide. In contrast to the bright red color of the oxygenated blood in the arteries, deoxygenated blood has a dark blue to purplish color. The term in this frame that means *low oxygen content* is _____.
	5–11 Label Figure 5–2 as you continue to identify and learn about the structures and functions of the circulatory system. The (8) **pulmonary trunk** is the only artery that carries deoxygenated blood. As deoxygenated blood is pumped from the right ventricle, it enters the pulmonary trunk. The pulmonary trunk runs diagonally upward, then divides abruptly to form the branches of the *right* and *left pulmonary arteries.* Each branch conveys deoxygenated blood to the lungs. The (9) **right lung** has three lobes; the (10) **left lung** has two lobes. Oxygen-rich blood returns to the heart via four pulmonary veins, which deposit the blood into the left atrium. There are two (11) **right pulmonary veins** and two (12) **left pulmonary veins.**

Competency Verification: Check your labeling of Figure 5–2 in Appendix B, Answer Key, page 514.

	5–12 Internally the heart is composed of four chambers. The upper chambers are the (1) **right atrium (RA)** and (2) **left atrium (LA).** The lower chambers are the (3) **right ventricle (RV)** and (4) **left ventricle (LV).** Locate and label the chambers of the heart in Figure 5–3.
atri/al Ā-trē-ăl	**5–13** The combining form **atri/o** refers to the *atrium.* A term that means *pertaining to the atrium* is _____ / _____.
atrium, left Ā-trē-ŭm	**5–14** The heart consists of two upper chambers, the right _____ and the _____ atrium.

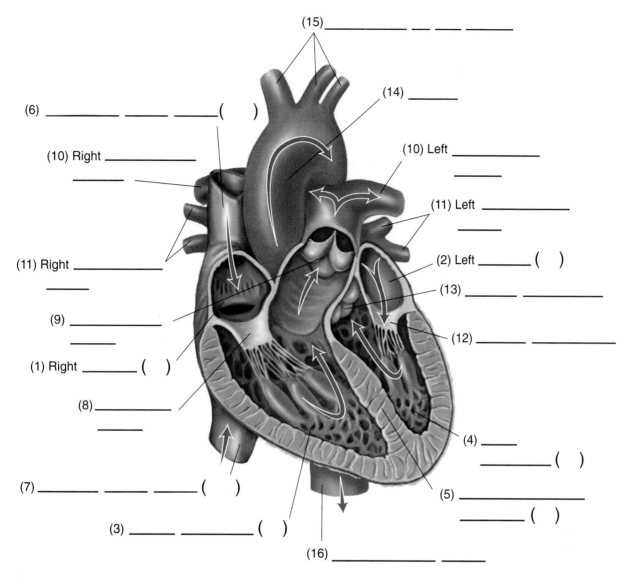

(15) _____ __ ___ _____

(6) _____ _____ _____ ( )

(14) _____

(10) Right _____
_____

(10) Left _____
_____

(11) Left _____
_____

(11) Right _____
_____

(2) Left _____ ( )

(13) _____ _____

(9) _____
_____

(12) _____ _____

(1) Right _____ ( )

(8)_____
_____

(4) _____
_____ ( )

(7) _____ ____ _____ ( )

(5) _____
_____ ( )

(3) _____ _____ ( )

(16) _____ _____

Figure 5-3 Internal structures of the heart. Red arrows designate oxygen-rich blood flow; blue arrows designate oxygen-poor blood flow.

	5-15 The combining form **ventricul/o** means *ventricle (of heart or brain)*. A ventricle is a small cavity, such as the right and left ventricles of the heart or one of the cavities filled with cerebrospinal fluid in the brain.
	Incisions are sometimes performed into these cavities. An incision of a
ventricul/o/tomy věn-trĭk-ū-LŎT-ō-mē	ventricle is known as a _____ / ____ / _____.
	5-16 The term atri/o/ventricul/ar (AV) refers to the atrium and the ventricle. It also pertains to a connecting conduction event between the atria and ventricles.
atrium Ă-trē-ŭm **ventricle** VĔN-trĭk-l	The singular form of atria is _____; the singular form of ventricles is _____.

ventricul/ar vĕn-TRĬK-ū-lăr	**5–17** A flutter is a rapid contraction of the atrium or ventricle of the heart. When the flutter occurs in the atrium, it is called an atri/al flutter. When the flutter occurs in the ventricle, it is called a _____ / _____ flutter.
right atrium Ā-trē-ŭm **left atrium** Ā-trē-ŭm	**5–18** An atri/al flutter may cause chest pain and shortness of breath (SOB), which is common in the elderly population. An atri/al flutter originates in the upper chambers of the heart, which are known as the right atrium (RA) and the left atrium (LA). RA flutter originates in the _____ _____. LA flutter originates in the _____ _____.
RV **LV**	**5–19** Write the abbreviations for the two lower chambers of the heart. right ventricle: _____ left ventricle: _____
atria Ā-trē-ă **cardia** KĂR-dē-ă **septa** SĔP-tă **bacteria** băk-TĒ-rē-ă	**5–20** The rule for forming plural words from singular words that end in -um is to drop -um and add -a. Practice modifying the singular terms below to their plural forms. | Singular	Plural
atrium	
cardium	
septum	
bacterium		
	5–21 A wall or partition dividing a body space or cavity is known as a *septum* (septa, plural). Some *septa* are membranous; others are composed of bone or cartilage. Each is named according to its location in the body. In the heart, there are several septa, one of which is the *interventricular septum* (IVS), the partition that divides the LV from the RV. Label the (5) **interventricular septum (IVS)** in Figure 5–3.
IVS **IAS**	**5–22** The ventricles are separated by a thick muscular IVS, whereas the atria are separated by a thinner muscular *interatrial septum (IAS)*. The abbreviation of the septum situated between the: ventricles is: _____. atria is: _____.

	5-23 Form singular words from the following plural words. Apply the rule that was covered in Frame 5-20.

	Plural	**Singular**
bacterium băk-TĒ-rē-ŭm	bacteria	
septum SĔP-tŭm	septa	
atrium Ā-trē-ŭm	atria	
cardium KĂR-dē-ŭm	cardia	

rapid	**5-24** The prefix tachy- is used in words to mean *rapid*. Tachy/cardia is a heart rate that is _____.

rapid eating	**5-25** Tachy/pnea refers to rapid breathing; tachy/phagia refers to rapid swallowing or _____ _____.

brady/cardia brād-ē-KĂR-dē-ă	**5-26** The prefix brady- is used in words to mean *slow*. People with symptoms of brady/cardia often have difficulty pumping an adequate supply of blood to the tissues of the body. The medical term that literally means *slow heart* is _____ / _____.

brady/pnea brād-ĭp-NĒ-ă **brady/phagia** brād-ē-FĂ-jē-ă	**5-27** Form medical words that literally mean slow breathing: _____ / _____. slow eating: _____ / _____.

tachy/pnea tăk-ĭp-NĒ-ă **tachy/phagia** tăk-ē-FĂ-jē-ă	**5-28** Construct medical words that mean rapid breathing: _____ / _____. rapid eating: _____ / _____.

RA **LA** **RV** **LV** **IVS**	**5-29** Review the chambers and structures of the heart (see Figure 5-3) by writing the abbreviation for the right atrium: _____. left atrium: _____. right ventricle: _____. left ventricle: _____. interventricular septum: _____.

Blood Flow Through the Heart

	5-30 Although general circulatory information was discussed previously, this section covers in greater detail the specific structures involved in the flow of blood through the heart. The heart's double pump serves two distinct circulations: *pulmonary circulation,* which is the short loop of blood vessels that runs from the heart to the lungs and back to the heart; *systemic circulation* routes blood through a long loop to all parts of the body before returning it to the heart.
	Continue to label Figure 5–3 as you read the following information. The right atrium receives oxygen-poor blood from all tissues except those of the lungs. The blood from the head and arms is delivered to the RA through the (6) **superior vena cava (SVC).** The blood from the legs and torso is delivered to the RA through the (7) **inferior vena cava (IVC).**
inferior **superior**	**5-31** Determine the directional words in Frame 5–30 that mean: below (another structure): _____. above (another structure): _____.
superior **inferior**	**5-32** Refer to Figure 5–3 and use the words superior or inferior to complete this frame. The left atrium is _____ to the left ventricle. The right ventricle is _____ to the right atrium.
	5-33 Blood flows from the right atrium through the (8) **tricuspid valve** and into the right ventricle. The leaflets (cusps) are shaped so that they form a one-way passage, which keeps the blood flowing in only one direction. Label the tricuspid valve in Figure 5–3.
tri/cuspid valve trī-KŬS-pĭd	**5-34** The prefix tri- means *three.* The valve that has three leaflets or flaps is the _____ / _____ _____.
three	**5-35** In the English language, a tri/angle is a figure that has _____ sides.
two	**5-36** The prefix bi- refers to *two.* A bi/cuspid valve has _____ leaflets or flaps.
three	**5-37** In the English language, a bi/cycle has two wheels; a tri/cycle has _____ wheels.
two, three	**5-38** By relating bi- and tri- to words in the English language, these prefixes should not be difficult to recall. bi- means _____; tri- means _____.

5-39 The ventricles are the pumping chambers of the heart. As the right ventricle contracts to pump oxygen-deficient blood through the (9) **pulmonary valve** into the pulmonary artery, the tri/cuspid valve remains closed, preventing a backflow of blood into the right atrium. When the blood passes through the main pulmonary artery, it branches into the (10) **right pulmonary artery** and the (10) **left pulmonary artery.** The pulmonary arteries carry the oxygen-deficient blood to the lungs. Label the structures introduced in this frame in Figure 5–3.

---

artery
Ăr-tĕr-ē

5-40 The combining form **arteri/o** refers to an *artery.* Arteri/al bleeding is bleeding from an _____.

---

arteries
Ăr-tĕr-ēs

5-41 Arteri/al circulation is movement of blood through the _____.

---

arteri/o/scler/osis
ăr-tē-rē-ō-sklĕ-RŌ-sĭs

5-42 Arteri/o/scler/osis is a disease characterized by thickening and loss of elasticity of arteri/al walls. A person with a disease or abnormal condition of arteri/al hardening has

_____ / _____ / _____ / _____.

---

stone

artery
Ăr-tĕr-ē

5-43 The suffix -lith refers to a stone or calculus. An arteri/o/lith, also called an arteri/al calculus, is a calculus or _____ in an

_____.

---

artery
Ăr-tĕr-ē

5-44 An arteri/al spasm is a spasm of an _____.

---

arteri/o/rrhexis
ăr-tē-rē-ō-RĔK-sĭs
arteri/o/rrhaphy
ăr-tē-rē-OR-ă-fē
arteri/o/pathy
ăr-tē-rē-ŎP-ă-thē
arteri/o/spasm
ăr-TĔ-rē-ō-spăzm

5-45 Develop medical words that mean

rupture of an artery: _____ / _____ / _____.

suture of an artery: _____ / _____ / _____.

disease of an artery: _____ / _____ / _____.

twitching of an artery: _____ / _____ / _____.

5-46 The right and left pulmonary arteries leading to the lungs branch and subdivide until ultimately they form capillaries around the alveoli. Carbon dioxide is passed from the blood into the alveoli and expelled out of the lungs. Oxygen inhaled in by the lungs is passed from the alveoli into the blood. (Refer to Chapter 4 to review the alveolar structure.) The left and right pulmonary arteries are identified in Figure 5–3 as

number _____.

10

	5-47 Oxygenated blood leaves the lungs and returns to the heart via the (11) **right pulmonary veins** and (11) **left pulmonary veins**. The four pulmonary veins empty into the LA. The LA contracts to force blood through the (12) **mitral valve** into the LV. Label the structures in Figure 5-3.
two	**5-48** The mitral valve, located between the LA and LV, is a bi/cuspid or bi/leaflet valve. This means that the number of leaflets or flaps that the mitral valve has is _____.
left atrium Ā-trē-ŭm **left ventricle** VĔN-trĭk-l **inter/ventricul/ar septum** ĭn-tĕr-vĕn-TRĬK-ū-lăr SĔP-tum **inter/atri/al septum** ĭn-tĕr-Ā-trē-ăl SĔP-tŭm	**5-49** Write the meaning for the following abbreviations: LA: _____ _____. LV: _____ _____. IVS: _____ / _____ / _____ _____. IAS: _____ / _____ / _____ _____.
vein vān	**5-50** **Ven/o** is a combining form meaning _____.
vein vān	**5-51** **Phleb/o** is another combining form for *vein*. Phleb/o/tomy is a procedure used to draw blood from a _____.
phleb/o/rrhaphy flĕb-ŎR-ă-fē **phleb/o/rrhexis** flĕb-ō-RĔK-sĭs **phleb/o/stenosis** flĕb-ō-stĕ-NŌ-sĭs	**5-52** Use **phleb/o** to construct words meaning suture of a vein: _____ / __ / _____. rupture of a vein: _____ / __ / _____. stricture or narrowing of a vein: _____ / __ / _____.
ven/o/scler/osis vēn-ō-sklĕ-RŌ-sĭs **ven/o/tomy** vē-NŎT-ō-mē **ven/o/spasm** VĒ-nō-spăzm	**5-53** Use **ven/o** to form words meaning hardening of a vein: _____ / __ / _____ / __. incision of a vein: _____ / __ / _____. contraction or twitching of a vein: _____ / __ / _____.
blood	**5-54** **Hemat/o** and **hem/o** mean _____.

hemat/o/logy hē-mă-TŎL-ō-jē **hemat/o/logist** hē-mă-TŎL-ō-jĭst	**5-55** Use **hemat/o** to form words meaning study of blood: _____ / ____ / _____. specialist in the study of blood: _____ / ____ / _____
lymph vessels	**5-56** The combining form **angi/o** means *vessel (usually blood or lymph)*. An angioma is a tumor consisting primarily of blood or _____ _____.
hemangi/oma hē-măn-jē-Ō-mă	**5-57** You can combine **hem/o** and **angi/o** into a new element that also means blood vessel. Use **hemangi/o** *(blood vessel)* to develop a word meaning tumor of blood vessels: _____ / _____.
expansion	**5-58** Hemangi/ectasis is a dilation or _____ of a blood vessel.
	5-59 Label the structures in Figure 5–3 as you continue to learn about the heart. Contractions of the LV send oxygenated blood through the (13) **aortic valve** and into the (14) **aorta**. The three ascending (15) **branches of the aorta** transport blood to the head and arms. The (16) **descending aorta** transports the blood to the legs and torso.
aort/o/pathy ā-ŏr-TŎP-ă-thē	**5-60** The aorta is the largest artery of the body and originates at the LV of the heart. The combining form **aort/o** refers to the *aorta*. Any disease of the aorta is called _____ / ____ / _____.
pulmon/ary PŬL-mō-nĕ-rē **vascul/ar** VĂS-kū-lăr **cardi/ac** KĂR-dē-ă	**5-61** Aortic stenosis, a narrowing or stricture of the aortic valve, may be due to congenital malformation or fusion of the cusps. The stenosis obstructs the flow of blood from the LV into the aorta, causing decreased cardi/ac output and pulmon/ary vascul/ar congestion. Treatment usually requires surgical repair. Identify the terms in this frame that mean pertaining to the lungs: _____ / _____. a vessel: _____ / _____. the heart: _____ / _____.
artery **small vein**	**5-62** The suffixes -ole and -ule refer to *small, minute*. An arteri/ole is a small _____; a ven/ule is a _____ _____.

arteries **arteri/oles** ăr-TĒ-rē-ōls	**5–63** Arteries are large vessels that convey blood away from the heart; they branch into smaller vessels called arteri/oles. The arteri/oles deliver blood to adjoining minute vessels called capillaries (see Figure 5–1). Large vessels that transport blood away from the heart are called _____. Smaller vessels that are formed from arteries are called _____ / _____.
arteri/oles ăr-TĒ-rē-ōls	**5–64** Arteries convey blood to adjacent smaller vessels called _____ / _____.
capillaries KĂP-ĭ-lă-rēz	**5–65** Arteri/oles are thinner than arteries and carry blood to minute vessels called _____ (see Figure 5–1).
arteri/o/scler/osis ăr-tē-ō-sklĕ-RŌ-sĭs	**5–66** Arteries carry blood under high pressure, so deterioration of their walls is part of the aging process. As a person ages, the arteries lose their elasticity, thicken, and become weakened. This process of deterioration is also known as an abnormal condition of artery hardening, or _____ / ____ / _____ / _____.
arteri/o/scler/osis ăr-tē-rē-ō-sklĕ-RŌ-sĭs	**5–67** High blood pressure and high-fat diets contribute greatly to early arteri/o/scler/osis. A healthy diet can decrease the risk for hardening of the arteries, also called _____ / ____ / _____ / _____.
superior vena cava VĒ-nă KĂ-vă **inferior vena cava** VĒ-nă KĂ-vă	**5–68** Capillaries carry blood from arteri/oles to ven/ules. Ven/ules form a collecting system to return oxygen-deficient blood to the heart through two large veins, the SVC and the IVC. Define the following abbreviations SVC: _____ _____ _____. IVC: _____ _____ _____.
6 7	**5–69** In Figure 5–3, the SVC is number _____; the IVC is number _____.
arteri/o/spasm ăr-TĒ-rē-ō-spăzm	**5–70** Combine **arteri/o** and -spasm to form a word meaning arterial spasm: _____ / ____ / _____.

Competency Verification: Check your labeling of Figure 5–3 in Appendix B, Answer Key, page 515.

Heart Valves

5-71   Label Figure 5–4 as you read the material about the heart valves and their cusps, also called flaps. Four heart valves maintain the flow of blood in one direction through the heart. The (1) **tricuspid valve** and the (2) **mitral valve** are situated between the upper and lower chambers and are attached to the heart walls by fibrous strands called (3) **chordae tendineae.** The (4) **pulmonary valve** and the (5) **aortic valve** are located at the exits of the ventricles.

Heart valves are composed of thin, fibrous cusps covered by a smooth membrane called *endocardium* reinforced by dense connective tissue. The aortic, pulmonary, and tricuspid valves contain (6) **three cusps;** the mitral valve contains (7) **two cusps.** The purpose of the cusps is to open and permit blood to flow through and seal shut to prevent backflow. The opening and closing of the cusps takes place with each heartbeat.

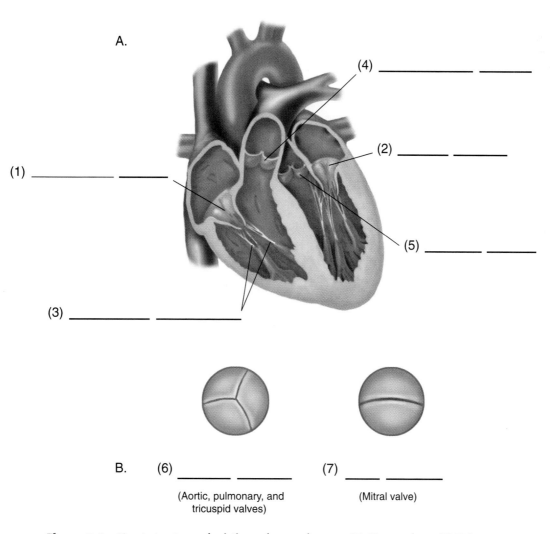

A.

(4) _____ _____

(2) _____ _____

(1) _____ _____

(5) _____ _____

(3) _____ _____

B.   (6) _____ _____   (7) ____ _____
       (Aortic, pulmonary, and   (Mitral valve)
          tricuspid valves)

Figure 5-4   Heart structures depicting valves and cusps. (A) Heart valves. (B) Valve cusps.

mitral valve
MĪ-trăl

5-72   To classify a heart abnormality, it is important to identify the part of the organ in which the disorder occurs. A mitral valve murmur is caused by an incompetent or faulty valve. This type of murmur occurs in the valvular structure of the heart known as the

_____ _____.

valve

5-73   Replacement surgery can be performed to replace a damaged heart valve. When the tri/cuspid valve is damaged, it is replaced at the level of the tri/cuspid _____.

cardi/o/rrhaphy
kăr-dē-OR-ă-fē

5-74   When valve replacement is performed, the heart must be opened. After the valve is inserted, sutures are required to repair the incision. The surgical procedure that literally means suture of the heart is

_____ / _____ / _____.

Competency Verification: Check your labeling of Figure 5–4 in Appendix B, Answer Key, page 521.

Listen and Learn, the audio CD-ROM that accompanies this book, will help you master the pronunciation of selected medical words. Use it to practice pronunciations _of_ selected _terms from frames 5–1 to 5–74_ and for instructions to complete the _Listen and Learn_ exercise on the CD-ROM for this section.

SECTION REVIEW 5-2

Using the following table, write the combining form, suffix, or prefix that matches its definition in the space provided to the left of the definition. There may be more than one word element that matches a definition.

Combining Forms		Suffixes		Prefixes
aort/o	my/o	-ectasis	-rrhaphy	bi-
arteri/o	phleb/o	-ole	-rrhexis	brady-
atri/o	scler/o	-osis	-spasm	epi-
cardi/o	ven/o	-pathy	-stenosis	peri-
hem/o	ventricul/o	-phagia	-ule	tachy-
hemat/o		-pnea		tri-

1. _____ abnormal condition; increase (used primarily with blood cells)
2. _____ above, on
3. _____ aorta
4. _____ around
5. _____ artery
6. _____ atrium
7. _____ blood
8. _____ breathing
9. _____ disease
10. _____ dilation, expansion
11. _____ hardening; sclera (white of eye)
12. _____ heart

13. _____ involuntary contraction, twitching
14. _____ muscle
15. _____ rapid
16. _____ rupture
17. _____ slow
18. _____ small, minute
19. _____ suture
20. _____ narrowing, stricture
21. _____ swallowing, eating
22. _____ three
23. _____ two
24. _____ vein
25. _____ ventricle (of heart or brain)

Competency Verification: Check your answers in Appendix B, Answer Key, page 515. If you are not satisfied with your level of comprehension, go back to Frame 5–1 and rework the frames.

Correct Answers _____ × 4 = _____% Score

Making a set of flash cards from key word elements in this chapter for each section review can help you remember the elements. Make a flash card by writing a word element on one side of a 3 × 5 or 4 × 6 index card. On the other side, write the meaning of the element. Do this for all word elements in the section reviews. Use your flash cards to review each section. You might also use the flash cards to prepare for the chapter review at the end of this chapter.

Conduction Pathway of the Heart

	5-75 The primary responsibility for initiating the heartbeat rests with the pacemaker of the heart or the (1) **sinoatrial (SA) node.** The SA node is a small region of specialized cardiac muscle tissue located on the posterior wall of the (2) **right atrium (RA).** Label the two structures in Figure 5–5.
SA **RA**	**5-76** Write the abbreviations for sinoatrial: _____. right atrium: _____.
electricity	**5-77** The combining form **electr/o** refers to *electricity*. Electric/al and electr/ic both mean pertaining to _____.
	5-78 The electric/al current generated by the heart's pacemaker causes the atrial walls to contract and forces the flow of blood into the ventricles. The wave of electricity moves to another region of the myo/cardi/um called the (3) **atrioventricular (AV) node.** Label the structure in Figure 5–5 to learn about the conduction pathway of the heart.
atri/o/ventricul/ar ā-trē-ō-věn-TRĬK-ū-lăr **electric/al** **atri/al** Ā-trē-ăl	**5-79** Identify the words in Frame 5–78 that mean pertaining to the atrium and ventricles: _____ / _____ / _____ / _____. pertaining to electricity: _____ / _____. pertaining to the atrium: _____ / _____.
AV **SA**	**5-80** Write the abbreviations for atri/o/ventricul/ar: _____. sino/atri/al: _____.
	5-81 The AV node instantaneously sends impulses to a bundle of specialized muscle fibers called the (4) **bundle of His,** which transmits them down the right and left (5) **bundle branches.** Label the structures in Figure 5–5.
	5-82 From the right and left bundle branches, impulses travel through the (6) **Purkinje fibers** to the rest of the ventricul/ar my/o/cardi/um and bring about ventricul/ar contraction. Label the Purkinje fibers in Figure 5–5.
	5-83 Use your medical dictionary to define *contraction*. _____ _____ _____ _____

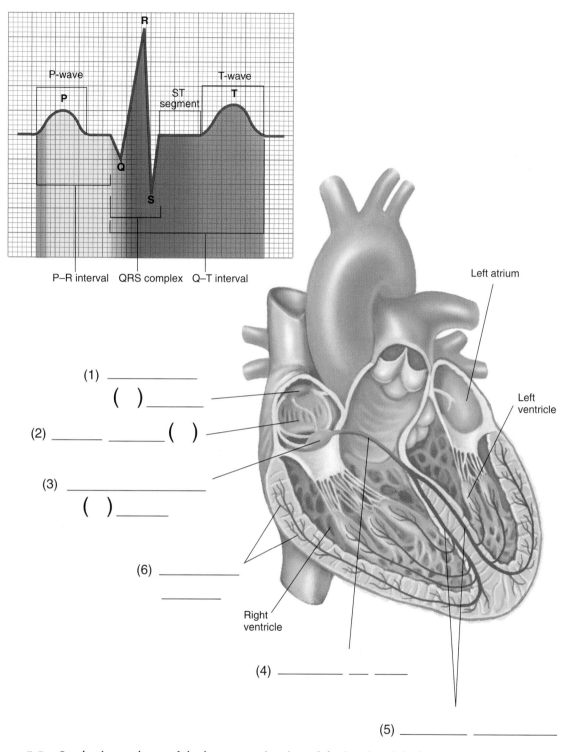

P-wave

T-wave

P

ST
segment

T

R

Q

S

P–R interval   QRS complex   Q–T interval

Left atrium

Left
ventricle

(1) _____
( )_____

(2) _____ _____ ( )

(3) _____
( )_____

(6) _____

_____

Right
ventricle

(4) _____ __ ___

(5) _____ _____

Figure 5-5   Conduction pathway of the heart. Anterior view of the interior of the heart. The electrocardiogram tracing is one normal heartbeat.

Competency Verification: Check your labeling of Figure 5–5 in Appendix B, Answer Key, page 515.

Cardiac Cycle and Heart Sounds

diastole dī-ĂS-tō-lē	**5-84** The cardi/ac cycle refers to the events of one complete heartbeat. Each contraction, or systole, of the heart is followed by a period of relaxation, or diastole. This occurs 60 to 100 times per minute in the normal functioning heart. The normal period of heart contraction is called systole; the normal period of heart relaxation is called _____.
systole SĬS-tō-lē **diastole** dī-ĂS-tō-lē **systole** SĬS-tō-lē	**5-85** When the heart is in the phase of relaxation, it is in diastole. When the heart is in the contraction phase, it is in _____. The pumping action of the heart consists of contraction and relaxation of the myocardial layer of the heart wall. During relaxation, *diastole,* blood fills the ventricles. The contraction that follows, *systole,* propels the blood out of the ventricles and into the circulation. Write the medical term relating to the cardi/ac cycle that is in the phase of relaxation: _____. contraction: _____.
-graphy **-gram**	**5-86** Recall the suffixes that mean process of recording: _____. record, writing: _____.
heart	**5-87** Electr/o/cardi/o/graphy is the process of recording electric/al activity generated by the _____.
record **heart**	**5-88** An electr/o/cardi/o/gram is a _____ of electric/al activity generated by the _____ (see Figure 5–5).
electr/o/cardi/o/gram ē-lĕk-trō-KĂR-dē-ō-grăm	**5-89** *ECG* and *EKG* are abbreviations for electr/o/cardi/o/gram. To evaluate an abnormal cardi/ac rhythm, such as tachy/cardia, an *EKG* may be helpful. The abbreviations *ECG* and *EKG* refer to _____ / ____ / _____ / ____ / _____.
tachy- **brady-**	**5-90** The prefix that means rapid is _____; the prefix that means slow is _____.
rapid **slow**	**5-91** Tachy/cardia is a heart rate that is _____; brady/cardia is a heart rate that is _____.

ALERT

The following summary provides a brief, general interpretation of an ECG. A more comprehensive explanation of ECG abnormalities is beyond the scope of this book. Refer to Figure 5–5 as you read the text that follows.

A normal heart rhythm or **sinus rhythm** shows five waves or deflections on the ECG strip, which represent electrical changes as they spread through the heart. The deflections are known as the **P, QRS**, and **T** waves.

The **P** wave, which represents the transmission of electrical impulses from the **SA** node, indicates atrial contraction. The **QRS** waves represent the electrical impulses through the bundle of His and the Purkinje fiber system and ventricular walls (during systole). The **T** wave represents the electrical recovery and relaxation of the ventricles (during diastole).

---

electr/o/cardi/o/gram ē-lĕk-trō-KĂR-dē-ō-grăm	**5-92** Although the heart itself generates the heartbeat, factors such as hormones, drugs, and nervous system stimulation also can influence the heart rate. To evaluate a patient's heart rate, a physician may order an *EKG*, which is an abbreviation for _____ / ____ / _____ / ____ / _____.
micro/cardia mī-krō-KĂR-dē-ă	**5-93** Micro/cardia, an abnormal smallness of the heart, is a condition that is not usually compatible with a normal life. A person diagnosed with an underdeveloped heart suffers from the condition called _____ / _____.
enlargement, heart	**5-94** Megal/o/cardia is an enlargement of the heart. Cardi/o/megaly also means _____ of the _____.
cardi/o/megaly kăr-dē-ō-MĔG-ă-lē **megal/o/cardia** mĕg-ă-lō-KĂR-dē-ă	**5-95** In patients with high blood pressure, the heart must work extremely hard. As a result, it enlarges, similar to any other muscle in response to excessive activity or exercise. A patient who develops an enlarged heart has a condition called _____ / ____ / _____ or _____ / ____ / _____.
	5-96 Use your medical dictionary to define *angina pectoris* and *lumen*. _____ _____ _____ _____

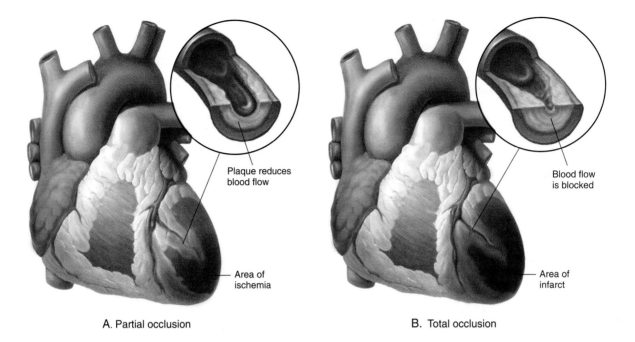

A. Partial occlusion   B. Total occlusion

Figure 5-6   Coronary artery disease. (A) Partial occlusion. (B) Total occlusion.

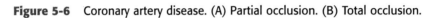

	5–97 Coronary artery disease is an abnormal condition that may affect the heart's arteries and produce various pathological effects, especially the reduced flow of oxygen and nutrients to the myocardium (see Figure 5–6). The most common kind of coronary artery disease is coronary ather/o/scler/osis, which is now the leading cause of death in the Western world.
	Identify the word elements in this frame that mean
-osis	abnormal condition: _____.
scler	hardening: _____.
ather/o	fatty plaque: _____ / _____.
	5–98 Arteri/o/scler/osis describes conditions that affect arteries and may lead to occlusive vascular disease. The lining of the artery and arteri/ole walls becomes thickened and hardened and loses elasticity.
	When the physician diagnoses a hardening of the arteries, the medical chart denotes the condition called
arteri/o/scler/osis ăr-tē-rē-ō-sklĕ-RŌ-sĭs	_____ / _____ / _____ / _____.
	5–99 *Ather/o/scler/osis*, a type of *arteri/o/scler/osis*, is characterized by an accumulation of plaque within the arterial wall (see Figure 5–6). Both conditions develop over a long period, usually occurring together.
	Review the word elements used to denote coronary artery disease.
ather/o	fatty plaque: _____ / _____.

arteri/o	artery: _____ / _____.
scler/o	hardening: _____ / _____.
my/o	muscle: _____ / _____.
cardi	heart: _____.

---

arteri/o/scler/osis
ăr-tē-rē-ō-sklĕ-RŌ-sĭs

ather/o/scler/osis
ăth-ĕr-ō-sklĕ-RŌ-sĭs

5-100 Build medical words that mean
abnormal condition of arterial hardening:

_____ / _____ / _____ / _____.

abnormal condition of fatty plaque hardening:

_____ / _____ / _____ / _____.

---

excision *or* removal

5-101 The combining form **necr/o** refers to *death or necrosis.*
Necr/ectomy is an _____ of dead tissue.

---

necr/o/phobia
nĕk-rē-FŌ-bē-ă

5-102 Use -phobia to form a word meaning fear of death.
_____ / _____ / _____.

---

cardi/ac
KĂR-dē-ăk
necr/osis
nĕ-KRŌ-sĭs

5-103 Necr/osis of the my/o/cardi/um occurs when there is insufficient blood supply to the heart. Eventually this may result in cardi/ac failure and death of the my/o/cardi/um.

Identify the words in this frame meaning

pertaining to the heart: _____ / _____.

abnormal condition of tissue death: _____ / _____.

5-104 A my/o/cardi/al infarction (MI), or infarct, is caused by
occlusion of one or more coronary arteries. *MI* is a medical emergency
requiring immediate attention. Using your medical dictionary, define
infarct.

_____

---

thromb/us
THRŎM-bŭs

5-105 The combining form **thromb/o** is used in words to refer to a
blood clot; the suffix -us means *condition, structure.*

Combine **thromb/o** and -us to form a word that means condition of a

blood clot: _____ / _____.

---

thromb/ectomy
thrŏm-BĔK-tō-mē

5-106 Thromb/osis is a condition in which a stationary blood clot
obstructs a blood vessel at the site of its formation.

The surgical excision of a blood clot is called

_____ / _____.

thrombi THRŎM-bī **anti-**	**5–107** Anti/coagulants are agents that prevent or delay blood coagulation; they are used in the prevention and treatment of a thrombus. The plural form of thrombus is _____. The element in this frame meaning against is _____.
thromb/o/genesis thrŏm-bō-JĔN-ĕ-sĭs	**5–108** Use -genesis to form a word meaning producing or forming a blood clot: _____ / _____ / _____.
clot	**5–109** If the anti/coagulant does not dissolve the clot, it may be surgically removed. A thromb/ectomy is an excision of a blood _____.
anti/coagulant ăn-tī-kō-ĂG-ū-lănt	**5–110** To prevent blood coagulation, the physician uses an agent known as an _____ / _____.
thromb/o/lysis thrŏm-BŎL-ĭ-sĭs	**5–111** Use the surgical suffix -lysis to form a word meaning destruction or dissolving of a thrombus: _____ / _____ / _____.
thromb/o/lysis thrŏm-BŎL-ĭ-sĭs	**5–112** The surgical procedure to destroy or remove a clot is thromb/ectomy or _____ / _____ / _____.
aneurysm ĂN-ū-rĭzm	**5–113** An aneurysm is an abnormal dilation of the vessel wall caused by weakness that causes the vessel to balloon and potentially rupture (see Figure 5–7). A ballooning out of the wall of the aorta is called an aort/ic _____.
aorta ā-ŎR-tă	**5–114** If a cerebr/al aneurysm ruptures, the hem/o/rrhage occurs in the cerebrum or brain. If an aort/ic aneurysm ruptures, the hem/o/rrhage occurs in the _____.
aort/ic ā-ŎR-tĭk **hem/o/rrhage** HĔM-ĕ-rĭj **cerebr/al** SĔR-ĕ-brăl **aneurysm** ĂN-ū-rĭzm	**5–115** Identify the words in Frame 5–114 that mean pertaining to the aorta: _____ / _____. bursting forth (of) blood: _____ / _____ / _____. pertaining to the cerebrum: _____ / _____. dilation of a vessel caused by weakness: _____.

Saccular

Fusiform

Dissecting

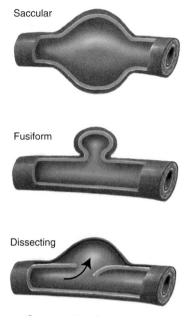

Figure 5-7   Aneurysm.

Listen and Learn, the audio CD-ROM that accompanies this book, will help you master the pronunciation of selected medical words. Use it to practice pronunciations *of* selected *terms from frames 5–75 to 5–115* and for instructions to complete the *Listen and Learn* exercise on the CD-ROM for this section.

Lymphatic System

The lymphatic system consists of lymph, lymph vessels, many lymphoid tissue masses known as lymph nodes, and three organs—the tonsils, thymus, and spleen. All of these organs, including bone marrow, play an important role in the immune response. An important function of the lymphatic system is to drain excess fluid from the tissues, to return the tissue fluid back to the bloodstream, to protect the body against infectious disease and foreign invaders, and to maintain a healthy internal environment in the body.

Lymph fluid originates from the blood. As certain constituents of blood plasma filtrate through the tiny capillaries into the spaces between cells, it becomes *interstitial fluid.* Most of the interstitial fluid is absorbed from the interstitial (or intercellular) spaces by thin-walled vessels called lymph capillaries. At this point, interstitial fluid becomes lymph and is passed through lymphatic tissue called lymph nodes. Eventually lymph reaches large lymph vessels in the upper chest and reenters the bloodstream (see Figure 5–1).

Word Elements

This section introduces combining forms related to the lymphatic system. Included are key suffixes; prefixes are defined in the right-hand column as needed. Review the following table, and pronounce each word in the word analysis column aloud before you begin to work the frames.

Word Element	Meaning	Word Analysis
COMBINING FORMS		
agglutin/o	clumping, gluing	agglutin/ation (ă-gloo-tĭ-NĀ-shŭn): process of cells clumping together *-ation:* process (of)
aden/o	gland	aden/o/pathy (ă-dĕ-NŎP-ă-thē): swelling and morbid change in lymph nodes; glandular disease *-pathy:* disease
lymph/o	lymph	lymph/o/poiesis (lĭm-fō-poy-Ē-sĭs): formation of lymphocytes or of lymphoid tissue *-poiesis:* formation, production
lymphaden/o	lymph gland (node)	lymphaden/itis (lĭm-făd-ĕn-Ī-tĭs): inflammation of one or more lymph nodes, usually caused by a primary focus of infection elsewhere in the body *-itis:* inflammation
lymphangi/o	lymph vessel	lymphangi/oma (lĭm-făn-jē-Ō-mă): tumor composed of lymphatic vessels *-oma:* tumor
splen/o	spleen	splen/o/megaly (splĕ-nō-MĔG-ă-lē): enlargement of the spleen *-megaly:* enlargement
immun/o	immune, immunity, safe	immun/o/gen (ĭ-MŪ-nō-jĕn): producing immunity *-gen:* forming, producing, origin *An immunogen is a substance capable of producing an immune response.*
phag/o	swallowing, eating	phag/o/cyte (FĂG-ō-sīt): cell that surrounds, engulfs, and digests microorganisms and cellular debris *-cyte:* cell
thym/o	thymus gland	thym/oma (thī-MŌ-mă): usually a benign tumor of the thymus gland *-oma:* tumor
SUFFIX		
-phylaxis	protection	ana/phylaxis (ăn-ă-fĭ-LĂK-sĭs): extreme allergic reaction characterized by a rapid decrease in blood pressure, breathing difficulties, hives, and abdominal cramps *ana-:* against; up; back

For the following medical terms, first write the suffix and its meaning. Then translate the meaning of the remaining elements starting with the first part of the word. The first word is an example that is completed for you.

Term	Meaning
1. agglutin/ation	-ation: process (of); clumping, gluing
2. thym/oma	
3. phag/o/cyte	
4. lymphaden/itis	
5. splen/o/megaly	
6. aden/o/pathy	
7. ana/phylaxis	
8. lymphangi/oma	
9. lymph/o/poiesis	
10. immun/o/gen	

Competency Verification: Check your answers in Appendix B, Answer Key, page 516. If you are not satisfied with your level of comprehension, review the vocabulary and retake the review.

Correct Answers _____ × 10 = _____% Score

5–116 Similar to blood capillaries, (1) **lymph capillaries** are thin-walled tubes that carry lymph from the tissue spaces to larger (2) **lymph vessels.** Label these structures in Figure 5–8.

5–117 Lymph/oma is a malignant tumor of lymph nodes and lymph tissue. Two main kinds of lymphomas are *Hodgkin disease* and *non-Hodgkin lymphoma.* These are covered in the pathology section of this chapter.

Use **lymph/o** to build terms that mean

tumor composed of lymph tissue:

_____ / _____.

lymph/oma
lĭm-FŌ-mă

cell present in lymph tissue:

_____ / _____ / _____.

lymph/o/cyte
LĬM-fō-sīt

formation or production of lymph:

_____ / _____ / _____.

lymph/o/poiesis
lĭm-fō-poy-Ē-sĭs

5–118 Recall that **angi/o** is used in words to denote a *vessel (usually blood or lymph).* Angio/card/itis is an inflammation of the heart and blood

vessel

_____.

5–119 Combine **lymph/o** and **angi/o** to form a new element meaning

lymphangi/o

lymph vessel: _____ / _____.

5–120 Use **lymphangi/o** to form a word meaning tumor composed of

lymphangi/oma
lĭm-făn-jē-Ō-mă

lymph vessels: _____ / _____

5–121 Use **angi/o** to develop medical words meaning

angi/o/rrhaphy
ăn-jē-OR-ă-fē

suture of a vessel: _____ / _____ / _____.

angi/o/plasty
ĂN-jē-ō-plăs-tē

surgical repair of a vessel: _____ / _____ / _____.

angi/o/rrhexis
ăn-jē-ō-RĔK-sĭs

rupture of a vessel: _____ / _____ / _____.

5–122 Similar to veins, lymph vessels contain valves that keep lymph flowing in one direction, toward the thorac/ic cavity.

chest

Thorac/ic means pertaining to the _____.

5–123 The (3) **thoracic duct** and the (4) **right lymphatic duct** carry lymph into veins in the upper thoracic region. Label these two ducts in Figure 5–8.

5–124 Use -oid to form a word meaning resembling lymph:

lymph/oid
LĬM-foyd

_____ / _____.

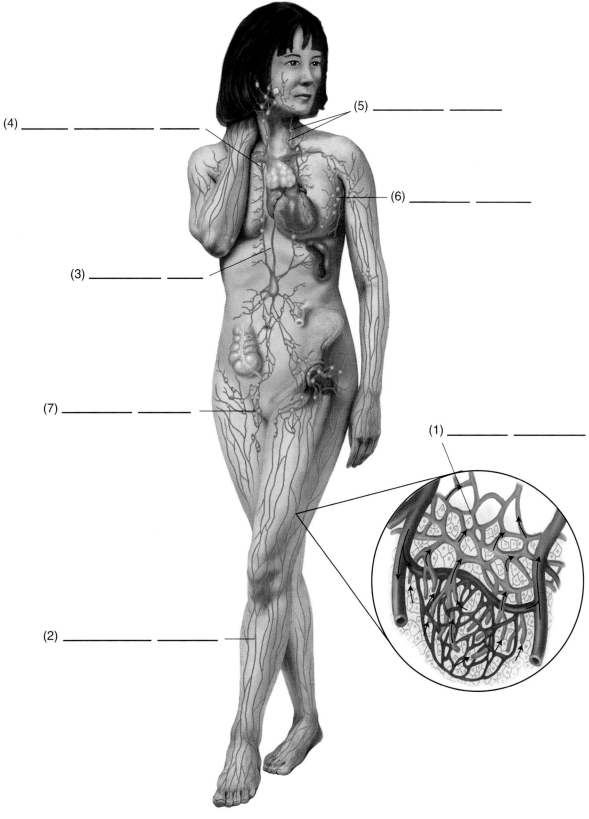

(4) _____ _____ _____

(5) _____ _____

(6) _____ _____

(3) _____ _____

(7) _____ _____

(1) _____ _____

(2) _____ _____

Figure 5-8   Lymphatic system.

lymph/o/pathy
lĭm-FŎP-ă-thē

5-125 The word meaning any disease of the lymphat/ic system is

_____ / ____ / _____.

lymph/o/cytes
LĬM-fō-sīts

5-126 Small round structures called *lymph nodes* not only produce lymph/o/cytes, but also filter and purify lymph by removing harmful substances such as bacteria or cancerous cells.

Lymph cells are known as _____ / ____ / _____.

5-127 The major lymph node sites are (5) the **cervical nodes**, (6) the **axillary nodes**, and (7) the **inguinal nodes**. Label the three major lymph node sites in Figure 5–8.

cervical
SĔR-vĭ-kăl
axillary
ĂK-sĭ-lăr-ē

inguinal
ĬNG-gwĭ-năl

5-128 Write the name of the lymph node located in

the neck: _____.

the armpit: _____.

the groin area (depression between the thigh and trunk):

_____.

Competency Verification: Check your labeling of Figure 5–8 in Appendix B, Answer Key, page 516.

Listen and Learn, the audio CD-ROM that accompanies this book, will help you master the pronunciation of selected medical words. Use it to practice pronunciations *of selected terms from frames 5–116 to 5–128* and from the word elements table. Listen for instructions to complete the *Listen and Learn* exercise on the CD-ROM for this section.

SECTION REVIEW 5 – 4

Using the following table, write the combining form or suffix that matches its definition in the space provided to the left of the definition. There may be more than one word element that matches a definition.

Combining Forms	Suffixes
angi/o	-al
aort/o	-cyte
cardi/o	-ic
cerebr/o	-gram
electr/o	-graphy
hem/o	-lysis
lymph/o	-megaly
my/o	-pathy
necr/o	-plasty
thromb/o	-rrhexis
	-stenosis

1. _____ aorta
2. _____ blood
3. _____ blood clot
4. _____ cell
5. _____ cerebrum
6. _____ death, necrosis
7. _____ disease
8. _____ electricity
9. _____ enlargement
10. _____ heart

11. _____ lymph
12. _____ muscle
13. _____ process of recording
14. _____ record, writing
15. _____ pertaining to, relating to
16. _____ rupture
17. _____ separation; destruction; loosening
18. _____ narrowing, stricture
19. _____ surgical repair
20. _____ vessel (usually blood or lymph)

Competency Verification: Check your answers in Appendix B, Answer Key, page 516. If you are not satisfied with your level of comprehension, go back to Frame 5–75 and rework the frames.

Correct Answers _____ × 5 = _____% Score

Abbreviations

This section introduces cardiovascular and lymphatic systems–related abbreviations and their meanings. Included are abbreviations contained in the medical record activities that follow.

Abbreviation	Meaning	Abbreviation	Meaning
CARDIOVASCULAR			
AS	aortic stenosis	IVC	inferior vena cava
ASD	atrial septal defect	IVS	interventricular septum
ASHD	arteriosclerotic heart disease	LA	left atrium
AV	atrioventricular, arteriovenous	LDL	low-density lipoprotein
BBB	bundle-branch block	LV	left ventricle
BP	blood pressure	MI	myocardial infarction
CABG	coronary artery bypass graft	MVP	mitral valve prolapse
CAD	coronary artery disease	RA	right atrium
CC	cardiac catheterization; chief complaint	RBC	red blood cell(s); red blood count
CHF	congestive heart failure	RV	right ventricle
CV	cardiovascular	SA	sinoatrial (node)
CVA	cerebrovascular accident	SVC	superior vena cava
ECG, EKG	electrocardiogram	VSD	ventricular septal defect
HF	heart failure	WBC	white blood cell(s); white blood count
IAS	interatrial septum		
LYMPHATIC			
AIDS	acquired immunodeficiency syndrome	HSV	herpes simplex virus
EBV	Epstein-Barr virus	KS	Kaposi sarcoma
HIV	human immunodeficiency virus	PCP	*Pneumocystis carinii* pneumonia

Pathological, Diagnostic, and Therapeutic Terms

The following are additional terms related to the cardiovascular and lymphatic systems. Recognizing and learning these terms will help you understand the connection between a pathological condition, its diagnoses, and the rationale behind the method of treatment selected for a particular disorder.

Pathological

Cardiovascular System

aneurysm (ĂN-ū-rĭzm): localized dilation of the wall of a blood vessel, introducing the risk of a rupture.

> *An aneurysm may rupture, causing hemorrhage, or thrombi may form in the dilation and give rise to emboli that may obstruct smaller vessels (see Figure 5–7).*

arrhythmia (ă-RĬTH-mē-ă): irregularity or loss of rhythm of the heartbeat; also called *dysrhythmia*.

arteriosclerosis (ăr-tē-rē-ō-sklē-RŌ-sĭs): thickening, hardening, and loss of elasticity of arterial walls.

> *Arteriosclerosis results in altered function of tissues and organs; also called hardening of the arteries.*

atherosclerosis (ăth-ĕ-rō-sklē-RŌ-sĭs): most common form of arteriosclerosis, caused by an accumulation of fatty substances within the walls of the arteries causing partial and eventually total occlusion (see Figure 5–6).

bruit (brwē): soft blowing sound heard on auscultation caused by turbulent blood flow.

coronary artery disease (KŌR-ō-nă-rē ĂR-tĕr-ē): abnormal condition that may affect the heart's arteries and produce various pathological effects, especially the reduced flow of oxygen and nutrients to the myocardium (see Figure 5–6).

> *The most common kind of coronary artery disease is coronary atherosclerosis, now the leading cause of death in the Western world.*

deep vein thrombosis (DĒP vān thrŏm-BŌ-sĭs): formation of a blood clot in a deep vein of the body, occurring most frequently in the iliac and femoral veins.

embolus (ĔM-bō-lŭs): mass of undissolved matter present in a blood or lymphatic vessel brought there by the blood or lymph current.

> *Emboli may be solid, liquid, or gaseous. Occlusion of vessels from emboli usually results in the development of infarcts.*

fibrillation (fĭ-brĭl-Ā-shŭn): irregular, random contraction of heart fibers.

> *Fibrillation commonly occurs in the atria or ventricles of the heart and is usually described by the part that is contracting abnormally, such as atrial fibrillation or ventricular fibrillation.*

heart failure: condition in which the heart cannot pump enough blood to meet the metabolic requirement of body tissues.

> *Heart failure (HF) includes myocardial infarction, ischemic heart disease, and cardiomyopathy. It also may be caused by the dysfunction of organs other than the heart, especially the lungs, kidneys, and liver. The term heart failure (HF) is currently replacing the term congestive heart failure (CHF).*

hypertension (hī-pĕr-TĔN-shŭn): consistently elevated blood pressure that is higher than normal causing damage to the blood vessels and ultimately the heart.

ischemia (ĭs-KĒ-mē-ă): decreased supply of oxygenated blood to a body part due to an interruption of blood flow. See the ischemic area of an occluded coronary artery in Figure 5–6.

Some causes of ischemia are arterial embolism, atherosclerosis, thrombosis, and vasoconstriction.

mitral valve prolapse (MĪ-trăl vălv prō-LĂPS): condition in which the leaflets of the mitral valve prolapse into the left atrium during systole, resulting in incomplete closure and backflow of blood.

murmur (MĔR-mĕr): abnormal sound heard on auscultation, caused by defects in the valves or chambers of the heart.

myocardial infarction (mī-ō-KĂR-dē-ăl ĭn-FĂRK-shŭn): necrosis of a portion of cardiac muscle caused by partial or complete occlusion of one or more coronary arteries; also called *heart attack.*

patent ductus arteriosus (PĂT-ĕnt DŬK-tŭs ăr-tē-rē-Ō-sĭs): failure of the ductus arteriosus to close after birth, resulting in an abnormal opening between the pulmonary artery and the aorta.

Raynaud phenomenon (rā-NŌ): numbness in fingers or toes due to intermittent constriction of arterioles in the skin.

This condition is typically caused by exposure to cold temperatures or emotional stress. It also may be an indicator of some other more serious problem.

rheumatic heart disease (rū-MĂT-ĭk): streptococcal infection that causes damage to the heart valves and heart muscle, most often seen in children and young adults.

stroke (strōk): damage to part of the brain due to interruption of its blood supply, commonly caused by blockage of an artery. Bleeding within brain tissue is another cause of strokes.

When the affected brain cells are deprived of oxygen, they cease to function. Movement, vision, and speech may be impaired; also called cerebrovascular accident (CVA).

transient ischemic attack (TRĂN-zhĕnt ĭs-KĒ-mĭk): temporary interference with blood supply to the brain, causing no permanent brain damage.

varicose veins (VĂR-ĭ-kōs vāns): swollen, distended veins caused by incompetent venous valves; most often seen in the lower legs.

Lymphatic System

acquired immunodeficiency syndrome (ă-KWĪRD ĭm-ū-nō-dē-FĬSH-ĕn-sē SĬN-drōm): deficiency of cellular immunity induced by infection with the human immunodeficiency virus (HIV), characterized by increasing susceptibility to infections, malignancies, and neurological diseases; also called *AIDS.*

HIV is transmitted from person to person in cell-rich body fluids (notably blood and semen) through sexual contact, sharing of contaminated needles (as by intravenous drug abusers), or other contact with contaminated blood (as in accidental needle sticks among health care workers).

Hodgkin disease (HŎJ-kĭn): malignant disease characterized by painless, progressive enlargement of lymphoid tissue, usually first evident in cervical lymph nodes, splenomegaly, and the presence of unique Reed-Sternberg cells in the lymph nodes.

Kaposi sarcoma (KĂP-ō-sē săr-KŌ-mă): malignancy of connective tissue including bone, fat, muscle, and fibrous tissue.

Kaposi sarcoma is closely associated with AIDS and is commonly fatal because the tumors readily metastasize to various organs.

lymphadenitis (lĭm-făd-ĕn-Ī-tĭs): inflammation and enlargement of the lymph nodes, usually as a result of infection.

mononucleosis (mŏn-ō-nū-klē-Ō-sĭs): acute infection caused by the Epstein-Barr virus (EBV) characterized by a sore throat, fever, fatigue, and enlarged lymph nodes.

non-Hodgkin lymphoma (non HŎJ-kĭn lĭm-FŌ-mă): any of a heterogeneous group of malignant tumors involving lymphoid tissue except for Hodgkin disease; previously called *lymphosarcoma*.

Diagnostic

Cardiovascular System

cardiac catheterization (KĂR-dē-ăk kăth-ĕ-tĕr-ĭ-ZĀ-shŭn): insertion of a small tube (catheter) through an incision into a large vein, usually of an arm (brachial approach) or leg (femoral approach), which is threaded through a blood vessel until it reaches the heart.

A contrast medium also may be injected and x-rays taken (angiography). This procedure can identify and assess accurately many conditions, including congenital heart disease, valvular incompetence, blood supply, and myocardial infarction.

cardiac enzyme studies (KĂR-dē-ăk ĔN-zīm): battery of blood tests performed to determine the presence of cardiac damage.

echocardiography (ĕk-ō-KĂR-dē-ŏ-grăf-ē): ultrasound, also called ultrasonography, to visualize internal cardiac structures and motion of the heart.

electrocardiography (ē-lĕk-trō-KĂR-dē-ŏ-grăf-ē): creation and study of graphic records (electrocardiograms) produced by electric activity generated by the heart muscle; also called *cardiography*.

Electrocardiography (ECG, EKG) is analyzed by a cardiologist and is valuable in diagnosing cases of abnormal rhythm and myocardial damage.

Holter monitor (HŌL-ter MŎN-ĭ-tĕr): monitoring device worn on the patient for making prolonged electrocardiograph recordings (usually 24 hours) on a portable tape recorder while conducting normal daily activities.

Holter monitoring is particularly useful in obtaining a record of cardiac arrhythmia that would not be discovered by means of an ECG of only a few minutes' duration. Also the patient may keep an activity diary to compare daily events with electrocardiograph tracings (see Figure 5–9).

stress test: method of evaluating CV fitness. While exercising, usually on a treadmill, the individual is subjected to steadily increasing levels of work. At the same time, the amount of oxygen consumed is measured while an ECG is administered.

troponin I (TRŌ-pō-nĭn): blood test that measures protein that is released into the blood by damaged heart muscle (but not skeletal muscle) and is a highly sensitive and specific indicator of recent MI.

ultrasonography (ŭl-tră-sŏn-Ŏ-grăf-ē): imaging technique that uses high-frequency sound waves (ultrasound) that bounce off body tissues and are recorded to produce an image of an internal organ or tissue. Ultrasonic echoes are recorded and interpreted by a computer, which produces a detailed image of the organ or tissue being evaluated (see Figure 2–5F).

Doppler ultrasonography measures blood flow in blood vessels. It allows the examiner to hear characteristic alterations in blood flow caused by vessel obstruction in various parts of an extremity.

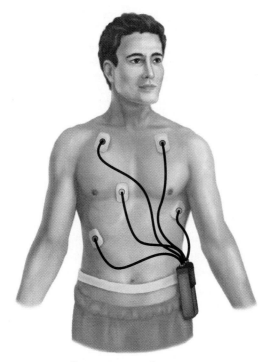

Figure 5-9   Holter monitor.

Lymphatic System

bone marrow aspiration biopsy (ăs-pĭ-RĀ-shŭn BĪ-ŏp-sē): removal of living tissue, usually taken from the sternum or iliac crest, for microscopic examination of bone marrow tissue.

Evaluates hematopoiesis by revealing the number, shape, and size of the red blood cells (RBCs) and white blood cells (WBCs) and platelet precursors.

lymphangiography (lĭm-făn-jē-Ŏ-grăf-ē): radiographic examination of lymph glands and lymphatic vessels after an injection of a contrast medium.

Lymphangiography is used to show the path of lymph flow as it moves into the chest region.

tissue typing: technique for determining the histocompatibility of tissues to be used in grafts and transplants with the recipient's tissues and cells; also known as *histocompatibility testing.*

Therapeutic

Cardiovascular System

angioplasty (ĂN-jē-ō-plăs-tē): any endovascular procedure that reopens narrowed blood vessels and restores forward blood flow. The blocked vessel is usually opened by balloon dilation.

coronary artery bypass graft (KOR-ă-năr-ē ĂHR-tă-rē BĪ-păss): surgery that involves bypassing one or more blocked coronary arteries to increase blood flow (see Figure 5–10).

Cardiac catheterization is used to identify blocked coronary arteries. After the blockages are identified, coronary artery bypass graft (CABG) surgery is often performed. The operation involves the use of one or more of the patient's arteries or veins. Generally, the saphenous vein from the leg or the right or left internal mammary artery from the chest wall is used to bypass the blocked section.

statins (STĂ-tĭnz): drugs that reduce low-density lipoprotein (LDL).

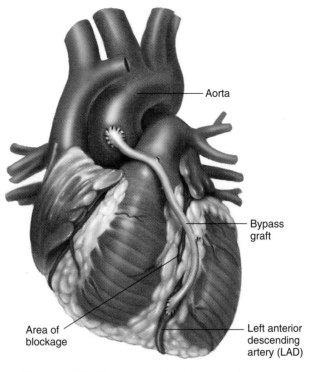

Aorta

Bypass graft

Area of blockage

Left anterior descending artery (LAD)

Figure 5-10   Coronary artery bypass graft.

thrombolytic therapy (thrŏm-bō-LĬT-ĭk THĔR-ă-pē): administration of drugs to dissolve a blood clot.

valvuloplasty (VĂL-vū-lō-plăs-tē): plastic or restorative surgery on a valve, especially a cardiac valve.

A special type of valvuloplasty is balloon valvuloplasty in which insertion of a balloon catheter to open a stenotic heart valve is performed. Inflating the balloon decreases the constriction.

 Listen and Learn, the audio CD-ROM that accompanies this book, will help you master the pronunciation of selected medical words. Use it to practice pronunciations of the above-listed medical terms and for instructions to complete the *Listen and Learn* exercise on the CD-ROM for this section.

PATHOLOGICAL, DIAGNOSTIC, AND THERAPEUTIC TERMS REVIEW

Match the medical term(s) below with the definitions in the numbered list.

AIDS
arrhythmia
atherosclerosis
bruit
CABG
DVT
embolus

fibrillation
heart failure (HF)
Hodgkin disease
Holter monitor
hypertension
ischemia
lymphadenitis

lymphangiography
mononucleosis
Raynaud phenomenon
rheumatic heart disease
stroke
thrombolytic therapy
tissue typing

TIA
troponin I
valvuloplasty
varicose veins

1. _____ are swollen, distended veins most often seen in the lower legs.

2. _____ is an acute infection caused by Epstein-Barr virus (EBV) characterized by a sore throat, fever, fatigue, and enlarged lymph nodes.

3. _____ refers to administration of drugs to dissolve a blood clot.

4. _____ is a mass of undissolved matter present in a blood vessel.

5. _____ is inflammation and enlargement of the lymph nodes.

6. _____ refers to formation of a blood clot in a deep vein of the body.

7. _____ refers to blood pressure that is consistently higher than normal.

8. _____ is irregularity or loss of heartbeat rhythm.

9. _____ refers to temporary interference of blood supply to the brain without permanent damage.

10. _____ is a soft blowing sound caused by turbulent blood flow.

11. _____ refers to partial brain damage due to interruption of its blood supply, commonly caused by blockage of an artery.

12. _____ is a streptococcal infection that causes damage to heart valves and heart muscle.

13. _____ is heart disease caused by an accumulation of fatty substances within the arterial walls.

14. _____ is a small portable device worn on a patient during normal activity to obtain a record of cardiac arrhythmia.

15. _____ is numbness in fingers or toes due to intermittent constriction of arterioles in the skin.

16. _____ refers to decreased supply of oxygenated blood to a body part due to an interruption of blood flow.

17. _____ refers to malignant solid tumors of the lymphatic system.

18. _____ is a transmissible infection caused by human immunodeficiency virus (HIV).

19. _____ is a condition in which the heart cannot pump enough blood to meet the metabolic requirement of body tissues.

20. _____ means irregular, random contraction of heart fibers.

21. _____ refers to plastic or restorative surgery on a valve, especially a cardiac valve.

22. _____ is a radiographic examination of lymph glands and lymphatic vessels after an injection of a contrast medium.

23. _____ also is known as histocompatibility testing.

24. _____ refers to blood test that measures protein that is released into the blood by damaged heart muscle.

25. _____ refers to surgery that involves bypassing one or more blocked coronary arteries to restore blood flow.

Competency Verification: Check your answers in Appendix B, Answer Key, page 516. If you are not satisfied with your level of comprehension, review the pathological, diagnostic, and therapeutic terms and retake the review.

Correct Answers: _____ × 4 = _____% Score

Medical Record Activities

The following medical records reflect common real-life clinical scenarios using medical terminology to document patient care. The physician who specializes in the treatment of cardiovascular disorders is a *cardiologist;* the medical specialty concerned in the diagnoses and treatment of cardiovascular disorders is *cardiology*. The physician who specializes in the surgical treatment of blood vessels and vascular disorders is a *vascular surgeon*.

✓ MEDICAL RECORD ACTIVITY 5–1. Myocardial Infarction (MI)

Terminology

The terms listed in the chart come from the medical record *Myocardial Infarction (MI)* that follows. Use a medical dictionary such as *Taber's Cyclopedic Medical Dictionary,* the appendices of this book, or other resources to define each term. Then practice reading the pronunciations aloud for each term.

Term	Definition
apnea ăp-NĒ-ă	
desiccated dĕs-ĭ-KĀ-tĕd	
dyspnea dĭsp-NĒ-ă	
EKG	
fibrillation fĭ-brĭl-Ā-shŭn	
malaise mă-LĀZ	
myocardial infarction mĭ-ō-KĂR-dē-ăl ĭn-FĂRK-shŭn	
ST-T wave (see Figure 5–5)	
syncope SĬN-kō-pē	
tachycardia tăk-ē-KĂR-dē-ă	
thyroidectomy thī-royd-ĔK-tō-mē	

Listen and Learn Online! will help you master the pronunciation of selected medical words from this medical record activity. Visit www.fadavis.com/gylys/simplified for instructions in completing the *Listen and Learn Online!* exercise for this section and then to practice pronunciations.

MYOCARDIAL INFARCTION (MI)

Reading

Practice pronunciation of medical terms by reading the following medical report aloud.

A 70-year-old white woman was admitted to the hospital for evaluation of a syncopal episode. She states that most recently she has experienced generalized malaise, increased shortness of breath while at rest, and dyspnea followed by periods of apnea and syncope.

Her past history includes recurrent episodes of thyroiditis, which led her to have a thyroidectomy 6 years ago while she was under the care of Dr. Knopp. At the time of surgery, the results of her EKG were interpreted as sinus tachycardia with nonspecific ST-T wave changes. The tachycardia was attributed to preoperative anxiety and thyroiditis. Postoperatively, under the direction of Dr. Knopp, the patient was treated with a daily dose of 50 mg of desiccated thyroid and has been symptom-free until this admission.

On clinical examination, the patient's radial pulse was found to be irregular, and the EKG showed uncontrolled atrial fibrillation with evidence of a recent myocardial infarction (MI).

Evaluation

Review the medical record to answer the following questions.

1. What symptoms did the patient experience before admission to the hospital?

   _____

   _____

2. What was found during clinical examination?

   _____

   _____

3. What is the danger of atrial fibrillation?

   _____

   _____

4. Did the patient have prior history of heart problems? If so, describe them.

   _____

   _____

5. Was the patient's prior heart problem related to her current one?

   _____

   _____

✓ MEDICAL RECORD ACTIVITY 5–2. Cardiac Catheterization

Terminology

The terms listed in the chart come from the medical record *Cardiac Catheterization* that follows. Use a medical dictionary such as *Taber's Cyclopedic Medical Dictionary,* the appendices of this book, or other resources to define each term. Then practice reading the pronunciations aloud for each term.

Term	Definition
angiography ăn-jē-ŎG-ră-fē	
angioplasty ĂN-jē-ō-plăs-tē	
catheter KĂTH-ĕ-tĕr	
heparin HĔP-ă-rĭn	
lidocaine LĪ-dō-kān	
sheath shēth	
ST elevations	
stenosis stĕ-NŌ-sĭs	

Listen and Learn Online! will help you master the pronunciation of selected medical words from this medical record activity. Visit www.fadavis.com/gylys/simplified for instructions in completing the *Listen and Learn Online!* exercise for this section and then to practice pronunciations.

CARDIAC CATHETERIZATION

Reading

Practice pronunciation of medical terms by reading the following medical report aloud.

PROCEDURE: The patient was prepared and draped in a sterile fashion and 20 mL of 1% lidocaine was infiltrated in the right groin. A No. 6 French Cordis right femoral arterial sheath was placed and a No. 6 French JL-5 and JR-4 catheter was used to engage the left and right coronary. A No. 6 French pigtail was used for left ventricular angiography. Angioplasty was made, and further dictation is under the angioplasty report. There were minor irregularities, with a maximal 25% stenosis just after the first diagonal. The remainder of the vessel was free of significant disease.

A 0.014, high-torque, floppy, extra-support, exchange-length wire was used to cross the stenosis in the distal right coronary artery. A 3.5 × 20-mm Track star balloon was inflated in the right coronary artery in the distal portion. The initial stenosis was 50% to 75% with an ulcerated plaque, and the final stenosis was 20% with no significant clot seen in the region. The patient had significant ST elevations in the inferior leads and severe throat tightness and shortness of breath. This would resolve immediately with the inflation of the balloon. The catheters were removed, and the sheath was changed to a No. 8 French Arrow sheath. The patient will be on heparin over the next 12 hours.

IMPRESSION: (1) Two-vessel coronary artery disease with a 75% obtuse marginal and a 75% right coronaryartery lesion; (2) normal left ventricular function; (3) successful angioplasty to right coronary artery with initial stenosis of 75% and a final stenosis of 20%.

Evaluation

Review the medical record to answer the following questions.

1. What coronary arteries were under examination?

_____

_____

2. Which surgical procedure was used to clear the stenosis?

_____

_____

3. What symptoms did the patient exhibit before balloon inflation?

_____

_____

4. Why was the patient put on heparin?

_____

_____

Chapter Review

Word Elements Summary

The following table summarizes combining forms, suffixes, and prefixes related to the cardiovascular and lymphatic systems.

Word Element	Meaning
COMBINING FORMS	
angi/o	vessel (usually blood or lymph)
aort/o	aorta
arteri/o	artery
atri/o	atrium
cardi/o	heart
electr/o	electric
lymph/o	lymph
phleb/o, ven/o	vein
thromb/o	blood clot
ventricul/o	ventricle (of heart or brain)
OTHER COMBINING FORMS	
cerebr/o	cerebrum
hem/o	blood
my/o	muscle
necr/o	death, necrosis
scler/o	hardening; sclera (white of eye)
SUFFIXES	
SURGICAL	
-ectomy	excision, removal
-lysis	separation; destruction; loosening
-plasty	surgical repair
-rrhaphy	suture
-tomy	incision
DIAGNOSTIC, SYMPTOMATIC, AND RELATED	
-cardia	heart condition
-cyte	cell

Word Element	Meaning
-ectasis	dilation, expansion
-genesis	forming, producing, origin
-gram	record, writing
-graphy	process of recording
-lith	stone, calculus
-malacia	softening
-megaly	enlargement
-oid	resembling
-ole, -ule	small, minute
-oma	tumor
-osis	abnormal condition; increase (used primarily with blood cells)
-pathy	disease
-phagia	swallowing, eating
-phobia	fear
-pnea	breathing
-rrhexis	rupture
-spasm	involuntary contraction, twitching
-stenosis	narrowing, stricture
-um	structure, thing

ADJECTIVE

-al, -ic	pertaining to, relating to

PREFIXES

anti-	against
bi-	two
brady-	slow
endo-	in, within
epi-	above, upon
micro-	small
peri-	around
tachy-	rapid
tri-	three

WORD ELEMENTS REVIEW

After you review the Word Elements Summary, complete this activity by writing the meaning of each element in the space provided.

Word Element	Meaning
COMBINING FORMS	
1. angi/o	
2. aort/o	
3. arteri/o	
4. atri/o	
5. cardi/o	
6. lymph/o	
7. phleb/o	
8. ven/o	
9. thromb/o	
10. ventricul/o	
OTHER COMBINING FORMS	
11. electr/o	
12. my/o	
13. necr/o	
14. hem/o	
15. scler/o	
SUFFIXES	
SURGICAL	
16. -ectomy	
17. -lysis	
18. -plasty	
19. -rrhaphy	
20. -tomy	

Word Element	Meaning
DIAGNOSTIC, SYMPTOMATIC, AND RELATED	
21. -cyte	
22. -ectasis	
23. -genesis	
24. -gram	
25. -graphy	
26. -lith	
27. -malacia	
28. -megaly	
29. -oid	
30. -ole, -ule	
31. -oma	
32. -osis	
33. -pathy	
34. -phagia	
35. -phobia	
36. -pnea	
37. -rrhexis	
38. -spasm	
39. -stenosis	
40. -um	
ADJECTIVE	
41. -al, -ic	

(Continued)

Word Element	Meaning *(Continued)*
PREFIXES	
42. anti-	
43. bi-	
44. brady-	
45. endo-	
46. epi-	
47. micro-	
48. peri-	
49. tachy-	
50. tri-	

Competency Verification: Check your answers in Appendix A, Glossary of Medical Word Elements, page 497. If you are not satisfied with your level of comprehension, review the word elements and retake the review.

Correct Answers _____ × 2 = _____% Score

Chapter 5 Vocabulary Review

Match the medical term(s) with the definitions in the numbered list.

agglutination	arteriosclerosis	EKG	pacemaker
anaphylaxis	capillaries	hemangioma	phagocyte
aneurysm	cardiomegaly	malaise	systole
angina pectoris	desiccated	MI	tachyphagia
arterioles	diastole	myocardium	tachypnea

1. _____ refers to the muscular layer of the heart.

2. _____ means rapid breathing.

3. _____ is disease characterized by an abnormal hardening of the arteries.

4. _____ is a cell that engulfs and digests cellular debris.

5. _____ refers to the contraction phase of the heart.

6. _____ refers to the relaxation phase of the heart.

7. _____ is a record of the electrical impulses of the heart.

8. _____ means a vague feeling of bodily discomfort, which may be the first indication of an infection or disease.

9. _____ means dried thoroughly; rendered free from moisture.

10. _____ means enlarged heart.

11. _____ refers to weakness in the vessel wall that balloons and eventually bursts.

12. _____ is severe pain and constriction about the heart caused by an insufficient supply of oxygenated blood to the heart.

13. _____ is necrosis of an area of muscular heart tissue after cessation of blood supply.

14. _____ is a process of cells clumping together.

15. _____ means rapid eating or swallowing.

16. _____ is a allergic reaction characterized by a rapid decrease in blood pressure.

17. _____ are the smallest vessels of the circulatory system.

18. _____ is a tumor composed of blood vessels.

19. _____ are small arteries.

20. _____ maintains primary responsibility for initiating the heartbeat.

Competency Verification: Check your answers in Appendix B, Answer Key, page 517. If you are not satisfied with your level of comprehension, review the chapter vocabulary and retake the review.

Correct Answers _____ × 5 = _____% Score

6

Digestive System

OBJECTIVES

Upon completion of this chapter, you will be able to:

■ Name the organs of the digestive system and discuss their primary functions.

■ Describe pathological, diagnostic, therapeutic, and other terms related to the digestive system.

■ Recognize, define, pronounce, and spell terms correctly by completing the audio CD-ROM exercises.

■ Demonstrate your knowledge of this chapter by successfully completing the frames, reviews, and medical report evaluations.

The digestive system, also known as the *gastrointestinal (GI) system,* consists of a digestive tube called the *GI tract,* or *alimentary canal.* The GI system includes several accessory organs whose primary function is to break down food, prepare it for absorption, and eliminate waste substances. The GI tract, extending from the oral cavity (mouth) to the anus, varies in size and structure in several distinct regions. It terminates at the anus, where solid wastes are eliminated from the body by means of defecation (see Figure 6–1).

Word Elements

This section introduces combining forms related to the oral cavity, esophagus, pharynx, and stomach. Included are key suffixes; prefixes are defined in the right-hand column as needed. Review the following table and pronounce each word in the word analysis column aloud before you begin to work the frames.

Word Element	Meaning	Word Analysis
COMBINING FORMS		
ORAL CAVITY		
dent/o	teeth	dent/ist (DĔN-tĭst): specialist who diagnoses and treats diseases and disorders of teeth and tissues of the oral cavity *-ist:* specialist
odont/o		orth/odont/ist (ŏr-thō-DŎN-tĭst): dental specialist in the prevention and correction of abnormally positioned or misaligned teeth *orth:* straight *-ist:* specialist
gingiv/o	gum(s)	gingiv/itis (jĭn-jĭ-VĪ-tĭs): inflammation of the gums *-itis:* inflammation
gloss/o	tongue	hypo/gloss/al (hī-pō-GLŎS-ăl): under the tongue *hypo-:* under, below, deficient *-al:* pertaining to, relating to
lingu/o		sub/lingu/al (sŭb-LĬNG-gwăl): under the tongue *sub-:* under, below *-al:* pertaining to, relating to
or/o	mouth	or/al (OR-ăl): pertaining to the mouth *-al:* pertaining to, relating to
stomat/o		stomat/o/pathy (stō-mă-TŎP-ă-thē): any disease of the mouth *-pathy:* disease
ptyal/o	saliva	ptyal/ism (TĪ-ă-lĭzm): excessive salivation *-ism:* condition
sial/o	saliva, salivary gland	sial/o/rrhea (sī-ă-lō-RĒ-ă): excessive flow of saliva; hypersalivation, ptyalism *-rrhea:* discharge, flow *Sialorrhea may be associated with various conditions, such as acute inflammation of the mouth, teething, malnutrition, and alcoholism.*
ESOPHAGUS, PHARYNX, AND STOMACH		
esophag/o	esophagus	esophag/o/scope (ē-SŎF-ă-gō-skōp): endoscope for examination of the esophagus *-scope:* instrument for examining

Word Element	Meaning	Word Analysis
pharyng/o	pharynx (throat)	pharyng/o/tonsill/itis (fă-rĭng-gō-tŏn-sĭ-LĪ-tĭs): inflammation of the pharynx and tonsils *tonsill:* tonsils *-itis:* inflammation
gastr/o	stomach	gastr/o/scopy (găs-TRŎS-kō-pē): visual inspection of the interior of the stomach by means of a flexible, fiberoptic gastroscope inserted through the esophagus *-scopy:* visual examination
pylor/o	pylorus	pylor/o/tomy (pī-lor-ŎT-ō-mē): incision of the pylorus, usually performed to remove an obstruction *-tomy:* incision *The pylorus is the lower portion of the stomach*

SUFFIXES

Word Element	Meaning	Word Analysis
-algia -dynia	pain	gastr/algia (găs-TRĂL-jē-ă): pain in the stomach *gastr:* stomach gastr/o/dynia (găs-trō-DĬN-ē-ă): pain in the stomach *gastr/o:* stomach
-emesis	vomiting	hyper/emesis (hī-pĕr-ĔM-ĕ-sĭs): excessive vomiting *hyper-:* excessive, above normal
-megaly	enlargement	gastr/o/megaly (găs-trō-MĔG-ă-lē): an abnormal enlargement of the stomach *gastr/o:* stomach
-ics	pertaining to, relating to	peri/odont/ics (pĕr-ē-ō-DŎN-tĭks): branch of dentistry dealing with treatment of diseases of the tissues around the teeth *peri-:* around *odont:* teeth
-orexia	appetite	an/orexia (ăn-ō-RĔK-sē-ă): loss of appetite *an-:* without, not *Anorexia can result from various conditions, such as side effects of medication or various physical or psychological causes.*
-pepsia	digestion	dys/pepsia (dĭs-PĔP-sē-ă): feeling of epigastric discomfort after eating; indigestion *dys-:* bad; painful; difficult
-phagia	swallowing, eating	dys/phagia (dĭs-FĀ-jē-ă): inability to swallow or difficulty in swallowing *dys-:* bad; painful; difficult
-rrhea	discharge, flow	dia/rrhea (dī-ă-RĒ-ă): abnormally frequent discharge or flow of watery stools from the bowel *dia-:* through, across

Listen and Learn, the audio CD-ROM that accompanies this book, will help you master the pronunciation of selected medical words. Use it to practice pronunciations of the above medical terms and for instructions to complete the *Listen and Learn* exercise on the CD-ROM for this section.

197

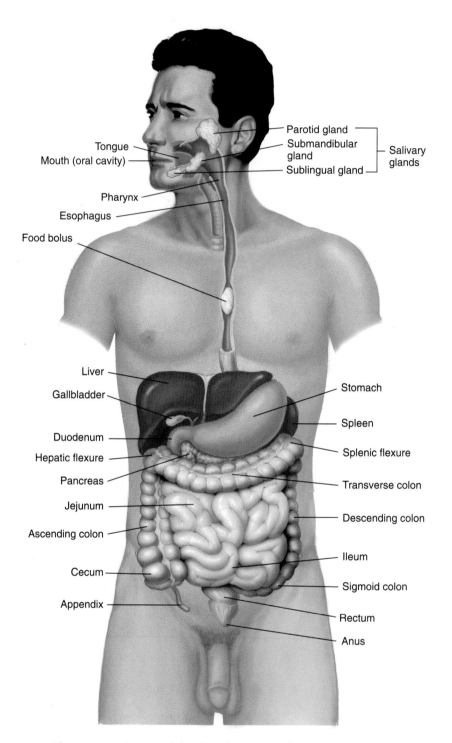

Figure 6-1   Organs of the digestive system shown in anterior view.

For the following medical terms, first write the suffix and its meaning. Then translate the meaning of the remaining elements starting with the first part of the word. The first word is an example that is completed for you.

Term	Meaning
1. gingiv/itis	-itis: inflammation; gum(s)
2. dys/pepsia	_____
3. pylor/o/tomy	_____
4. dent/ist	_____
5. esophag/o/scope	_____
6. gastr/o/scopy	_____
7. dia/rrhea	_____
8. hyper/emesis	_____
9. an/orexia	_____
10. sub/lingu/al	_____

Competency Verification: Check your answers in Appendix B, Answer Key, page 518. If you are not satisfied with your level of comprehension, review the vocabulary and retake the review.

Correct Answers _____ × 10 = _____% Score

Oral Cavity, Esophagus, Pharynx, and Stomach

6-1   Label the structures in Figure 6–2 as you read the material in the following frames.

The chemical and mechanical process of digestion begins in the (1) **oral cavity** or mouth, when food is chewed to make it easier to swallow.

6-2   The combining forms for the mouth are **or/o** and **stomat/o**.

From stomat/itis, construct the combining form for mouth:

_____ / _____.

stomat/o

or/o

From or/al, construct the combining form for mouth: _____ / _____.

6-3   The suffix -itis refers to *inflammation*. It is used in all body systems to describe an inflammation of a particular organ. Use **stomat/o** to form a word meaning inflammation of the mouth:

_____ / _____.

stomat/itis
stō-mă-TĪ-tĭs

199

pain, mouth **pain, mouth**	**6-4** The suffixes -dynia and -algia refer to *pain*. Stomat/o/dynia is a _____ in the _____. Stomat/algia is a _____ in the _____.
combining form *or* **combining vowel**	**6-5** The suffixes -dynia and -algia are used interchangeably. Because -algia begins with a vowel, use a word root to link the suffix. Because -dynia begins with a consonant, use a _____ _____ to link the suffix.
stomat/o/dynia stō-mă-tō-DĬN-ē-ă, **stomat/algia** stō-mă-TĂL-jē-ă	**6-6** Use **stomat/o** to develop a word that means pain in the mouth: _____ / ____ / _____ or _____ / _____.
	6-7 There are three pairs of salivary glands: the (2) sublingual gland, the (3) submandibular gland, and the (4) parotid gland. The salivary glands, whose primary function is to secrete saliva into the oral cavity, is richly supplied with blood vessels and nerves. Label the salivary glands in Figure 6–2.
sial/o	**6-8** During the chewing process, salivary secretions begin the chemical breakdown of food. The combining form **sial/o** refers to *saliva* or the *salivary glands*. From sial/ic (pertaining to saliva), construct the combining form for saliva or salivary gland: _____ / ____.
sial/itis sī-ă-LĪT-tĭs	**6-9** Use **sial/o** + -itis to form a word meaning inflammation of a salivary gland: _____ / _____.
-rrhea	**6-10** The suffix -rrhea is used in words to mean *discharge* or *flow*. From sial/o/rrhea, write the element that means discharge, flow: _____.
saliva **flow** **saliva** **condition**	**6-11** Sial/o/rrhea, more commonly called *ptyal/ism* and *hyper/salivation*, refers to excessive secretion of saliva. Analyze sial/o/rrhea by defining the elements. **Sial/o** refers to the salivary glands or _____. -rrhea refers to discharge or _____. **ptyal/o** refers to _____. -ism refers to _____.
tongue	**6-12** The combining form **lingu/o** refers to the *tongue;* the prefix sub- means *under*. Sub/lingu/al means pertaining to under or below the _____.

jaw	**6-13** The combining form **maxill/o** refers to the *jaw*. Sub/maxill/ary is a positional term that means pertaining to under the _____.
below below above	**6-14** Refer to Figure 6–1 and use the directional words *below* or *above* to complete this frame. The sub/lingu/al gland is located _____ the tongue. The sub/mandibul/ar gland is located _____ the parotid gland. The tongue is located _____ the esophagus.
lingu/o	**6-15** From sub/lingu/al, construct the combining form for tongue: _____ / ____.
pertaining to tongue	**6-16** Lingu/o/dent/al means _____ ____ the _____ and teeth.
dent	**6-17** From lingu/o/dent/al, determine the root for teeth: _____.
abnormal condition mouth	**6-18** The suffix -osis refers to *abnormal condition, increase (used primarily with blood cells)*. Stomat/osis literally means _____ _____ of the _____ .
stomat/osis stō-mă-TŌ-sĭs **stomat/itis** stō-mă-TĪ-tĭs	**6-19** Use **stomat/o** to form medical words meaning abnormal condition of the mouth: _____ / _____. inflammation of the mouth: _____ / _____.
myc	**6-20** Stomat/o/myc/osis is an abnormal condition of a mouth fungus. From stomat/o/myc/osis, identify the root meaning fungus: _____.
abnormal condition fungus	**6-21** Myc/osis literally means an _____ _____ of a _____.
abnormal condition fungus	**6-22** Whenever you see -osis in a word, you will know it means an _____ _____ or increase (used primarily with blood cells). Whenever you see **myc/o** in a word, you will know it refers to a _____.
myc/osis mī-KŌS-sĭs	**6-23** Two types of mycoses are *athlete's foot* and *candidiasis*. Change mycoses (plural) to a singular form: _____ / _____

-logist	**6–24** The combining form **log/o** means *study of*. Combine **log/o** and -ist to form a new suffix meaning specialist in study of: _____.
gastr/o/logist găs-TRŎL-ō-jĭst **enter/o/logist** ĕn-tĕr-ŎL-ō-jĭst **gastr/o/enter/o/logist** găs-trō-ĕn-tĕr-ŎL-ō-jĭst	**6–25** Recall that -logist means *specialist in study of*. Specialists who treat digestive disorders are the gastr/o/logist, enter/o/logist, and gastr/o/enter/o/logist. Build medical words meaning specialist who treats stomach disorders: _____ / _____ / _____ intestin/al disorders: _____ / _____ / _____ stomach and intestin/al disorders: _____ / _____ / _____ / _____ / _____.
gastr/o/logy găs-TRŎL-ō-jē **gastr/o/enter/o/logist** găs-trō-ĕn-tĕr-ŎL-ō-jĭst	**6–26** Use -logy or -logist to form medical words meaning study of the stomach: _____ / _____ / _____. specialist in the study of the stomach and intestines: _____ / _____ / _____ / _____ / _____.
gastr/o/logist găs-TRŎL-ō-jĭst	**6–27** The specialist who diagnoses and treats stomach disorders is a _____ / _____ / _____.
bowel movement **fasting blood sugar** **diagnosis** dī-ăg-NŌ-sĭs **gastr/o/intestin/al** găs-trō-ĭn-TĔS-tĭn-ăl	**6–28** Standardized abbreviations are commonly used in medical reports and insurance claims. Abbreviations are summarized at the end of each chapter and in Appendix E, Abbreviations. If needed, use one of those references to complete this frame. BM: _____ _____ FBS: _____ _____ _____ Dx: _____ GI: _____ / _____ / _____ / _____
dent/o **odont/o**	**6–29** Most of us take our teeth for granted and do not think about the important mechanical function they perform in the first step of the digestive process—breaking food down into its component parts. The combining forms for teeth are _____/ _____ and _____ / _____.
teeth, gums	**6–30** A dent/ist specializes in the prevention, diagnosis, and treatment of disease of the teeth and gums. Dentistry is the branch of medicine dealing with the care of the _____ and _____.

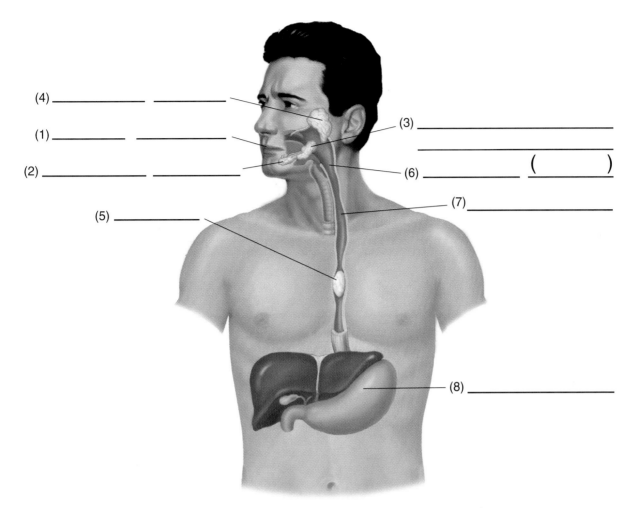

(4) _____ _____

(1) _____ _____

(2) _____ _____

(3) _____

_____

(6) _____ (_____)

(5) _____

(7) _____

(8) _____

Figure 6–2   The oral cavity, esophagus, pharynx, and stomach

pain, tooth **odont/algia** ō-dŏn-TĂL-jē-ă	**6-31** Odont/algia literally means _____ in a _____. A toothache is another word for odont/o/dynia or _____ / _____.
specialist, teeth	**6-32** An orth/odont/ist is a dent/al specialist who corrects and prevents irregularities and malocclusions (abnormal contacts) of the teeth. **Orth/o** refers to *straight.* Orth/odont/ist literally means _____ in straight _____.
odont **orth** **-ist**	**6-33** From orth/odont/ist, determine the following root for teeth: _____. root for straight: _____. element meaning specialist: _____.

orth/odont/ist ŏr-thō-DŎN-tĭst	**6-34** A person with crooked, or misaligned teeth, needs the dental services of an _____ / _____ / _____ to correct the deformity.
orth/odont/ist ŏr-thō-DŎN-tĭst	**6-35** A person who needs to be fitted with braces to straighten his or her teeth should see a specialist known as an _____ / _____ / _____.
specialist **around** **teeth**	**6-36** Another dental specialist, the peri/odont/ist, treats abnormal conditions of the tissues surrounding the teeth. (Use Appendix A, Glossary of Medical Word Elements, whenever you need help to work the frames.) -ist refers to _____. (suffix) peri- refers to _____. (prefix) **odont** refers to _____. (root)
gingiv/o	**6-37** Gingiv/itis, a general term for inflammation of the gums, is usually caused by an accumulation of food particles in the crevices between the gums and teeth. From gingiv/itis, construct the combining form for gums: _____ / ____.
gingiv/itis jĭn-jĭ-VĪ-tĭs	**6-38** Form a word that means an inflammation of the gums: _____ / _____.
inflammation, teeth **inflammation, gums**	**6-39** One of the primary symptoms of gingiv/itis is bleeding of the gums. This condition can lead to a more serious disorder, peri/odont/itis. Gingiv/itis is best prevented by correct brushing of the teeth and proper gum care. Peri/odont/itis is an _____ around the _____. Gingiv/itis means _____ of the _____.
gingiv/osis jĭn-jĭ-VŌ-sĭs **dent/ist** DĔN-tĭst **orth/odont/ist** ŏr-thō-DŎN-tĭst	**6-40** Develop words to mean abnormal condition of the gums: _____ / _____. specialist in teeth: _____ / _____. specialist in straightening teeth: _____ / _____/ _____.
tooth **pain, tooth**	**6-41** Dent/algia is a toothache. Literally, it means pain in a _____. Dent/o/dynia also means _____ in a _____.

	6-42 Continue labeling Figure 6-2 as you read the material in this frame. After food is chewed in the mouth, it is formed into a round, sticky mass called a (5) **bolus.** The bolus is pushed by the tongue into the (6) **pharynx (throat),** where it begins its descent down the (7) **esophagus** to the (8) **stomach.**
esophagus ē-SŎF-ă-gŭs	**6-43** In the stomach, undigested food is mixed with gastric juices to break it down further into a liquid mass called *chyme.* Name the structure that transports food from the mouth to the stomach: _____

Competency Verification: Check your labeling of Figure 6-2 with the answers in Appendix B, Answer Key, page 518.

esophag/o	**6-44** Esophag/itis can be caused by excessive acid production in the stomach. From esophag/itis, construct the combining form for esophagus: _____ / _____.
muc/ous MŪ-kŭs	**6-45** An ulcer is a lesion of the skin or muc/ous membrane marked by inflammation, necr/osis, and sloughing of damaged tissue. A wide variety of aggravations may produce ulcers, including trauma, drugs, infectious agents such as *Helicobacter pylori* bacterium, smoking, and alcohol. A term that means pertaining to mucus is: _____ / _____.
necr/osis nĕ-KRŌ-sĭs	**6-46** An insufficient blood supply may result in necr/osis of the ulcerated tissue. The combining form necr/o refers to *death, necrosis.* An abnormal condition of (tissue) death is called _____ / _____.
gastr/ic ulcers GĂS-trĭk	**6-47** Peptic ulcers that occur in the small intestine are called *duoden/al ulcers;* peptic ulcers that occur in the stomach are called _____ / _____ _____.
gastr/itis găs-TRĪ-tĭs	**6-48** Gastr/ic ulcers may cause severe pain and inflammation of the stomach. A medical term meaning inflammation of the stomach is: _____ / _____.
gastr/algia găs-TRĂL-jē-ă	**6-49** Gastr/o/dynia is the medical term for pain in the stomach. Another term that means pain in the stomach is: _____ / _____.
stomach	**6-50** Gastr/o/megaly and megal/o/gastr/ia means enlargement of the _____.

megal/o/gastr/ic mĕg-ă-lō-GĂS-trĭk	**6–51**　In megal/o/gastr/ia the suffix -ia is a noun ending that denotes a *condition*. Use -ic to change this word to an adjective: _____ / ___ / _____ / ___
endo/scopy ĕn-DŎS-kō-pē	**6–52**　Endo/scopy is a visual examination of a hollow organ or cavity using a rigid or flexible fiberoptic tube and lighted optical system (see Figure 2–6). The term in this frame that means visual examination in or within is: _____ / _____.
duoden/o/scopy* dū-ŏd-ĕ-NŎS-kō-pē	**6–53**　The device used to perform an endo/scopy is called an *endo/scope*. The organ being examined dictates the name of the endoscopic procedure: visual examination of the esophagus (esophagoscopy), stomach (gastroscopy), and duodenum (duodenoscopy). Endo/scopy is used for biopsy, aspirating fluids, and coagulating bleeding areas. A laser can also be passed through the endo/scope, which permits endoscopic surgery. A camera or video recorder is often used during endoscopic procedures to provide a permanent record for later reference (see Figure 2–6). When the physician visually examines the duodenum, the endoscopic procedure is called _____ / ___ / _____.
esophag/o/scopy ē-sŏf-ă-GŎS-kō-pē	**6–54**　Gastr/o/scopy is the visual examination of the stomach. Build another term with -scopy that means visual examination of the esophagus: _____ / ___ / _____.
esophag/o/gastr/o/ **duoden/o/scopy** ĕ-SŎF-ă-gō-găs-trō- dū-ŏd-ĕ-NŎS-kō-pē	**6–55**　Upper GI tract endoscopy includes the visualization of the esophagus, stomach, and duodenum. The abbreviation for this procedure is EGD. Use Appendix E to determine the medical term for this procedure: _____ / ___ / _____ / ___ / _____ / ___ / _____
gastr/ectomy găs-TRĔK-tō-mē	**6–56**　Surgery is the branch of medicine concerned with diseases and trauma requiring operative procedures. The operative procedure to remove either all or part of the stomach is called _____ / _____.
mouth	**6–57**　The surgical suffix -plasty is used in words to mean surgical repair. Stomat/o/plasty is a surgical repair of the _____.

* Terms that include "duoden" may be pronounced as "dū-ŏd-ĕn" or "dū-ō-dĕn." Both dū-ŏd-ĕ-NŎS-kō-pē and dū-ōd-ĕ-NŎS-kō-pē are correct pronunciations. Throughout this text, pronunciations of "duoden" are listed as "dū-ŏd-ĕn."

esophag/o/plasty ē-SŎF-ă-gō-plăs-tē **gastr/o/plasty** GĂS-trō-plăs-tē	**6-58** Form medical words that mean surgical repair of the esophagus: _____ / ____ / _____ . surgical repair of the stomach: _____ / ____ / _____ .
	6-59 Some common surgical suffixes that refer to cutting are summarized below. Review and use them to complete subsequent frames related to operative procedures. **Surgical Suffix** **Meaning** -ectomy excision, removal -tome instrument to cut -tomy incision
esophagus ē-SŎF-ă-gŭs	**6-60** Whenever you see a suffix or word with **tom** in it, relate it to an incision. Esophag/o/tomy is an incision through the wall of the of the _____ .
esophag/o/tome ē-SŎF-ă-gō-tōm	**6-61** When surgery of the esophagus necessitates an incision, the physician will ask for an instrument called an _____ / ____ / _____ .
gastr/ectomy găs-TRĔK-tō-mē	**6-62** The surgical procedure to remove all, or more commonly, part of the stomach is called a _____ / _____ .
gastr **-ectomy**	**6-63** Partial or total gastr/ectomy is often performed for stomach cancer. From gastr/ectomy, identify the element meaning stomach: _____ . excision or removal: _____ .
gastr/ectomy găs-TRĔK-tō-mē	**6-64** A perforated (punctured) stomach ulcer also may require a partial _____ / _____ .
stomach	**6-65** A gastr/o/tome is an instrument to cut or incise the _____ .
gastr/o/tome GĂS-trō-tōm	**6-66** When there is a need to incise the stomach, the physician uses an instrument called a _____ / ____ / _____ .

esophagus ē-SŎF-ă-gŭs	**6–67** Esophag/o/tomy is an incision of the _____.
gastr/o/tomy găs-TRŎT-ō-mē	**6–68** Develop a word meaning incision of the stomach: _____ / ____ / _____.
carcin/oma kăr-sĭ-NŌ-mă	**6–69** Cancer (CA) is a general term used to indicate various types of malignant neoplasms. Most cancers invade surrounding tissues and metastasize (spread) to other sites in the body. The combining form for *cancer* is **carcin/o**. Combine **carcin/o** + -oma to build a word that means tumor that is cancer: _____ / _____.
cancer	**6–70** CA, especially sarc/oma, can recur even though the tumor is excised and ultimately may cause death. Whenever you see CA in a medical report, you will know that it refers to _____.
-ous	**6–71** Cancer/ous means pertaining to cancer. Identify the adjective element meaning pertaining to: _____.
cancerous *or* **malignant**	**6–72** A carcin/oma is a tumor that is _____.
cancer **tumor**	**6–73** Often a patient has an organ removed because of a carcin/oma. Analyze carcin/oma by defining the elements: **carcin/o** refers to _____. -oma refers to _____.
gastr/itis găs-TRĪ-tĭs **epi/gastr/ic** ĕp-ĭ-GĂS-trĭk	**6–74** Epi- is a prefix meaning *above, upon*. An epi/gastr/ic pain may result from an acute form of gastr/itis. Identify the words in this frame meaning inflammation of the stomach: _____ / _____. pertaining to above the stomach: _____ / _____ / ____.
hyper/emesis hī-pĕr-ĔM-ĕ-sĭs	**6–75** *Emesis* is a term that means vomiting, but it also may be used as a suffix. A symptomatic term that means excessive vomiting is hyper/_____.
hyper- **-emesis**	**6–76** *Hyper/emesis* is characterized by excessive vomiting. Unless treated, it can lead to malnutrition. Determine the elements in this frame that mean excessive, above normal: _____. vomiting: _____.

hemat/emesis hĕm-ăt-ĔM-ĕ-sĭs	**6-77** **Hemat/o** refers to *blood*. A person with acute gastr/itis or a peptic ulcer may vomit blood. Build a word meaning vomiting blood: _____ / _____.
hemat/emesis hĕm-ăt-ĔM-ĕ-sĭs	**6-78** Bleeding in the stomach may be due to a gastric ulcer and may cause the patient to vomit blood. The diagnosis of vomiting blood would be entered in the medical record as _____ / _____.
epi/gastr/ic ĕp-ĭ-GĂS-trĭk	**6-79** The most common symptom of gastr/ic disease is pain. When pain occurs in the region above the stomach, it is called epi/gastr/ic pain. Form a word that means pertaining to above or on the stomach: _____ / _____ / _____.
-pepsia **dys-**	**6-80** Dys/pepsia literally means painful or difficult digestion and is a form of gastric indigestion. It is not a disease in itself but may be symptomatic of other diseases or disorders. Determine the word elements in this frame that mean digestion: _____. bad, painful, difficult: _____.
dys/pepsia dĭs-PĔP-sē-ă	**6-81** Over-the-counter antacids (agents that neutralize acidity) usually provide prompt relief of pain from _____ / _____.
dys/phagia dĭs-FĀ-jē-ă **bad, painful, difficult** **swallowing, eating**	**6-82** The suffix -phagia means *swallowing, eating.* Use dys- and -phagia to form a word meaning difficult or painful swallowing: _____ / _____. Analyze dys/phagia by defining the word elements: dys- means _____, _____, _____. -phagia means _____, _____.
aer/o	**6-83** A person who swallows air, usually followed by belching and gaxric distention, suffers from a condition called *aerophagia*. _____ / _____.
aer/o/phagia ĕr-ō-FĀ-jē-ă	**6-84** Infants have a tendency to swallow air as they suck milk from a bottle. This condition is called _____ / _____ / _____.

Listen and Learn, the audio CD-ROM that accompanies this book, will help you master the pronunciation of selected medical words. Use it to practice pronunciations *of selected term from frames 6–1 to 6–84* for instructions to complete the *Listen and Learn* exercise on the CD-ROM for this section.

SECTION REVIEW 6 – 2

Using the following table, write the combining form, suffix, or prefix that matches its definition in the space provided to the left of the definition. There may be more than one word element that matches a definition.

Combining Forms		Suffixes		Prefixes
dent/o	odont/o	-al	-oma	an-
gastr/o	or/o	-ary	-orexia	dia-
gingiv/o	orth/o	-algia	-pepsia	dys-
gloss/o	pylor/o	-dynia	-phagia	hyper-
lingu/o	sial/o	-ic	-rrhea	hypo-
myc/o	stomat/o	-ist	-scope	peri-
			-tomy	

1. _____ tumor

2. _____ pertaining to, relating to

3. _____ around

4. _____ under, below, deficient

5. _____ discharge, flow

6. _____ fungus

7. _____ gum(s)

8. _____ pylorus

9. _____ bad; painful; difficult

10. _____ excessive, above normal

11. _____ saliva, salivary gland

12. _____ stomach

13. _____ specialist

14. _____ straight

15. _____ teeth

16. _____ through, across

17. _____ tongue

18. _____ instrument for examining

19. _____ incision

20. _____ appetite

21. _____ mouth

22. _____ pain

23. _____ swallowing, eating

24. _____ without, not

25. _____ digestion

Competency Verification: Check your answers in Appendix B, Answer Key, page 518. If you are not satisfied with your level of comprehension, go back to Frame 6–1 and rework the frames.

Correct Answers _____ × 4 = _____% Score

Making a set of flash cards from key word elements in this chapter for each section review can help you remember the elements. Make a flash card by writing a word element on one side of a 3 × 5 or 4 × 6 index card. On the other side, write the meaning of the element. Do this for all word elements in the section review. Use your flash cards to review each section. You also might use the flash cards to prepare for the chapter review at the end of this chapter.

Word Elements

This section introduces combining forms related to the small intestine and colon. Key suffixes are defined in the right-hand column as needed. Review the following table, and pronounce each word in the word analysis column aloud before you begin to work the frames.

Word Element	Meaning	Word Analysis
COMBINING FORMS		
SMALL INTESTINE		
duoden/o	duodenum (first part of small intestine)	duoden/o/scopy (dū-ŏd-ĕ-NŎS-kō-pē): visual examination of the duodenum *-scopy:* visual examination
enter/o	intestine (usually small intestine)	enter/o/pathy (ĕn-tĕr-ŎP-ă-thē): any intestinal disease *-pathy:* disease
jejun/o	jejunum (second part of small intestine)	jejun/o/rrhaphy (jĕ-joo-NOR-ă-fē): suture of the jejunum *-rrhaphy:* suture
ile/o	ileum (third part of small intestine)	ile/o/stomy (ĭl-ē-ŎS-tō-mē): creation of an opening between the ileum and the abdominal wall *-stomy*:* forming an opening (mouth) *An ileostomy creates an opening in the abdomen, which is attached to the ileum to allow fecal matter to discharge into a pouch worn on the abdomen.*
LARGE INTESTINE		
append/o	appendix	append/ectomy (ăp-ĕn-DĔK-tō-mē): removal of the appendix *-ectomy:* excision, removal *An appendectomy is performed to remove a diseased appendix that is in danger of rupturing*
appendic/o		appendic/itis (ă-pĕn-dĭ-SĪ-tĭs): inflammation of the appendix *-itis:* inflammation
col/o	colon	col/o/stomy (kō-LŎS-tō-mē): creation of an opening between the colon and the abdominal wall *-stomy*:* forming an opening (mouth) *A colostomy creates a place for fecal matter to exit the body other than through the anus. It may be temporary or permanent.*
colon/o		colon/o/scopy (kō-lŏn-ŎS-kō-pē): visual examination of the inner surface of the colon using a long, flexible endoscope *-scopy:* visual examination

(Continued)

Word Element	Meaning	Word Analysis *(Continued)*
sigmoid/o	sigmoid colon	sigmoid/o/tomy (sĭg-moyd-ŎT-ō-mē): incision of the sigmoid colon *-tomy:* incision
rect/o	rectum	rect/o/cele (RĔK-tō-sēl): herniation or protrusion of the rectum; also called *proctocele* *-cele:* hernia, swelling
proct/o	anus, rectum	proct/o/logist (prŏk-TŎL-ō-jĭst): physician who specializes in treating disorders of the colon, rectum, and anus *-logist:* specialist in study of

*When the suffix -stomy is used with a combining form that denotes an organ, it refers to a surgical opening to the outside of the body.

Listen and Learn, the audio CD-ROM that accompanies this book, will help you master the pronunciation of selected medical words. Use it to practice pronunciations of the above-listed medical terms and for instructions to complete the *Listen and Learn* exercise on the CD-ROM for this section.

For the following medical terms, first write the suffix and its meaning. Then translate the meaning of the remaining elements starting with the first part of the word. The first word is an example that is completed for you.

Term	Meaning
1. duoden/o/scopy	-scopy: visual examination; duodenum (first part of small intestine)
2. appendic/itis	_____
3. enter/o/pathy	_____
4. col/o/stomy	_____
5. rect/o/cele	_____
6. sigmoid/o/tomy	_____
7. proct/o/logist	_____
8. jejun/o/rrhaphy	_____
9. append/ectomy	_____
10. ile/o/stomy	_____

Competency Verification: Check your answers in Appendix B, Answer Key, page 519. If you are not satisfied with your level of comprehension, review the vocabulary and retake the review.

Correct Answers _____ × 10 = _____ % Score

Small and Large Intestine

6-85 The small intestine is a continuation of the GI tract. It is where digestion of food is completed as nutrients are absorbed into the bloodstream through tiny, finger-like projections called **villi**. Any unabsorbed material is passed on to the large intestine to be excreted from the body. There are three parts of the small intestine: the (1) **duodenum**, the (2) **jejunum**, and the (3) **ileum**. Label these parts in Figure 6–3.

6-86 Here is a review of the parts of the small intestine.

duoden/o refers to the first part of the small intestine. This is called the _____.

duodenum
dū-ŎD-ĕ-nŭm

jejun/o refers to the second part of the small intestine. This is called the _____.

jejunum
jē-JŪ-nŭm

ile/o refers to the third part of the small intestine. This is called the _____.

ileum
ĬL-ē-ŭm

duoden/ectomy
dū-ŏd-ĕ-NĔK-tō-mē
jejun/ectomy
jē-jū-NĔK-tō-mē
ile/ectomy
ĭl-ē-ĔK-tō-mē

6-87 Duoden/ectomy, jejun/ectomy, and ile/ectomy are total or partial excisions of the denoted section of the small intestine. Build a word that means

excision of the duodenum: _____ / _____.

excision of the jejunum: _____ / _____.

excision of the ileum: _____ / _____.

---

duodenum, duoden/o
dū-ŎD-ĕ-nŭm
jejunum, jejun/o
jē-JŪ-nŭm
ileum, ile/o
ĪL-ē-ŭm

6-88 Name the three parts of the small intestine and their combining forms.

Part	Combining Form
1. _____	_____
2. _____	_____
3. _____	_____

---

duodenum
dū-ŎD-ĕ-nŭm

6-89 Another surgical procedure called a *duoden/o/stomy* is performed to form an opening (mouth) into the _____.

-stomy

6-90 Identify the element in Frame 6–89 that means forming an opening (mouth): _____.

---

opening, jejunum
jē-JŪ-nŭm

6-91 The surgical procedure jejun/o/stomy means forming an _____ into the _____.

---

opening, ileum
ĪL-ē-ŭm

6-92 When the colon is removed because of colon cancer, an ile/o/stomy is performed. The patient must wear an ile/o/stomy bag to collect the fecal material from the ileum.

The surgical procedure ile/o/stomy means forming

an _____ into the _____.

-stomy

6-93 The suffix meaning forming an opening (mouth) is _____.

It also means mouth because the opening is shaped like a mouth.

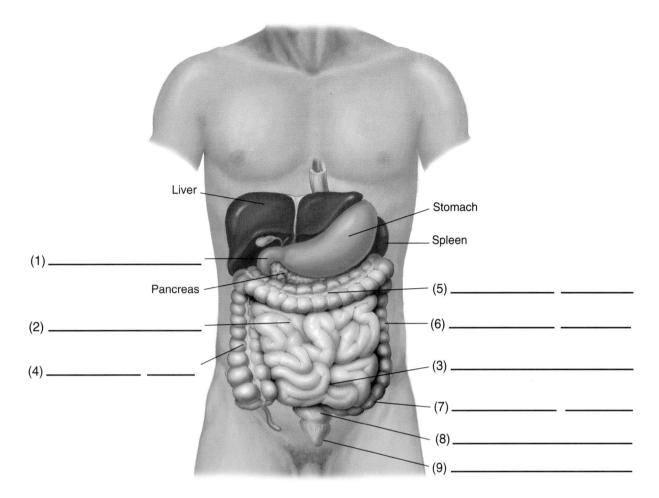

Liver

Stomach

Spleen

(1) _____

Pancreas

(5) _____ _____

(2) _____

(6) _____ _____

(4) _____ _____

(3) _____

(7) _____ _____

(8) _____

(9) _____

Figure 6–3   The small intestine and colon.

	6–94 For people who cannot eat by mouth, a jejun/al (pertaining to the jejunum) feeding tube is often placed through a jejun/o/tomy incision.
-tomy	The surgical suffix meaning incision is _____.
	An incision of the jejunum is called a
jejun/o/tomy jē-jū-NŎT-ō-mē	_____ / _____ / _____.
	6–95 An incision of the duodenum is called a
duoden/o/tomy dū- ŏd-ĕ-NŎT-ō-mē	_____ / _____ / _____.
	6–96 An incision of the ileum is called an
ile/o/tomy ĭl-ē-ŎT-ō-mē	_____ / _____ / _____.

ileum
ĬL-ē-ŭm
suture

6–97 The surgical suffix -rrhaphy refers to *suture* (sew). An ile/o/rrhaphy is performed to surgically repair the ileum. Analyze ile/o/rrhaphy by defining the elements:

ile/o means _____.

-rrhaphy means _____.

---

duoden/ectomy
dū-ŏd-ĕ-NĔK-tō-mē

duoden/o/rrhaphy
dū-ŏ-dĕ-NOR-ă-f ē

6–98 In a bleeding duoden/al ulcer, a suture over the bleeding portion often can prevent performing duoden/ectomy. Develop surgical words meaning

excision of the duodenum: _____ / _____.

suture of the duodenum:

_____ / _____ / _____.

---

jejun/o/rrhaphy
jĕ-joo-NOR-ă-f ē
ile/o/rrhaphy
ĭl-ē-OR-ă-f ē

6–99 Form surgical words meaning

suture of the jejunum:

_____ / _____ / _____.

suture of the ileum: _____ / _____ / _____.

---

opening

(mouth)

6–100 The suffix -stomy means forming an _____

(_____)

---

stomach, duodenum
dū-ŎD-ĕ-nŭm

6–101 A gastr/o/duoden/o/stomy is the formation of a new opening between the _____ and _____.

---

stomach, ileum
ĬL-ē-ŭm

6–102 A gastr/o/ile/o/stomy is the formation of a new opening between the _____ and _____.

---

stomach, small intestine

6–103 In a surgical anastomosis, a connection between two vessels, bowel segments, or ducts is performed to allow flow from one to another. Gastr/o/enter/o/anastomosis is a surgical anastomosis between the

_____ and _____ _____.

---

gastr/o/enter/o/
anastomosis
găs-trō-ĕn-tĕr-ō-
ă-năs-tō-MŌ-sĭs
gastr/o/enter/o/stomy
găs-trō-ĕn-tĕr-ŎS-tō-mē

6–104 *Gastr/o/enter/o/anastomosis*, also called *gastr/o/enter/o/stomy*, may be performed for a variety of malignant and benign gastroduodenal diseases. Terms in this frame that mean creation of a passage between the stomach and some part of the small intestine are:

_____ / _____ / _____ / _____ /

_____ and

_____ / _____ / _____ / _____ / _____.

-stomy	**6-105** Another type of anastomosis, *gastr/o/duoden/o/stomy* (see Figure 2–7), is a procedure in which the lower part of the stomach is excised, and the remainder is anastomosed to the duodenum. The element in this frame that means *forming an opening (mouth)* is _____ .
ileum ĬL-ē-ŭm	**6-106** Most of the absorption of food takes place in the third part of the small intestine, which is the _____ .
inflammation, ileum ĬL-ē-ŭm	**6-107** *Crohn disease*, a chronic inflammation of the ileum, may affect any part of the intestinal tract. It is distinguished from closely related bowel disorders by its inflammatory pattern; it is also called *regional ile/itis*. Ile/itis is a(n) _____ of the _____ .
enter/o	**6-108** *Enter/al* is a word meaning pertaining to the intestine (usually the small intestine). From enter/al, construct the combining form for intestine: _____ / _____ .
enter/ectomy ĕn-tĕr-ĔK-tō-mē **enter/o/rrhaphy** ĕn-tĕr-OR-ă-f ē	**6-109** Build the following surgical terms meaning excision of the intestine (usually small): _____ / _____ . suture of the intestine (such as an intestinal wound): _____ / _____ / _____ .
inflammation **intestine**	**6-110** Enter/itis is an _____ of the _____ (usually small).
enter/itis ĕn-tĕr-Ī-tĭs	**6-111** Crohn disease is distinguished from closely related bowel disorders by its inflammatory pattern. It is also known as regional enter/itis. Form a word meaning inflammation of the intestine: _____ / _____ .
	6-112 Continue labeling Figure 6–3 as you read the following: The large intestine, also called the colon, extends from the ileum of the small intestine to the anus. The colon consists of four segments: (4) **ascending colon,** (5) **transverse colon,** (6) **descending colon,** and (7) **sigmoid colon.**
col/ectomy kō-LĔK-tō-mē **col/itis** kō-LĪ-tĭs **col/o/tomy** kō-LŎT-ō-mē	**6-113** The combining form **col/o** refers to the *colon.* Form medical words that mean excision of the colon: _____ / _____ . inflammation of the colon: _____ / _____ . incision into the colon: _____ / _____ / _____ .

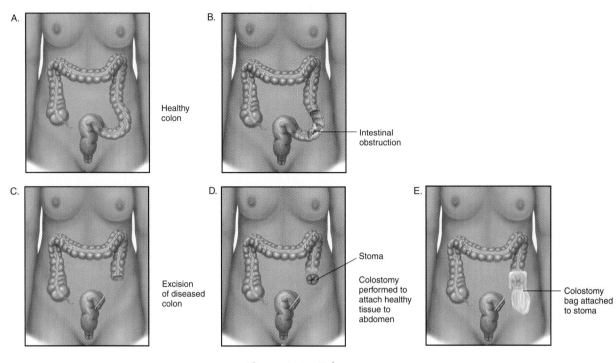

A.

B.
Healthy
colon

Intestinal
obstruction

C.

D.
Excision
of diseased
colon

Stoma

Colostomy
performed to
attach healthy
tissue to
abdomen

E.

Colostomy
bag attached
to stoma

Figure 6–4   Colostomy.

	6-114 A colostomy is the surgical creation of an opening into the colon (through the surface of the abdomen). It may be temporary or permanent and is performed as treatment for cancer or diverticulitis. A colostomy allows elimination of the feces into a bag attached to the skin. (See Figure 6–4).
	Write the surgical term meaning
	forming an opening (mouth) into the colon:
col/o/stomy kō-LŎS-tō-mē **col/o/rrhaphy** kō-LOR-ă-fē	_____ / ____ / _____.
	suture of the colon: _____ / ____ / _____.
	6-115 The absorption of water by the colon changes the intestinal contents from a fluid to a more solid consistency known as *feces* or *stool*. Use your medical dictionary to define *feces*.
	_____ _____
ascending, transverse **descending**	**6-116** Locate and name the three main parts of the colon as illustrated in Figure 6–1: _____, _____, and _____.
	6-117 The sigmoid colon is *S*-shaped and extends from the descending colon into the (8) **rectum**. The rectum terminates in the lower opening of the gastrointestinal tract, the (9) **anus**. Label Figure 6–3 to identify and locate the sigmoid colon and rectum.

sigmoid SĬG-moyd	**6-118** Sigmoid/ectomy, an excision of all or part of the sigmoid colon, is most commonly performed to remove a malignant tumor. A large percentage of cancers of the lower bowel occur in the sigmoid colon. From sigmoid/ectomy, determine the root for the sigmoid colon: _____.
sigmoid/itis sĭg-moyd-Ī-tĭs	**6-119** Form a term that means inflammation of the sigmoid colon: _____ / _____.
inflammation, rectum RĔK-tŭm	**6-120** The combining form **rect/o** refers to the *rectum*. Rect/itis is a(n) _____ of the _____.
inflammation **rectum, colon** RĔK-tŭm, KŌ-lŏn	**6-121** Rect/o/col/itis is a(n) _____ of the _____ and _____.
pain	**6-122** Rect/algia is a _____ in the rectum.
surgical repair **rectum** RĔK-tŭm	**6-123** Rect/o/plasty is a _____ _____ of the _____.
pertaining to *or* **relating to** **rectum** RĔK-tŭm	**6-124** Rect/o/vagin/al means _____ _____ the _____ and vagina.
through, across **discharge, flow**	**6-125** Dia- is a prefix meaning *through, across*. Dia/rrhea is a frequent passage of watery bowel movements. Analyze dia/rrhea by defining the elements: dia- means _____, _____. -rrhea means _____, _____.
dia/rrhea dī-ă-RĒ-ă	**6-126** A person with an irritable bowel may experience frequent passage of watery bowel movements or have symptoms of a condition called _____ / _____.
dia/rrhea dī-ă-RĒ-ă	**6-127** Some foods, such as prunes, are likely to cause _____ / _____.

Competency Verification: Check your labeling of Figure 6–3 with the answers in Appendix B, Answer Key, page 519.

stenosis stĕ-NŌ-sĭs	**6-128** *Stenosis* is a word that means narrowing or stricture of a passageway or orifice. This condition may result in an obstruction. *Stenosis* also can be used as a suffix. A narrowing or stricture of the pylorus is called pyloric _____.
rect/o **-stenosis**	**6-129** Rect/o/stenosis is a narrowing or stricture of the rectum. Determine the elements in this frame that mean rectum: _____ / _____. narrowing, stricture: _____.
proct/itis prŏk-TĪ-tĭs	**6-130** The combining form **proct/o** refers to the *anus* and *rectum*. Locate the anus and rectum in Figure 6–1. An inflammation of the anus and rectum is known as _____ / _____.
rectum, RĔK-tŭm **anus** Ā-nŭs	**6-131** Proct/o/dynia is a pain in the _____ and _____.
proct/algia prŏk-TĂL-jē-ă	**6-132** Use -algia to form another word meaning pain in the rectum and anus: _____ / _____.
rectum RĔK-tŭm **rectum, anus** RĔK-tŭm, Ā-nŭs	**6-133** Spasm means involuntary contraction or twitching. It is also used in words as a suffix. Rect/o/spasm is an involuntary contraction of the _____. Proct/o/spasm is an involuntary contraction of the _____ and _____.
path/o/log/ical păth-ō-LŎJ-ĭ-kăl	**6-134** Endo/scopy is an important tool in establishing or confirming a diagnosis or detecting a path/o/log/ical condition (see Figure 2–6). A video recorder is often used during an endoscopic procedure to guide the endo/scope and prevent perforation of the vessel. Can you determine the word in this frame that means study of disease? _____ / _____ / _____ / _____

colon/o/scopy
kō-lŏn-ŎS-kō-pē

proct/o/scopy
prŏk-TŎS-kō-pē

6-135 The organ being examined dictates the name of the endoscopic procedure.

Visual examination of the colon is called

_____ / ____ / _____.

Visual examination of the anus and rectum is called

_____ / ____ / _____.

sigmoid colon
SĬG-moyd KŌ-lŏn
visual examination

6-136 Sigmoid/o/scopy is used to screen for colon cancer (see Figure 6–5). The American Cancer Society recommends a first sigmoid/o/scopy after age 50. It is done sooner if there is a family history (FH) of colon cancer.

Analyze sigmoid/o/scopy by defining the elements:

sigmoid/o means _____ _____.

-scopy means _____ _____.

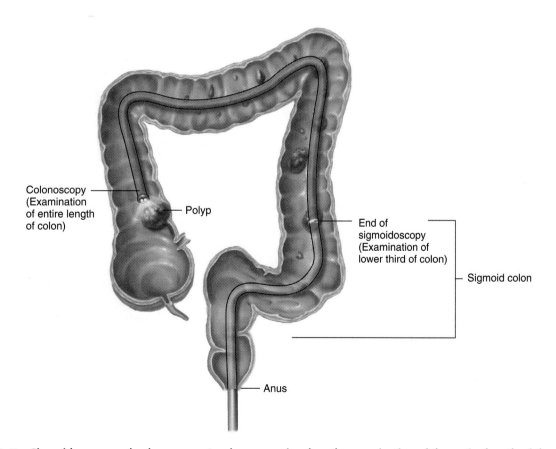

Figure 6–5 Sigmoidoscopy and colonoscopy. A colonoscopy involves the examination of the entire length of the colon; a sigmoidoscopy involves the examination of only the lower third of the colon.

sigmoid/o/scopy sĭg-moy-DŎS-kō-pē	**6-137** To examine an abnormality in the colon, the physician performs a visual examination of the sigmoid colon called _____ / ____ / _____.
sigmoid/o/scope sĭg-MOY-dō-skōp	**6-138** A sigmoid/o/scope, a flexible fiberoptic tube (permits transmission of light to visualize images around curves and corners), is placed through the anus to visualize part of the gastro/intestin/al tract. When the physician examines the colon, the physician uses a flexible fiberoptic instrument called a _____ / ____ / _____.
sigmoid/ectomy sĭg-moyd-ĔK-tō-mē **carcin/oma** kăr-sĭ-NŌ-mă	**6-139** The sigmoid colon is S-shaped and is the last part of the colon (see Figure 6–5). Sigmoid/ectomy most often is performed for carcin/oma of the sigmoid colon. Identify the words in this frame that mean excision of the sigmoid colon: _____ / _____. cancerous tumor: _____ / _____.
examination, colon KŌ-lŏn	**6-140** A col/o/scopy is commonly referred to as a colon/o/scopy. Both terms mean a visual _____ of the _____.
colon/itis kō-lŏn-Ī-tĭs **colon/o/scope** kō-LŎN-ō-skōp **colon/o/scopy** kō-lŏn-ŎS-kō-pē	**6-141** Use **colon/o** to form medical words meaning inflammation of the colon: _____ / _____. instrument to examine the colon: _____ / ____ / _____. visual examination of the colon: _____ / ____ / _____.
enter/o/scopy ĕn-tĕr-ŎS-kō-pē	**6-142** Enter/o/scopy is used to examine the small intestine. A visual examination of the intestines is known as a(n) _____ / ____ / _____.
enter/o/scope ĔN-tĕr-ō-skōp	**6-143** When there is a need to view the intestine, the physician uses a(n) _____ / ____ / _____.

6–144 Use -scopy to form medical words meaning visual examination of the

duoden/o/scopy
dū-ŏd-ĕ-NŎS-kō-pē

sigmoid/o/scopy
sĭg-moy-DŎS-kō-pē

gastr/o/scopy
găs-TRŎS-kō-pē

duodenum: _____ / ____ / _____.

sigmoid colon: _____ / ____ / _____.

stomach: _____ / ____ / _____.

Listen and Learn, the audio CD-ROM that accompanies this book, will help you master the pronunciation of selected medical words. Use it to practice pronunciations *of selected term from frames 6–85 to 6–144* for instructions to complete the *Listen and Learn* exercise on the CD-ROM for this section.

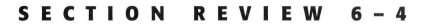

Using the following table, write the combining form or suffix that matches its definition in the space provided to the left of the definition. There may be more than one word element that matches a definition.

Combining Forms	Suffixes
col/o	-rrhaphy
colon/o	-scopy
duoden/o	-spasm
enter/o	-stenosis
ile/o	-stomy
jejun/o	-tome
proct/o	-tomy
rect/o	
sigmoid/o	

1. _____ intestine (usually small intestine)

2. _____ instrument to cut

3. _____ rectum

4. _____ involuntary contraction, twitching

5. _____ ileum (third part of small intestine)

6. _____ visual examination

7. _____ jejunum (second part of small intestine)

8. _____ colon

9. _____ duodenum (first part of small intestine)

10. _____ forming an opening (mouth)

11. _____ anus, rectum

12. _____ narrowing, stricture

13. _____ suture

14. _____ incision

15. _____ sigmoid colon

Competency Verification: Check your answers in Appendix B, Answer Key, page 519. If you are not satisfied with your level of comprehension, go back to frame 6–85 and rework the frames

Correct Answers _____ × 6.67 = _____ % Score

Word Elements

This section introduces combining forms related to the accessory organs of digestion. Included are key suffixes; prefixes are defined in the right-hand column as needed. Review the following table and pronounce each word in the word analysis column aloud before you begin to work the frames.

Word Elements	Meaning	Word Analysis
COMBINING FORMS		
cholangi/o	bile vessel	cholangi/ole (kō-LĂN-jē-ōl): small terminal portion of the bile duct *-ole:* small, minute
chol/e*	bile, gall	chol/e/lith (kō-lē-LĬTH): gallstone *-lith:* stone, calculus
cholecyst/o	gallbladder	cholecyst/ectomy (kō-lē-sĭs-TĔK-tō-mē): removal of the gallbladder by laparoscopic or open surgery *-ectomy:* excision, removal
choledoch/o	bile duct	choledoch/o/tomy (kō-lĕd-ō-KŎT-ō-mē): incision into the common bile duct *-tomy:* incision
hepat/o	liver	hepat/itis (hĕp-ă-TĪ-tĭs): inflammation of the liver *-itis:* inflammation
pancreat/o	pancreas	pancreat/o/lysis (păn-krē-ă-TŎL-ĭ-sĭs): destruction of the pancreas by pancreatic enzymes *-lysis:* separation; destruction; loosening
SUFFIXES		
-iasis	abnormal condition (produced by something specified)	chol/e/lith/iasis (kō-lē-lĭ-THĪ-ă-sĭs): presence or formation of gallstones *chol/e:* bile, gall *-lith:* stone, calculus
-megaly	enlargement	hepat/o/megaly (hĕp-ă-tō-MĔG-ă-lē): enlargement of the liver *hepat/o:* liver *Hepatomegaly may be caused by infection; fatty infiltration, as in alcoholism; biliary obstruction; or malignancy.*
-prandial	meal	post/prandial (pōst-PRĂN-dē-ăl): following a meal *post-:* after, behind

*The combining vowel *e* is used instead of *o*. This is an exception to the rule.

Listen and Learn, the audio CD-ROM that accompanies this book, will help you master the pronunciation of selected medical words. Use it to practice pronunciations of the above-listed medical terms and for instructions to complete the *Listen and Learn* exercise on the CD-ROM for this section.

For the following medical terms, first write the suffix and its meaning. Then translate the meaning of the remaining elements starting with the first part of the word. The first word is an example that is completed for you.

Term	Meaning
1. hepat/itis	-itis: inflammation; liver
2. hepat/o/megaly	
3. chol/e/lith	
4. cholangi/ole	
5. cholecyst/ectomy	
6. post/prandial	
7. chol/e/lith/iasis	
8. choledoch/o/tomy	
9. pancreat/o/lith	
10. pancreat/o/lysis	

Competency Verification: Check your answers in Appendix B, Answer Key, page 520. If you are not satisfied with your level of comprehension, review the vocabulary and retake the review.

Correct Answers _____ × 10 = _____ % Score

Accessory Organs of Digestion: Liver, Gallbladder, and Pancreas

6–145   Label Figure 6–6 as you learn about the accessory organs of digestion.

Even though food does not pass through the (1) **liver,** (2) **gallbladder,** and (3) **pancreas,** these organs play a vital role in the proper digestion and absorption of nutrients. The gallbladder serves as a storage site for bile, which is produced by the liver. When bile is needed for digestion, the gallbladder releases it through ducts into the (4) **duodenum** through the (5) **common bile duct.**

The three accessory organs of digestion are the _____,
_____, and _____.

liver
gallbladder, pancreas

6–146   From hepat/itis, construct the combining form for liver:
_____ / ____.

hepat/o

cholecyst/o	**6-147** From cholecyst/itis, construct the combining form for gallbladder: _____ / ____.
pancreat/o	**6-148** From pancreat/itis, construct the combining form for pancreas: _____ / ____.
hepat/itis hĕp-ă-TĪ-tĭs	**6-149** Hepat/itis, inflammatory condition of the liver, may be caused by bacteri/al or viral infection, parasitic infestation, alcohol, drugs, toxins, or transfusion of incompatible blood. It may be mild and brief or severe and life-threatening. When a person has inflammation of the liver caused by a virus, the diagnosis most likely is _____ / _____.
hepat/o/megaly hĕp-ă-tō-MĔG-ă-lē	**6-150** Hepat/itis may be characterized by an enlarged liver. The medical term for enlarged liver is _____ / ____ / _____.
hepat/oma hĕp-ă-TŌ-mă	**6-151** Hepat/o/megaly may be a symptom of a rare malignant tumor of the liver called *hepat/oma*. The tumor occurs most frequently in association with hepat/itis or cirrhosis of the liver. The diagnosis of a person with a tumor of the liver is _____ / _____.
hepat/itis hĕp-ă-TĪ-tĭs	**6-152** Hepatitis B, the most common infectious hepatitis seen in hospitals, is transferred by blood and body secretions. As a preventative measure, hospital personnel are usually required to be vaccinated. The medical term for inflammation of the liver is _____ / _____.
hepat/ectomy hĕp-ă-TĔK-tō-mē **hepat/o/dynia** hĕp-ă-tō-DĬN-ē-ă **hepat/algia** hĕp-ă-TĂL-jē-ă **hepat/o/rrhaphy** hĕp-ă-TŌR-ă-fē	**6-153** Form medical words meaning excision of a portion of the liver: _____ / _____. pain in the liver: _____ / ____ / _____ or _____ / _____. suture of the liver: _____ / ____ / _____.
hepat/o/cyte HĔP-ă-tō-sīt	**6-154** Combine **hepat/o** and -cyte to form a word that means liver cell: _____ / ____ / _____.

	6–155 Identify and label the following structures in Figure 6–6 as you read about the accessory organs of digestion. Besides being released from the gallbladder, bile also is drained directly from the liver through the (6) **right hepatic duct** and the (7) **left hepatic duct.** These two ducts eventually form the (8) **hepatic duct.** The (9) **cystic duct** of the gallbladder merges with the hepatic duct to form the common bile duct and the (10) **pancreatic duct** (carries digestive juices) to carry their digestive products into the duodenum.
hepat/ic hĕ-PĂT-ĭk **cyst/ic** SĬS-tĭk **pancreat/ic** păn-krē-ĂT-ĭk	**6–156** Use -ic to form medical words that mean pertaining to the liver: _____ / _____. bladder: _____ / _____. pancreas: _____ / _____.

Competency Verification: Check your labeling of Figure 6–6 in Appendix B, Answer Key, page 520.

hepat/ic, cyst/ic, hĕ-PĂT-ĭk, SĬS-tĭk, **pancreat/ic** păn-krē-ĂT-ĭk	**6–157** Refer to Frame 6–156 to write the names of the ducts responsible for transporting digestive juices: _____ / _____, _____ / _____, _____ / _____, and the common bile duct.
vomiting	**6–158** The combining form **chol/e** refers to *bile, gall.* Chol/emesis means _____ bile.
chol/e/cyst/o	**6–159** Bile or gall is a bitter secretion produced by the liver and stored in the gallbladder. It passes into the small intestine via the bile ducts when needed for digestion. Combine **chol/e** and **cyst/o** to develop a new combining form _____ / ____ / _____ / ____.
gallbladder	**6–160** Cholecyst/itis is an inflammation of the _____.
o	**6–161** The combining form **e** in **chol/e** is an exception to the rule of using an _____ as a connecting vowel.
bile, gall **vomiting**	**6–162** When a person vomits bile, the condition is called *chol/emesis.* Analyze chol/emesis by defining the elements: **chol/e** refers to _____ or _____. -emesis refers to _____.

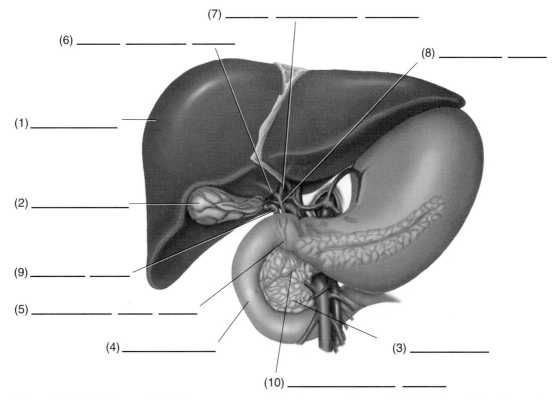

Figure 6–6 The liver, gallbladder, pancreas, and duodenum with associated ducts and blood vessels.

liver	**6–163** The suffix -lith is used in words to mean stone or calculus. A hepat/o/lith is a stone or calculus in the _____.
pancreat/o/lith păn-krē-ĂT-ō-lĭth **cholecyst/o/lith** kō-lē-SĬS-tō-lĭth **hepat/o/lith** hĕp-Ă-tō-lĭth	**6–164** Form medical words meaning stone or calculus in the pancreas: _____ / ____ / _____. gallbladder: _____ / ____ / _____. liver: _____ / ____ / _____.
chol/e	**6–165** A chol/e/lith is a gallstone. Unless a gallstone obstructs a biliary duct, the stones may or may not cause symptoms. The exact cause of gallstones is unknown, but they occur more frequently in women, elderly people, and obese persons. Figure 6–7 illustrates the sites of gallstones. From chol/e/lith, determine the combining form meaning bile, gall: _____ / ____.
chol/e/lith kō-lĕ-LĬTH	**6–166** The most common type of gallstone contains cholesterol. These calculi are formed in the gallbladder or bile ducts. The calculi may cause jaundice, right upper quadrant pain, obstruction, and inflammation of the gallbladder. The medical name for gallstone is _____ / ____ / _____.

cholang/itis kō-lăn-JĪ-tĭs	**6-167** A biliary duct, also called a *bile duct,* may become inflamed from a chol/e/lith. The combining form cholangi/o refers to a bile vessel. Inflammation of the bile vessel is called _____ / _____ .
cholangi/o/graphy kō-lăn-jē-ŎG-ră-f ē	**6-168** Diagnosis of cholang/itis is determined by ultrasound evaluation and cholangi/o/graphy. The radiographic procedure in this frame for outlining the major bile vessel is _____ / _____ / _____ .
bile duct	**6-169** **Choledoch/o** is a combining form for bile duct. A choledoch/o/lith is a stone in the _____ _____ .
choledoch/o	**6-170** Choledoch/o/lith/iasis refers to the formation of a stone in the common bile duct as illustrated in Figure 6–7. The combining form for bile duct is _____ / _____ .
choledoch/itis kō-lĕ-dō-KĪ-tĭs **choledoch/o/rrhaphy** kō-lĕd-ō-KŌR-ă-f ē **choledoch/o/plasty** kō-LĔD-ō-kō-plăs-tē	**6-171** Use **choledoch/o** *(bile duct)* to develop medical words meaning inflammation of the bile duct: _____ / _____ . suture of a bile duct: _____ / _____ / _____ . surgical repair of a bile duct: _____ / _____ / _____ .
stone **calculus, bile duct**	**6-172** Choledoch/o/lith is a _____ or _____ in the common _____ _____ .
choledoch/o/lith kō-LĔD-ŏ-kō-lĭth **choledoch/o/rrhaphy** kō-lĕd-ō-KŌR-ă-f ē **choledoch/o/tomy** kō-lĕd-ō-KŎT-ō-mē	**6-173** When a stone is trapped in the common bile duct, the duct may be incised to remove it, then the duct is sutured. Form medical words meaning stone in the bile duct: _____ / _____ / _____ . suture of the bile duct: _____ / _____ / _____ . incision of the bile duct: _____ / _____ / _____ .
gallbladder	**6-174** Locate the gallbladder, also called *cholecyst,* in Figure 6–6. This pouchlike structure is used to store bile, which is produced by the liver. Cholecyst is the medical name for the _____ .
cholecyst/itis kō-lē-sĭs-TĪ-tĭs	**6-175** An inflammation of the gallbladder may be caused by the presence of gallstones. The diagnosis "inflammation of gallbladder" is medically known as _____ / _____ .

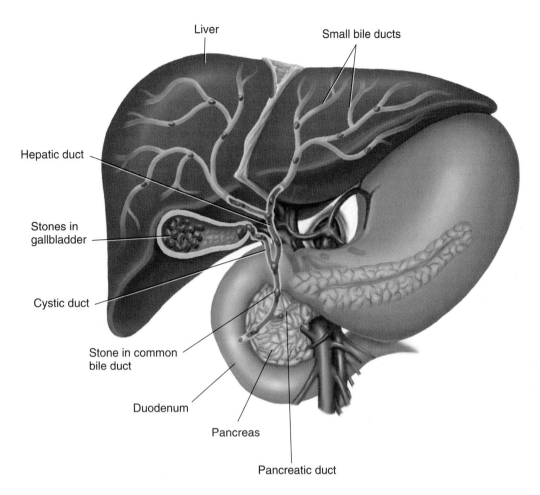

Liver   Small bile ducts

Hepatic duct

Stones in gallbladder

Cystic duct

Stone in common bile duct

Duodenum

Pancreas

Pancreatic duct

Figure 6–7   Cholelithiasis and choledocholithiasis.

gallstone	**6-176** A chole/lith is a _____.
stone, calculus KĂL-kū-lŭs	**6-177** The pancreat/ic duct transports pancreatic juices to the duodenum to help the digestive process. A pancreat/o/lith is a _____ or _____ within the pancreas.
pancreat/o -lith	**6-178** From pancreat/o/lith, identify the combining form for pancreas: _____ / _____. element meaning stone or calculus: _____.
stone, calculus KĂL-kū-lŭs	**6-179** **Lith/o** also is used in words as a combining form meaning *stone* or *calculus*. Whenever you see -lith or **lith/o,** you will know that both elements mean _____ or _____.

stone, calculus KĂL-kū-lŭs	**6-180** The suffixes -osis and -iasis are used to indicate an abnormal condition or diseased condition. The difference between the two suffixes is that -osis is used as a common suffix to denote a disorder but usually does not indicate the specific cause of the abnormal condition. In contrast, the suffix -iasis is attached to a word root to identify an abnormal condition that is produced by something that is specified.* For example, lith/iasis is an abnormal condition produced by a _____ or _____.
liver	**6-181** Hepat/osis is an abnormal or diseased condition of the _____. The cause of the abnormality is not specified and could be the result of any number of liver diseases.
lith/iasis lĭth-Ī-ă-sĭs **pancreat/o/lith/iasis** păn-krē-ă-tō-lĭ-THĪ-ă-sĭs	**6-182** When you form a word meaning an abnormal condition of stones or calculi, use -iasis because the abnormal or diseased condition is produced by something specified (stones). Use -iasis to construct medical words that mean an abnormal condition of stones: _____ / _____. an abnormal condition of pancreat/ic stones: _____ / ____ / _____ / _____.
chol/e/lith/iasis kō-lē-lĭ-THĪ-ă-sĭs	**6-183** Chol/e/lith/iasis is most common in obese women who are older than age 40 (see Figure 6–7). A person who has an abnormal or diseased condition of gallstones has _____ / ____ / _____ / _____.

!
ALERT
In some instances, you will find that -osis and -iasis are interchangeable. Whenever you are in doubt about which suffix to use, refer to your medical dictionary.

inflammation **gallbladder**	**6-184** Acute cholecyst/itis often leads to infection of the gallbladder and duct. Analyze cholecyst/itis by defining the elements: -itis refers to _____. **cholecyst/o** refers to the _____.
cholecyst/o/dynia kō-lē-sĭs-tō-DĬN-ē-ă **cholecyst/algia** kō-lē-sĭs-TĂL-jē-ă	**6-185** Most acute cholecyst/itis cases are the result of gallstones lodged in the bile ducts, which causes pain. Use **cholecyst/o** to form medical words meaning pain in the gallbladder: _____ / ____ / _____ or _____ / _____.

*There are a few exceptions to this rule.

cholecyst/o/lith/iasis kō-lē-sĭs-tō-lĭ-THĪ-ă-sĭs	abnormal condition of gallbladder stone(s): _____ / ____ / _____ / _____.
cholecyst/ectomy kō-lē-sĭs-TĔK-tō-mē	**6-186**　Sometimes the gallbladder is removed because the presence of gallstones causes a severe inflammation. The surgical procedure to excise the gallbladder is a _____ / _____.
pancreat/ectomy păn-krē-ă-TĔK-tō-mē	**6-187**　Because of its critical function of producing insulin and digestive enzymes, a complete excision of the pancreas is almost never performed. When an excision of the pancreas is indicated, the surgeon performs a _____ / _____.
pancreat/ectomy păn-krē-ă-TĔK-tō-mē	**6-188**　Pancreat/ic cancer is an extremely lethal CA, and surgery is performed for relief, but it is not a cure for the cancer. When the surgeon removes either part or all of the pancreas, the surgeon performs a _____ / _____.
cholecyst/ectomy kō-lē-sĭs-TĔK-tō-mē	**6-189**　Because the gallbladder performs no function except storage, it is not essential for life. When the surgeon removes a gallbladder, the surgical procedure is called a _____ / _____.
esophag/o/plasty ē-SŎF-ă-gō-plăs-tē **choledoch/o/plasty** kō-LĔD-ō-kō-plăs-tē	**6-190**　Plastic surgery is the surgical specialty for the restoration, repair, or reconstruction of body structures. Develop operative terms meaning surgical repair of the esophagus: _____ / ____ / _____. surgical repair of the bile duct: _____ / ____ / _____.
discharge, flow	**6-191**　The suffix -rrhea refers to a _____ or _____.
dia/rrhea dī-ă-RĒ-ă	**6-192**　Dia/rrhea is an abnormally frequent discharge of semisolid or fluid fecal matter from the intestine. A continuous passage of loose, watery stools most likely would be diagnosed as _____ / _____.
dia/rrhea dī-ă-RĒ-ă	**6-193**　When a person experiences a frequent passage of watery bowel movements, he or she has a condition known as _____ / _____.

dia/rrhea
dī-ă-RĒ-ă

6-194   Dia/rrhea is usually a symptom of some underlying disorder. *Irritable bowel syndrome,* GI tumors, or an inflammatory bowel disease may cause _____ / _____.

---

therm/o/meter
thĕr-MŎM-ĕ-tĕr

6-195   A therm/o/meter is an instrument for measuring the degree of heat or cold. The normal temperature taken orally ranges from about 97.6° F to 99.6° F. Infection, malignancy, severe trauma, and drugs may cause fever, but there are other conditions that also may cause an elevated temperature.

The combining form **therm/o** refers to *heat.* The instrument used to determine a patient's temperature is called a _____ / _____ / _____.

---

poison

6-196   Poison is any substance taken into the body by ingestion, inhalation, injection, or absorption that interferes with normal physiological function. The three elements commonly used to refer to poison are **tox/o, toxic/o,** and -toxic. Whenever you see any of these elements in a word, you will know that the element refers to _____.

---

toxic/o/logy
tŏks-ĭ-KŎL-ō-jē

6-197   Virtually any substance can be poisonous if consumed in sufficient quantity; the term *poison* more often implies an excessive degree of dosage rather than a specific group of substances. Aspirin is not usually thought of as a poison, but overdoses of this drug kill more children accidentally each year than any of the traditional poisons. Form a word that means study of poisons: _____ / _____ / _____.

---

abnormal condition

poison

toxic/o, tox/o

6-198   Toxic/osis literally means an _____ _____ of _____.

The combining form for poison is _____ / _____ or _____ / _____.

---

poisonous

6-199   When a person swallows a tox/ic substance, it means he or she has swallowed a substance that is _____.

---

ultra/son/o/graphy
ŭl-tră-sŏn-ŎG-ră-fē

6-200   The suffix -gram is used in words to mean *record, writing;* the suffix -graphy is used in words to mean the *process of recording.*

Ultra/son/o/graphy (US) is a process of imaging deep structures of the body by recording the reflection of high-frequency sound waves (ultrasound) and displaying the reflected echoes on a monitor. US also is called ultrasound and echo.

When confirmation of a suspected disease or tumor is needed, the physician may order the radi/o/graph/ic imaging procedure called ultrasound, also known as _____ / _____ / _____ / _____ (US).

6-201   Adjective and noun suffixes are attached to roots to indicate a part of speech. Some adjective suffixes that mean *pertaining to, relating to* (-eal, -ior, -ous) were introduced in Chapter 1. Some noun suffixes that mean *condition* (-ia, -ism, -y) also were introduced in Chapter 1. See if you can identify the part of speech for the following terms. The first one is completed for you.

pen/ile _____   *adjective* _____

adjective   cutane/ous _____

noun   hepat/o/megaly _____

noun   thyroid/ism _____

noun   pneumon/ia _____

adjective   poster/ior _____

6-202   Use -megaly to build a word meaning enlargement of the stomach

gastr/o/megaly
găs-trō-MĔG-ă-lē

_____ / ____ / _____ .

6-203   Hepat/o/megaly may be caused by hepat/itis or other infection; fatty infiltration, as in alcoholism; biliary obstruction; or malignancy. When there is an abnormal enlargement of the liver, the term used in the

hepat/o/megaly
hĕp-ă-tō-MĔG-ă-lē

diagnosis is _____ / ____ / _____ .

Listen and Learn, the audio CD-ROM that accompanies this book, will help you master the pronunciation of selected medical words. Use it to practice pronunciations *of selected terms from frames 6–145 to 6–203* for instructions to complete the *Listen and Learn* exercise on the CD-ROM for this section.

SECTION REVIEW 6 – 6

Using the following table, write the combining form or suffix that matches its definition in the space provided to the left of the definition. There may be more than one word element that matches a definition.

Combining Forms		Suffixes		
chol/e	pancreat/o	-algia	-graphy	-plasty
cholecyst/o	therm/o	-dynia	-iasis	-rrhaphy
choledoch/o	toxic/o	-ectomy	-lith	-stomy
cyst/o	tox/o	-emesis	-megaly	-toxic
hepat/o		-gram	-osis	

1. _____ abnormal condition; increase (used primarily with blood cells)
2. _____ abnormal condition (produced by something specified)
3. _____ bile duct
4. _____ bile, gall
5. _____ bladder
6. _____ enlargement
7. _____ excision, removal
8. _____ forming an opening (mouth)
9. _____ gallbladder
10. _____ heat
11. _____ liver
12. _____ pain
13. _____ pancreas
14. _____ poison
15. _____ process of recording
16. _____ record, writing
17. _____ stonc, calculus
18. _____ surgical repair
19. _____ suture
20. _____ vomiting

Competency Verification: Check your answers in Appendix B, Answer Key, page 520. If you are not satisfied with your level of comprehension, go back to Frame 6–145 and rework the frames.

Correct Answers _____ × 5 = _____ % Score

Abbreviations

This section introduces digestive system–related abbreviations and their meanings. Included are abbreviations contained in the medical record activities that follow.

Abbreviations	Meaning	Abbreviations	Meaning
Ba	barium	GTT	glucose tolerance test
BaE, BE	barium enema	HCl	hydrochloric acid
cm	centimeter	IBD	inflammatory bowel disease
CT scan, CAT scan	computed tomography scan	IVC	intravenous cholangiography
Dx	diagnosis	UGI	upper gastrointestinal
EGD	esophagogastroduodenoscopy	UGIS	upper gastrointestinal series
ERCP	endoscopic retrograde cholangiopancreatography	US	ultrasonography, ultrasound
FBS	fasting blood sugar		

OTHER ABBREVIATIONS RELATED TO THE DIGESTIVE SYSTEM			
BM	bowel movement	HBV	hepatitis B virus
cm	centimeter	PE	physical examination
GI	gastrointestinal	RUQ	right upper quadrant
HAV	hepatitis A virus		

Pathological, Diagnostic, and Therapeutic Terms

The following are additional terms related to the digestive system. Recognizing and learning these terms will help you understand the connection between a pathological condition, its diagnoses, and the rationale behind the method of treatment selected for a particular disorder.

Pathological

appendicitis (ă-pĕn-dĭ-SĪ-tĭs): inflammation of the appendix, usually acute and caused by blockage of the appendix that is followed by infection. When left untreated, it rapidly leads to perforation and peritonitis.

Treatment for acute appendicitis is appendectomy within 48 hours of the first symptom. Any further delay in treatment results in rupture and peritonitis as fecal matter is released into the peritoneal cavity (see Figure 6–8).

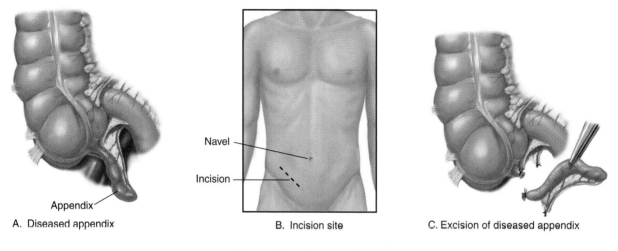

Navel

Incision

Appendix

A. Diseased appendix

B. Incision site

C. Excision of diseased appendix

Figure 6–8   Appendectomy.

ascites (ă-SĪ-tēz): abnormal accumulation of serous fluid in the abdomen.

Ascites occurs when fluid drains out of the bloodstream and accumulates in the peritoneal cavity. It may be a symptom of inflammatory disorders in the abdomen, venous hypertension caused by liver disease, or heart failure.

borborygmus (bŏr-bō-RĬG-mŭs): gurgling or rumbling sound heard over the large intestine, caused by gas moving through the intestines.

cirrhosis (sĭ-RŌ-sĭs): chronic liver disease characterized pathologically by destruction of liver cells that eventually leads to ineffective liver function and jaundice.

colonic polyposis (kō-LŎN-ĭk pŏl-ē-PŌ-sĭs): polyps, which are small benign growths, that project from the mucous membrane of the colon.

Polyps have the potential of becoming cancerous, so they are checked frequently or removed to detect any abnormalities at an early stage. Colonic polyps have a high likelihood of becoming colorectal cancer.

Crohn disease (krōn): chronic inflammatory bowel disease, usually affects the ileum, but may affect any portion of the intestinal tract. It is distinguished from closely related bowel disorders by its inflammatory pattern, which tends to be patchy or segmented; also called *regional colitis*.

diverticular disease (dī-vĕr-TĬK-ū-lăr): condition in which bulging pouches (diverticula) in the gastrointestinal (GI) tract push the mucosal lining through the surrounding muscle

When disease occurs on the left side of the colon, it may be referred to as "left-sided appendicitis." (See Figure 6–9).

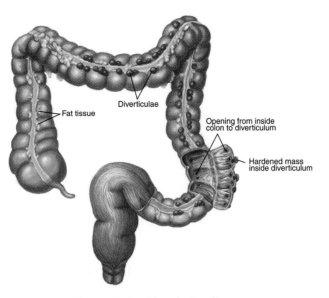

Fat tissue

Diverticulae

Opening from inside colon to diverticulum

Hardened mass inside diverticulum

Figure 6–9   Diverticular disease.

dysentery (DĬS-ĕn-tĕr-ē): term applied to many intestinal disorders, especially of the colon, characterized by inflammation of the mucous membrane, diarrhea, and abdominal cramps.

fistula (FĬS-tū-lă): abnormal passage from one organ to another, or from a hollow organ to the surface. An anal fistula is located near the anus and may open into the rectum.

hematochezia (hĕm-ă-tō-KĒ-zē-ă): passage of stools containing bright red blood.

hemorrhoid (HĔM-ō-royd): mass of enlarged, twisted varicose veins in the mucous membrane inside (internal) or just outside (external) the rectum; also known as *piles.*

hernia (HĔR-nē-ă): protrusion or projection of an organ or a part of an organ through the wall of the cavity that normally contains it (see Figure 6–10).

inflammatory bowel disease (ĭn-FLĂM-ă-tŏr-ē bou-ăl): ulceration of mucosa of the colon. Ulcerative colitis and Crohn disease are forms of inflammatory bowel disease; also known as *IBD.*

irritable bowel syndrome (ĬR-ĭ-tă-bl bou-ăl SĬN-drōm): abnormal increase in the motility of the small and large intestines that generally is associated with emotional stress. No pathological lesions are found in the intestine.

In diagnosing irritable bowel syndrome (IBS), other, more serious conditions, such as dysentery, lactose intolerance, and inflammatory bowel disease, must be ruled out because there is no organic disease present in IBS; also called spastic colon.

jaundice (JAWN-dĭs): yellow discoloration of the skin, mucous membranes, and sclerae of the eyes, caused by excessive levels of bilirubin in the blood *(hyperbilirubinemia).*

polyp (PŎL-ĭp): small, tumor-like benign growth that projects from a mucous membrane surface.

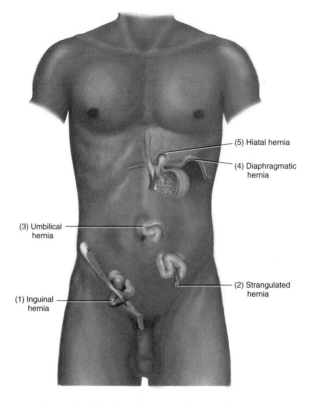

Figure 6–10 Common locations of hernias.

polyposis (pŏl-ē-PŌ-sĭs): general term for a condition in which polyps develop in the intestinal tract.

ulcer (UL-sĕr): open sore or lesion of the skin or mucous membrane, accompanied by sloughing of inflamed necrotic tissue.

An ulcer may be shallow, involving only the epidermis, or it may be deep, involving multiple layers of the skin. Some examples of ulcers are peptic ulcer, duodenal ulcer, and decubitus ulcer.

volvulus (VŎL-vū-lŭs): twisting of the bowel on itself, causing obstruction. Usually requires surgery to untwist the loop of bowel.

Diagnostic

barium enema (BĂ-rē-ŭm ĔN-ĕ-mă): radiographic examination of the rectum and colon after administration of barium sulfate (radiopaque contrast medium) into the rectum.

This procedure is used for diagnosis of obstructions, tumors, or other abnormalities, such as ulcerative colitis.

barium swallow (BĂ-rē-ŭm): radiographic examination of the esophagus, stomach, and small intestine after oral administration of barium sulfate (radiopaque contrast medium).

Structural abnormalities of the esophagus and vessels, such as esophageal varices, may be diagnosed by use of this technique; also called upper GI series.

computed tomography (CT) scan (kŏm-PŪ-tĕd tō-MŎG-ră-fē): radiographic technique that uses a narrow beam of x-rays, which rotates in a full arc around the patient to image the body in cross-sectional slices. A scanner and detector send the images to a computer, which consolidates all of the data it receives from the multiple x-ray views (see Figure 2–5D).

In the digestive system, CT scans are used to view the gallbladder, liver, bile ducts, and pancreas. CT scan is used to diagnose tumors, cysts, inflammation, abscesses, perforation, bleeding, and obstructions. A contrast material may be used to enhance the structures.

magnetic resonance imaging (măg-NĔT-ĭc RĔZ-ĕn-ăns ĬM-ĭj-ĭng): radiographic technique that uses electromagnetic energy to produce multiplanar cross-sectional images of the body (see Figure 2–5E).

In the digestive system, magnetic resonance imaging (MRI) is particularly useful in detecting abdominal masses and viewing images of abdominal structures.

stool guaiac (GWĪ-ăk): test performed on feces using the reagent gum guaiac to detect the presence of blood in the feces that is not apparent on visual inspection; also called *Hemoccult test.*

ultrasonography (ŭl-tră-sŏn-ŎG-ră-fē): imaging technique that uses high-frequency sound waves (ultrasound) that bounce off body tissues and are recorded to produce an image of an internal organ or tissue. Ultrasonic echoes are recorded and interpreted by a computer, which produces a detailed image of the organ or tissue being evaluated (see Figure 2–5B).

In the digestive system, ultrasound visualization includes, but is not limited to, the liver, gallbladder, bile ducts, and pancreas. It is used to diagnose and locate cysts, tumors, and other digestive disorders and to guide the insertion of instruments during surgical procedures.

Therapeutic

extracorporeal shock-wave lithotripsy (ĕks-tră-kor-POR-ē-ăl LĬTH-ō-trĭp-sē): use of shock waves as a noninvasive method to destroy stones in the gallbladder and biliary ducts.

Ultrasound is used to locate the stones and to monitor their destruction. After extracorporeal shock-wave lithotripsy (ESWL), a course of oral dissolution drugs is used to ensure complete removal of all stones and stone fragments.

lithotripsy (LĬTH-ō-trĭp-sē): procedure for eliminating a calculus in the gallbladder, renal pelvis, ureter, or bladder.

Stones may be crushed surgically or by using a noninvasive method, such as hydraulic, or high-energy, shock-wave or a pulsed-dye laser. The fragments may be expelled or washed out.

nasogastric intubation (nā-zō-GĂS-trĭk ĭn-tū-BĀ-shŭn): insertion of a nasogastric tube through the nose into the stomach.

Nasogastric intubation is used to relieve gastric distention by removing gas, gastric secretions, or food. It also is used to instill medication, food, or fluids or to obtain a specimen for laboratory analysis.

 Listen and Learn, the audio CD-ROM that accompanies this book, will help you master the pronunciation of selected medical words. Use it to practice pronunciations of the above-listed medical terms and for instructions to complete the *Listen and Learn* exercise on the CD-ROM for this section.

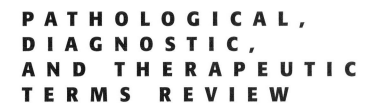

PATHOLOGICAL, DIAGNOSTIC, AND THERAPEUTIC TERMS REVIEW

Match the medical term(s) below with the definitions in the numbered list.

ascites	Crohn disease	irritable bowel syndrome (IBS)
barium enema	fistula	jaundice
barium swallow	hematochezia	lithotripsy
cirrhosis	hemoccult	nasogastric intubation
colonic polyposis	inflammatory bowel disease (IBD)	volvulus

1. _____ is a test performed on feces; detects presence of blood that is not apparent on visual inspection.

2. _____ refers to insertion of a tube through the nose into the stomach for therapeutic and diagnostic purposes.

3. _____ are small benign growths that project from the mucous membrane of the large intestine.

4. _____ is an abnormal accumulation of serous fluid in the abdomen.

5. _____ refers to chronic inflammatory bowel disease, usually affects the ileum.

6. _____ refers to surgically crushing a stone.

7. _____ is an abnormal tubelike passage from one organ to another or from one organ to the surface.

8. _____ is a yellow discoloration of the skin caused by hyperbilirubinemia.

9. _____ is a radiographic examination of the rectum and colon after administration of barium sulfate.

10. _____ refers to ulceration of mucosa of the colon, as seen in *Crohn disease.*

11. _____ refers to passage of stools containing red blood rather than tarry stools.

12. _____ means twisting of the bowel on itself, causing obstruction.

13. _____ refers to a chronic liver disease characterized pathologically by destruction of liver cells and jaundice.

14. _____ is a radiographic examination of the esophagus, stomach, and small intestine after oral administration of barium sulfate.

15. _____ means abnormally increased motility of the small and large intestines; also called spastic colon.

Competency Verification: Check your answers in Appendix B, Answer Key, page 520. If you are not satisfied with your level of comprehension, review the pathological, diagnostic, and therapeutic terms and retake the review.

Correct Answers _____ × 6.67 = _____% Score

Medical Record Activities

The two medical records included in the following activities reflect common real-life clinical scenarios to show how medical terminology is used to document patient care. The physician who specializes in the treatment of gastrointestinal disorders is a *gastroenterologist;* the medical specialty concerned in the diagnoses and treatment of gastrointestinal disorders is called *gastroenterology.* Gastroenterologists usually do not perform surgeries, but under the broad classification of surgery, they do perform such procedures as endoscopic examinations and biopsies.

✓ MEDICAL RECORD ACTIVITY 6–1. Rectal Bleeding

Terminology

The terms listed in the chart come from the medical record *Rectal Bleeding* that follows. Use a medical dictionary such as *Taber's Cyclopedic Medical Dictionary,* the appendices of this book, or other resources to define each term. Then practice reading the pronunciations aloud for each term.

Term	Definition
angulation ăng-ū-LĀ-shŭn	
anorectal ā-nō-RĔK-tăl	
carcinoma kăr-sĭ-NŌ-mă	
cm	
diarrhea dī-ă-RĒ-ă	
diverticulum dī-věr-TĬK-ū-lŭm (see Figure 6–9)	
dysphagia dĭs-FĀ-jē-ă	
emesis ĔM-ĕ-sĭs	
enteritis ĕn-těr-Ī-tĭs	
hematemesis hĕm-ăt-ĔM-ĕ-sĭs	
ileostomy ĬL-ē-ŎS-tō-mē	

Term	Definition
nausea NAW-sē-ă	
polyp PŎL-ĭp	
postprandial pōst-PRĂN-dē-ăl	
sigmoidoscopy sĭg-moy-DŎS-kō-pē	

Listen and Learn Online! will help you master the pronunciation of selected medical words from this medical record activity. Visit www.fadavis.com/gylys/simplified for instructions in completing the *Listen and Learn Online!* exercise for this section and then to practice pronunciations.

RECTAL BLEEDING

Reading

Practice pronunciation of medical terms by reading the following medical report aloud.

This 50-year-old white man has lost approximately 40 pounds since his last examination. The patient says he has had no dysphagia or postprandial distress, and there is no report of diarrhea, nausea, emesis, hematemesis, or constipation. The patient has had a history of regional enteritis, appendicitis, and colonic bleeding.

The regional enteritis resulted in an ileostomy with appendectomy about 6 months ago. On 5/30/XX, a sigmoidoscopy using a 10-cm scope showed no evidence of bleeding at the anorectal area. A 35-cm scope was then inserted to a level of 13 cm. At this point, angulation prevented further passage of the scope. No abnormalities had been encountered, but there was dark blood noted at that level.

My impression is that the rectal bleeding could be due to a polyp, bleeding diverticulum, or rectal carcinoma.

Evaluation

Review the medical record above to answer the following questions.

1. What is the patient's symptom that made him seek medical help?

2. What surgical procedures were performed on the patient for regional enteritis?

3. What abnormality was found with the sigmoidoscopy?

4. What is causing the rectal bleeding?

_____

_____

5. Write the plural form of diverticulum.

_____

_____

✓ MEDICAL RECORD ACTIVITY 6–2. Carcinosarcoma of the Esophagus

Terminology

The terms listed in the chart come from the medical record _Carcinosarcoma of the Esophagus_ that follows. Use a medical dictionary such as _Taber's Cyclopedic Medical Dictionary,_ the appendices of this book, or other resources to define each term. Then practice reading the pronunciations aloud for each term.

Term	Definition
aortic arch ā-OR-tĭk	
carcinosarcoma kăr-sĭ-nō-săr-KŌ-mă	
esophagoscopy ē-sŏf-ă-GŎS-kō-pē	
friable FRĪ-ă-bl	
intraluminal ĭn-tră-LŪ-mĭ-năl	
malignant mă-LĬG-nănt	
mediastinal mē-dē-ăs-TĪ-năl	
OR	
polypoid PŎL-ē-poyd	
reanastomosis rē-ăn-ăs-tō-MŌ-sĭs (see Figure 2–7)	

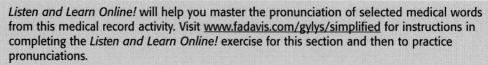

Listen and Learn Online! will help you master the pronunciation of selected medical words from this medical record activity. Visit www.fadavis.com/gylys/simplified for instructions in completing the _Listen and Learn Online!_ exercise for this section and then to practice pronunciations.

CARCINOSARCOMA OF THE ESOPHAGUS

Reading

Practice pronunciation of medical terms by reading the following medical report aloud.

ADMITTING DIAGNOSIS: Carcinosarcoma of the esophagus.

DISCHARGE DIAGNOSIS: Carcinosarcoma of the esophagus.

HISTORY OF PRESENT ILLNESS: Patient had been complaining of dysphagia over the last 4 months with a worsening recently in symptoms.

SURGERY: Esophagoscopy was performed, and a small friable biopsy specimen was obtained. Pathology tests confirmed it to be malignant. A barium x-ray study revealed polypoid, intraluminal, esophageal obstruction. Surgical findings revealed an infiltrating tumor of the middle third of the esophagus with intraluminal, friable, polypoid masses, each 3 cm in diameter. A resection of the esophagus was performed with reanastomosis of the stomach at the aortic arch. An adjacent mediastinal lymph node was excised. There were no complications during the procedure. Patient left the OR in stable condition.

Evaluation

Review the medical record above to answer the following questions.

1. What surgery was performed on this patient?

_____

_____

2. What diagnostic testing confirmed malignancy?

_____

_____

3. Where was the carcinosarcoma located?

_____

_____

4. Why was the adjacent lymph node excised?

_____

_____

Chapter Review

Word Elements Summary

The following table summarizes combining forms, suffixes, and prefixes related to the digestive system.

Word Element	Meaning
COMBINING FORMS	
chol/e	bile, gall
cholecyst/o	gallbladder
choledoch/o	bile duct
col/o, colon/o	colon
dent/o, odont/o	teeth
duoden/o	duodenum (first part of small intestine)
enter/o	intestine (usually small intestine)
esophag/o	esophagus
gastr/o	stomach
gingiv/o	gum(s)
gloss/o, lingu/o	tongue
hepat/o	liver
ile/o	ileum (second part of small intestine)
jejun/o	jejunum (third part of small intestine)
or/o, stomat/o	mouth
pancreat/o	pancreas
proct/o	anus, rectum
ptyal/o, sial/o	saliva, salivary gland
rect/o	rectum
sigmoid/o	sigmoid colon
OTHER COMBINING FORMS	
aer/o	air
carcin/o	cancer
hemat/o	blood
lith/o	stone, calculus
maxill/o	maxilla (upper jaw bone)

Word Element	Meaning
myc/o	fungus
orth/o	straight
ptyal/o	saliva
therm/o	heat
tox/o, toxic/o	poison
SUFFIXES	
SURGICAL	
-ectomy	excision, removal
-plasty	surgical repair
-rrhaphy	suture
-stomy	forming an opening (mouth)
-tome	instrument to cut
-tomy	incision
DIAGNOSTIC, SYMPTOMATIC, AND RELATED	
-algia, -dynia	pain
-emesis	vomiting
-gram	record, writing
-graphy	process of recording
-iasis	abnormal condition (produced by something specified)
-itis	inflammation
-lith	stone, calculus
-logist	specialist in study of
-logy	study of
-megaly	enlargement
-oma	tumor
-osis	abnormal condition; increase (used primarily with blood cells)
-pepsia	digestion
-phagia	swallowing, eating
-rrhea	discharge, flow
-scope	instrument for examining

(Continued)

Word Element	Meaning *(Continued)*
-scopy	visual examination
-spasm	involuntary contraction, twitching
-stenosis	narrowing, stricture
ADJECTIVE	
-al, -ar, -ary, -ic	pertaining to, relating to
NOUN	
-ia	condition
-ist	specialist
PREFIXES	
ab-	from, away from
dys-	bad; painful; difficult
epi-	above, upon
hyper-	excessive, above normal
hypo-	under, below, deficient
peri-	around
sub-	under, below

WORD ELEMENTS REVIEW

After you review the Word Elements Summary, complete this activity by writing the meaning of each element in the space provided.

Word Element	Meaning
COMBINING FORMS	
DIGESTIVE SYSTEM STRUCTURES	
1. col/o, colon/o	
2. dent/o, odont/o	
3. duoden/o	
4. enter/o	
5. esophag/o	
6. gastr/o	
7. gingiv/o	
8. ile/o	
9. jejun/o	
10. lingu/o	
11. maxill/o	
12. ptyal/o	
13. rect/o	
14. sial/o	
15. sigmoid/o	
OTHER COMBINING FORMS	
16. carcin/o	
17. hemat/o	
18. myc/o	
19. orth/o	
20. tox/o, toxic/o	

(Continued)

Word Element	Meaning *(Continued)*
SUFFIXES	
SURGICAL	
21. -ectomy	
22. -plasty	
23. -rrhaphy	
24. -stomy	
25. -tomy	
DIAGNOSTIC, SYMPTOMATIC, AND RELATED	
26. -algia, -dynia	
27. -emesis	
28. -gram	
29. -graphy	
30. -iasis	
31. -itis	
32. -lith	
33. -megaly	
34. -oma	
35. -osis	
36. -pepsia	
37. -phagia	
38. -rrhea	
39. -scope	
40. -scopy	
41. -spasm	
42. -stenosis	

Word Element	Meaning
NOUN	
43. -ia	
PREFIXES	
44. dia-	
45. dys-	
46. epi-	
47. hyper-	
48. hypo-	
49. peri-	
50. sub-	

Competency Verification: Check your answers in Appendix A, Glossary of Medical Word Elements, page 497. If you are not satisfied with your level of comprehension, review the word elements and retake the review.

Correct Answers _____ × 2 = _____% Score

Chapter 6 Vocabulary Review

Match the medical word(s) below with the definitions in the numbered list.

alimentary canal	duodenotomy	hematemesis	sigmoid colon
anastomosis	dyspepsia	hepatomegaly	sigmoidotomy
cholecystectomy	dysphagia	ileostomy	stomach
choledochal	friable	rectoplasty	stomatalgia
cholelithiasis	gastroscopy	salivary glands	ultrasound

1. _____ refers to visual examination of the stomach.

2. _____ means bad, painful, difficult digestion.

3. _____ means vomiting blood.

4. _____ refers to use of high-frequency sound waves to produce internal images of the body.

5. _____ are glands that secrete saliva.

6. _____ is another term for the GI tract.

7. _____ means pain in the mouth.

8. _____ is an incision of the duodenum.

9. _____ means enlargement of the liver.

10. _____ refers to inability to swallow or difficulty or painful swallowing.

11. _____ means removal of the gallbladder.

12. _____ is a surgical connection between two vessels, bowel segments, or ducts to allow flow from one to another.

13. _____ is an incision of the sigmoid colon.

14. _____ refers to surgical repair of the rectum.

15. _____ is the organ to which the esophagus transports food.

16. _____ refers to formation of an opening (mouth) into the ileum.

17. _____ refers to presence or formation of gallstones.

18. _____ means easily broken or pulverized.

19. _____ means pertaining to the bile duct.

20. _____ is the S-shaped lower end of the colon.

Competency Verification: Check your answers in Appendix B, Answer Key, page 521. If you are not satisfied with your level of comprehension, review the chapter vocabulary and retake the review.

Correct Answers _____ × 5 = _____ % Score

Urinary System

The primary function of the urinary system is to remove waste products and other potentially harmful substances from the blood by excreting them in the urine. Organs of the urinary system are the kidneys, ureters, bladder, and urethra. The formation of urine is performed by the function of the kidneys. Other important functions of the kidneys are to regulate the body's tissue fluid and maintain a balance of electrolytes (potassium, sodium, and calcium) and an acid-base balance in the blood. The rest of the urinary structures are responsible for storing and eliminating urine. Review Figure 7–1, which illustrates the location of urinary structures in the body.

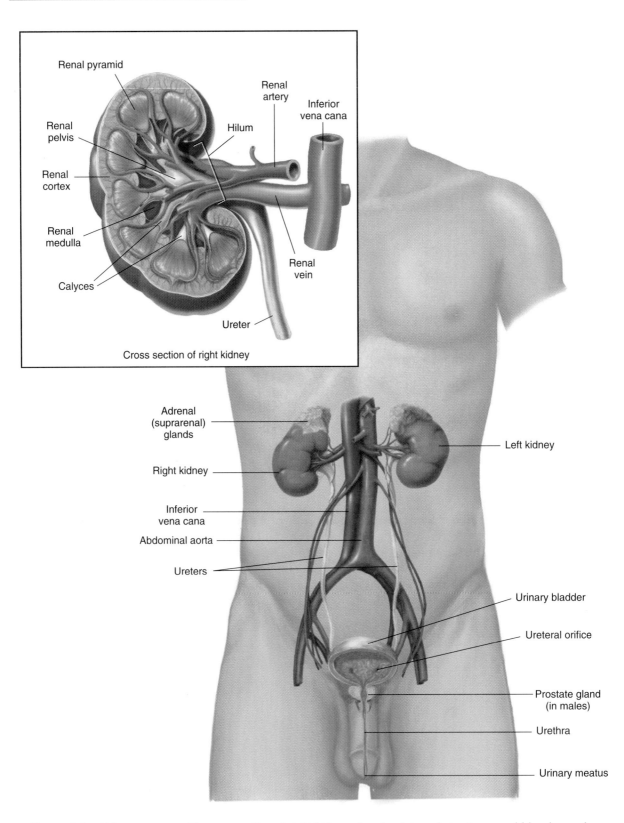

Figure 7-1 Urinary system with cross section of right kidney showing internal structures and blood vessels.

Word Elements

This section introduces combining forms related to the urinary system. Included are key suffixes; prefixes are defined in the right-hand column as needed. Review the following table, and pronounce each word in the word analysis column aloud before you begin to work the frames.

Word Element	Meaning	Word Analysis
COMBINING FORMS		
cyst/o	bladder	cyst/o/scopy (sĭs-TŎS-kō-pē): visual examination of the urinary tract by means of a cystoscope inserted into the urethra 　　*-scopy:* visual examination *A cystoscopy is usually performed with the patient under sedation or anesthesia. It also is performed to obtain biopsy specimens of tumors or other growths and for removing polyps.*
vesic/o		vesic/o/cele (VĔS-ĭ-kō-sēl): hernial protrusion of the urinary bladder; also called cystocele 　　*-cele:* hernia, swelling
glomerul/o	glomerulus	glomerul/o/scler/osis (glō-mĕr-ū-lō-sklē-RŌ-sĭs): hardening or scarring within the glomeruli 　　*scler:* hardening; sclera (white of eye) 　　*-osis:* abnormal condition, increase (used primarily with blood cells) *A degenerative process occurring in association with renal arteriosclerosis and diabetes; glomerular function of blood filtration is lost as fibrous scar tissue replaces the glomeruli.*
meat/o	opening, meatus	meat/us (mē-Ā-tŭs): opening or tunnel through any part of the body, such as the external opening of the urethra 　　*-us:* condition, structure
nephr/o	kidney	nephr/oma (nĕ-FRŌ-mă): tumor of the kidney 　　*-oma:* tumor
ren/o		ren/al (RĒ-năl): pertaining to the kidney 　　*-al:* pertaining to, relating to
pyel/o	renal pelvis	pyel/o/plasty (PĪ-ĕ-lō-plăs-tē): surgical repair of the renal pelvis 　　*-plasty:* surgical repair
ur/o	urine	ur/emia (ū-RĒ-mē-ă): excessive urea and other nitrogenous waste products in the blood; also called azotemia 　　*-emia:* blood condition *The waste products are normally excreted by healthy kidneys. Uremia occurs in renal failure.*
urin/o		urin/ary (Ū-rĭ-năr-ē): pertains to urine or formation of urine 　　*-ary:* pertaining to, relating to
ureter/o	ureter	ureter/o/stenosis (ū-rē-tĕr-ō-stĕ-NŌ-sĭs): narrowing or stricture of a ureter 　　*-stenosis:* narrowing, stricture

(Continued)

Word Element	Meaning	Word Analysis
urethr/o	urethra	urethr/o/cele (ū-RĒ-thrō-sēl): hernial protrusion of the urethra *-cele:* hernia, swelling *Urethrocele may be congenital or acquired and secondary to obesity, parturition, and poor muscle tone.*

SUFFIXES

Word Element	Meaning	Word Analysis
-emia	blood condition	azot/emia (ăz-ō-TĒ-mē-ă): excessive amounts of nitrogenous compounds in the blood *azot:* nitrogenous compounds *Azotemia is a toxic condition that is caused by failure of the kidneys to remove urea from the blood and is characteristic of uremia.*
-iasis	abnormal condition (produced by something specified)	lith/iasis (lĭth-Ī-ă-sĭs): abnormal condition or presence of stones or calculi *lith:* stone, calculus *Lithiasis occurs most commonly in the kidney, lower urinary tract, and gallbladder.*
-lysis	separation; destruction; loosening	dia/lysis (dī-ĂL-ĭ-sĭs): process of removing toxic materials from the blood when the kidneys are unable to do so *dia-:* through, across
-pathy	disease	nephr/o/pathy (nĕ-FRŎP-ă-thē): any disorder of the kidneys, including inflammatory, degenerative, and sclerotic conditions *nephr:* kidney
-pexy	fixation (of an organ)	nephr/o/pexy (NĔF-rō-pĕks-ē): surgical procedure to fixate a floating kidney *nephr/o:* kidney
-ptosis	prolapse, downward displacement	nephr/o/ptosis (nĕf-rŏp-TŌ-sĭs): downward displacement or dropping of a kidney *nephr/o:* kidney
-tripsy	crushing	lith/o/tripsy (LĬTH-ō-trĭp-sē): crushing of a stone in the bladder or urethra *lith/o:* stone, calculus
-uria	urine	poly/uria (pŏl-ē-Ū-rē-ă): excessive urination *poly-:* many, much

Listen and Learn, the audio CD-ROM that accompanies this book, will help you master the pronunciation of selected medical words. Use it to practice pronunciations of the above-listed medical terms and for instructions to complete the *Listen and Learn* exercise on the CD-ROM for this section.

For the following medical terms, first write the suffix and its meaning. Then translate the meaning of the remaining elements starting with the first part of the word. The first word is an example that is completed for you.

Term	Meaning
1. glomerul/o/scler/osis	-osis: abnormal condition, increase (used primarily with blood cells); glomerulus; hardening, sclera (white of eye)
2. cyst/o/scopy	_____
3. poly/uria	_____
4. lith/o/tripsy	_____
5. dia/lysis	_____
6. ureter/o/stenosis	_____
7. meat/us	_____
8. ur/emia	_____
9. nephr/oma	_____
10. ureter/o/cele	_____

Competency Verification: Check your answers in Appendix B, Answer Key, page 522. If you are not satisfied with your level of comprehension, review the vocabulary and retake the review.

Correct Answers _____ × 10 = _____% Score

Kidneys

7-1 Label the urinary structures in Figure 7–2 as you read the following material. The urinary system is composed of a (1) **right kidney** and a left kidney. These are the primary structural units of the urinary system that are responsible for the formation of urine. Each kidney is composed of an outer layer, called the (2) **renal cortex,** and an inner region, called the (3) **renal medulla.** Blood enters the kidneys through the (4) **renal artery** and leaves through the (5) **renal vein.** When inside the kidney, the renal artery branches into smaller arteries called *arterioles* that lead into microscopic filtering units called *nephrons*. Each (6) **nephron** is designed to filter urea and other waste products effectively from the blood.

7-2 Two combining forms that refer to the kidneys are **nephr/o** and **ren/o.** Whenever you see terms such as nephr/itis and ren/al, you will know they refer to the _____.

kidney(s)

kidney(s)	**7-3** The term *ren/al* is used frequently as an adjective to modify a noun. Some examples are ren/al dialysis and ren/al biopsy. Both of these terms refer to the _____.
nephr/ectomy nĕ-FRĔK-tō-mē	**7-4** A diseased kidney or *renal failure* may necessitate its removal. Use **nephr/o** to form a word meaning excision of a kidney: _____ / _____.
nephr/ectomy nĕ-FRĔK-tō-mē	**7-5** Renal failure also may result in extreme hypertension. If this occurs, both kidneys may have to be removed. Nevertheless, the surgical procedure to remove either one or both kidneys is still known as a _____ / _____.
nephr/o/megaly nĕf-rō-MĔG-ă-lē	**7-6** When nephr/ectomy is performed, the remaining kidney most likely will become enlarged. Build a word meaning enlargement of a kidney: _____ / ____ / _____.

ALERT If you had difficulty in deciding whether to use **nephr/o** or **ren/o** in the previous frames, refer to your medical dictionary. Until you master the language of medicine, the dictionary will help you identify commonly used terms in medicine.

lith/iasis lĭth-Ī-ă-sĭs	**7-7** The suffix -iasis is used to describe an *abnormal condition (produced by something specified)*. An abnormal condition of stones is called _____ / _____.
nephr/o/lith NĔF-rō-lĭth **nephr/o/lith/iasis** nĕf-rō-lĭth-Ī-ă-sĭs	**7-8** Use **nephr/o** to construct medical words meaning stone (in the) kidney: _____ / ____ / _____. abnormal condition of kidney stone(s): _____ / ____ / _____ / _____.
nephr/algia nĕ-FRĂL-jē-ă **nephr/itis** nĕf-RĪ-tĭs	**7-9** When kidney stones (see Figure 7–3) are present, they can be extremely painful. A person with kidney stones may suffer from pain in the kidney caused by an inflammation of a kidney. Use **nephr/o** to build a word meaning pain in the kidney: _____ / _____. inflammation of the kidney: _____ / _____.

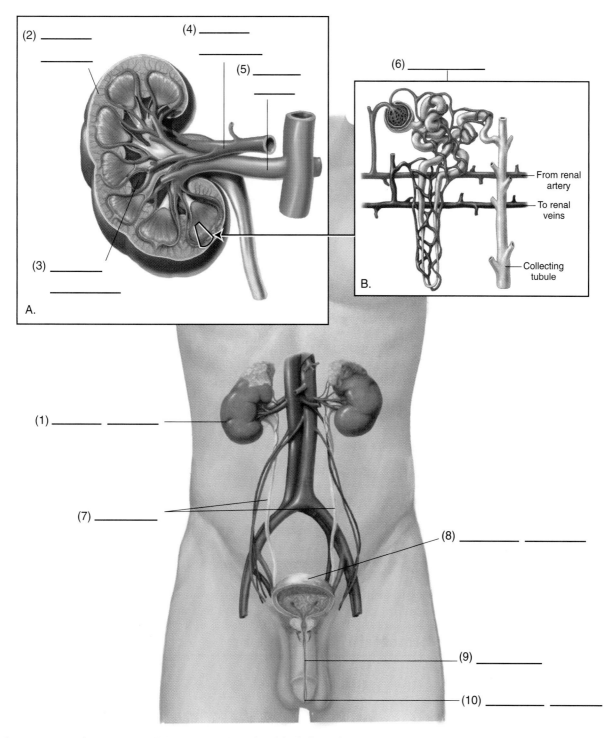

(2) _____

(4) _____

(5) _____

(6) _____

From renal artery

To renal veins

Collecting tubule

B.

(3) _____

A.

(1) _____ _____

(7) _____

(8) _____ _____

(9) _____

(10) _____ _____

Figure 7-2 Urinary system. (A) Cross section of a right kidney showing internal structures and blood vessels. (B) A single nephron with a collecting duct and associated blood vessels.

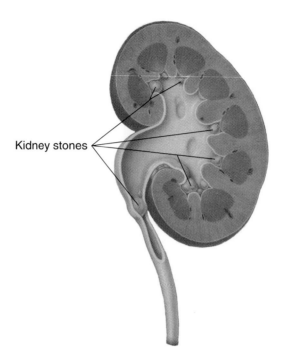

Figure 7-3   Kidney stones shown in the calices and ureter.

stone **calculus**	**7-10** Nephr/o/lith, renal calculus, and ren/al stone all are terms that mean a person suffers from a kidney _____ or _____.
nephr/o/lith/iasis nĕf-rō-lĭth-Ī-ă-sĭs	**7-11** A disorder that literally means abnormal condition of a kidney stone is: _____ / ____ / _____ / _____.
	7-12 The surgical suffixes -ectomy, -tomy, and -tome are often confusing to beginning medical terminology students. To reinforce your understanding of their meanings, review them in the following chart. <table><tr><td>**Surgical Suffix**</td><td>**Meaning**</td></tr><tr><td>-ectomy</td><td>excision, removal</td></tr><tr><td>-tomy</td><td>incision</td></tr><tr><td>-tome</td><td>instrument to cut</td></tr></table>
incision **stone** *or* **calculus**	**7-13** Stones that are trapped in the kidney or ureter may need to be removed surgically. Nephr/o/lith/o/tomy is an _____ to remove a ren/al _____.

	7-14 Ren/al hyper/tension produced by kidney disease is the most common type of hyper/tension caused by an abnormal condition, such as glomerul/o/nephr/itis or ren/al artery stenosis.
	Identify the terms in this frame that mean
ren/al RĒ-năl	pertaining to the kidney(s): _____ / _____.
sten/osis stĕ-NŌ-sĭs	narrowing, stricture: _____ / _____.
	inflammation of the glomerulus of the kidney:
glomerul/o/nephr/itis glō-mĕr-ū-lō-nĕ-FRĪ-tĭs	_____ / ____ / _____ / _____.
hyper/tension hī-pĕr-TĔN-shŭn	high blood pressure: _____ / _____.
	7-15 *Nephr/o/tic syndrome*, a group of symptoms characterized by chronic loss of protein in the urine (protein/uria), leads to depletion of body protein, especially albumin. Normally, albumin and other serum proteins maintain fluid within the vascular space. When levels of these proteins are low, fluid leaks from the blood vessels into tissues, resulting in edema. The syndrome may occur as a result of other disease processes.
	A chronic loss of protein in the urine is called
protein/uria prō-tē-ĭn-Ū-rē-ă	_____ / _____.
	7-16 Although there are many disorders that manifest fluid retention (excess fluid in tissues), a person with nephr/o/tic syndrome usually exhibits edema or swelling, especially around the ankles, feet, and eyes.
swelling	The term edema indicates a _____.
	7-17 When body tissues contain an excessive amount of fluid that causes swelling, the term designated in a medical report for this condition would be _____.
edema ĕ-DĒ-mă	
	7-18 Diuretics are agents or drugs prescribed to control edema and stimulate the flow of urine. Edema around the ankles and feet also may be due to a diet that is high in sodium. When this occurs, the physician may recommend a low-sodium diet and prescribe an agent known as a
diuretic dī-ū-RĔT-ĭc	_____.
	7-19 Coffee increases the production of urine, which means that
diuretic dī-ū-RĔT-ĭc	coffee is a _____ agent.

supra- **ren** **-al**	**7-20** *Supra/ren/al* is a directional term that means above the kidney. Identify the elements in this frame that mean above, excessive, superior: _____. kidney: _____. pertaining to, relating to: _____.
scler/o	**7-21** The combining form **scler/o** is used in words to indicate a hardening of a body part. It also refers to the sclera (white of eye) (see Chapter 11). To indicate a hardening, use the combining form _____ / _____.
hardening	**7-22** Scler/osis is an abnormal condition of _____.
nephr/osis něf-RŌ-sĭs **nephr/o/scler/osis** něf-rō-sklĕ-RŌ-sĭs **nephr/o/lith** NĚF-rō-lĭth **nephr/o/lith/iasis** něf-rō-lĭth-Ī-ă-sĭs	**7-23** Hyper/tension damages the kidneys by causing sclerotic changes, such as arteriosclerosis with thickening and hardening of the renal blood vessels *(nephr/o/scler/osis)*. Use **nephr/o** to form medical words meaning abnormal condition of a kidney: _____ / _____. abnormal condition of kidney hardening: _____ / _____ / _____ / _____. stone in a kidney: _____ / _____ / _____. abnormal condition of kidney stone(s): _____ / _____ / _____ / _____.
-megaly	**7-24** The suffix for enlargement is _____.
nephr/o/megaly něf-rō-MĚG-ă-lē	**7-25** When the kidneys become diseased, an enlargement of one or both kidneys may result. Use **nephr/o** to create a word meaning enlargement of a kidney: _____ / _____ / _____
kidney **stone *or* calculus**	**7-26** A lith/o/tomy is an incision to remove a stone or calculus. A nephr/o/lith/o/tomy is an incision of the _____ to remove a _____.

nephr/ectomy ně-FRĚK-tō-mē **nephr/o/rrhaphy** něf-ROR-ă-fē **nephr/o/tomy** ně-FRŎT-ō-mē **nephr/o/lith/o/tomy** něf-rō-lǐth-ŎT-ō-mē	**7-27** Many kidney disorders can be treated surgically. Learn these procedures by building surgical terms with **nephr/o** that mean excision of a kidney: _____ / _____ . suture of a kidney: _____ / ___ / _____ . incision of the kidney: _____ / ___ / _____ . incision (to remove a) kidney stone: _____ / ___ / _____ / ___ / _____ .
nephr/o/ptosis něf-rŏp-TŌ-sǐs	**7-28** A kidney may prolapse or drop from its normal position because of a birth defect or injury. The downward displacement may occur because the kidney supports are weakened due to the sudden strain or blow. Nephr/o/ptosis occurs, also called a floating kidney. A person who has a prolapsed kidney is suffering from a condition called _____ / ___ / _____ .
-ptosis **nephr/o**	**7-29** Determine the element in nephr/o/ptosis that means prolapse, downward displacement: _____ . kidney: _____ / ___ .
nephr/o/ptosis něf-rŏp-TŌ-sǐs	**7-30** A downward displacement of a kidney, or kidneys, because of a congenital defect or injury also is called _____ / ___ / _____ .
nephr/o/pexy NĚF-rō-pěks-ē	**7-31** Nephr/o/ptosis can be treated surgically. Use -pexy to build a surgical procedure that means fixation of the kidney: _____ / ___ / _____

Using the following table, write the combining form, suffix, or prefix that matches its definition in the space provided to the left of the definition. There may be more than one word element that matches a definition.

Combining Forms	Suffixes	Prefixes
lith/o	-iasis	dia-
nephr/o	-megaly	poly-
ren/o	-osis	supra-
scler/o	-pathy	
	-pexy	
	-ptosis	
	-rrhaphy	
	-tome	
	-tomy	

1. _____ abnormal condition; increase (used primarily with blood cells)

2. _____ abnormal condition (produced by something specified)

3. _____ above; excessive; superior

4. _____ disease

5. _____ enlargement

6. _____ through, across

7. _____ fixation (of an organ)

8. _____ hardening; sclera (white of eye)

9. _____ instrument to cut

10. _____ incision

11. _____ kidney

12. _____ prolapse, downward displacement

13. _____ stone, calculus

14. _____ suture

15. _____ many, much

Competency Verification: Check your answers in Appendix B, Answer Key, page 522. If you are not satisfied with your level of comprehension, go back to Frame 7–1 and rework the frames.

Correct Answers _____ × 6.67 = _____% Score

Making a set of flash cards from key word elements in this chapter for each section review can help you remember the elements. Make a flash card by writing a word element on one side of a 3 × 5 or 4 × 6 index card. On the other side, write the meaning of the element. Do this for all word elements in the section reviews. Use your flash cards to review each section. You also might use the flash cards to prepare for the chapter review at the end of this chapter.

Ureters, Bladder, Urethra

	7–32 When urine is formed, it is conveyed from each kidney through the (7) **ureters** and stored in the (8) **urinary bladder** until it is expelled from the body through the (9) **urethra** and (10) **urinary meatus**. Label Figure 7–2 to locate the urinary structures.
ureters Ū-rĕ-tĕrs	**7–33** Locate the two pencil-like tubes in Figure 7–2 that transport urine from the kidneys to the urinary bladder. These are the _____.
enlargement, ureter(s) Ū-rĕ-tĕr	**7–34** The combining form **ureter/o** refers to the *ureter.* Ureter/o/megaly is an _____ of the _____.
ureter/o **-ectasis**	**7–35** Ureter/ectasis is a dilation of the ureter. The combining form for ureter is _____ /_____. The element that denotes dilation or expansion is _____.
calculi KĂL-kū-lī	**7–36** A renal calculus (see Figure 7–3), also called kidney stone, is a concretion occurring in the kidney. If the stone is large enough to block the ureter and stop the flow of urine from the kidney, it must be removed. When there is one stone, it is referred to as a calculus, but multiple stones are referred to as _____.
crushing	**7–37** When stones are found in the kidneys, the condition is called *nephr/o/lith/iasis.* A person with this condition may experience pain or other difficulties. Lith/o/tripsy therapy may be used to break the stones into smaller parts that can be removed or expelled in the urine. There are different forms of lith/o/tripsy, but the term literally means stone or calculus _____.
ureter/o/lith ū-RĒ-tĕr-ō-lĭth **ureter/o/lith/iasis** ū-rē-tĕr-ō-lĭth-Ī-ă-sĭs	**7–38** Ureter/itis may be caused by infection or by the mechanical irritation of a stone. Develop some applicable terms related to ureter stones by building words that mean stone or calculus in the ureter: _____ /_____ /_____. abnormal condition (produced by something specified) of a ureter(al) stone: _____ /_____ /_____ /_____.
incision **ureter, stone *or* calculus**	**7–39** Ureter/o/lith/o/tomy is an _____ of a _____ to remove a _____.

dilation **ureter** DĪ-lā-shŭn, Ū-rĕ-tĕr	**7–40** Ureter/ectasis is an expansion or _____ of a _____.
ureter/ectasis ū-rē-tĕr-ĔK-tă-sĭs	**7–41** When kidney stones get trapped in the ureter, the urine is blocked, causing pressure on the walls of the ureter. This blockage results in an expansion or dilation of the ureter, which is called _____ / _____.

Competency Verification: Check your labeling of Figure 7–2 with Appendix B, Answer Key, page 522.

cyst/o/lith SĬS-tō-lĭth **cyst/o/lith/iasis** sĭs-tō-lĭ-THĪ-ă-sĭs **cyst/o/lith/o/tomy** sĭs-tō-lĭth-ŎT-ō-mē	**7–42** The urinary bladder, which is a muscular sac, stores urine until it is voided. The combining forms **cyst/o** and **vesic/o** are used in words to refer to the *bladder.* Use **cyst/o** to form words meaning stone in the bladder: _____ / ____ / _____. abnormal condition of a bladder stone: _____ / ____ / _____ / _____. incision of the bladder to remove a stone: _____ / ____ / _____ / ____ / _____.
instrument **ureter(s)**	**7–43** A ureter/o/cyst/o/scope is a special _____ for examining the _____ and bladder.
ureter/algia ū-rē-tĕr-ĂL-jē-ă	**7–44** When ureter/o/liths become trapped in the ureter, a person may experience ureter/o/dynia or _____ / _____.
ureter/o/liths ū-RĒ-tĕr-ō-lĭths **ureter/o/cyst/o/scope** ū-rē-tĕr-ō-SĬS-tō-skōp **ureter/o/cyst/o/scopy** ū-rē-tĕr-ō-sĭs-TŎS-kō-pē	**7–45** Form medical words to mean stones in the ureter: _____ / ____ / _____. an instrument to view the ureter and bladder: _____ / ____ / _____ / ____ / _____. visual examination of the ureter and bladder: _____ / ____ / _____ / ____ / ____.
suture SŪ-chūr	**7–46** The surgical suffix -rrhaphy is used in words to mean _____.

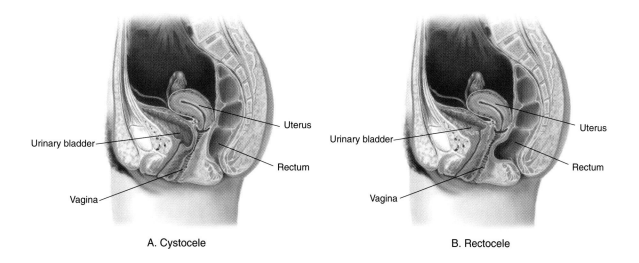

A. Cystocele   B. Rectocele

Figure 7-4   Herniations. (A) Cystocele. (B) Rectocele.

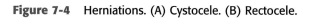

ureter/o/rrhaphy ū-rē-tĕr-OR-ră-fē **cyst/o/rrhaphy** sĭs-TOR-ă-fē	**7-47** Construct surgical words meaning suture of the ureter: _____ / ____ / _____. suture of the bladder: _____ / ____ / _____.
vesic/o, cyst/o	**7-48** The combining forms for bladder are _____ / ____ and _____ / ____.
bladder **intestine**	**7-49** Vesic/o/enter/ic means pertaining to the _____ and _____.
	7-50 A *hernia,* also referred to as a *rupture,* is a protrusion of an anatomical structure through the wall that normally contains it. Hernias may develop in several parts of the body. Two examples of hernias, a cyst/o/cele and a rect/o/cele, are illustrated in Figure 7–4. A cyst/o/cele is the herniation of part of the urinary bladder through the vaginal wall caused by weakened pelvic muscles. A rect/o/cele is the herniation of a portion of the rectum toward the vagina through weakened vaginal wall muscles (see Figure 7–4). Define the following word elements in this frame:
bladder **hernia, swelling** **rectum** RĔK-tŭm	**cyst/o:** _____. -cele: _____, _____. **rect/o:** _____.

cyst/o/cele SĬS-tō-sēl	**7-51** *Cyst/o/cele* develops over years as vaginal wall muscles weaken and no longer can support the weight of the urine in the urinary bladder. This condition usually occurs after a woman has delivered several infants. It also occurs in elderly persons because of weakened pelvic muscles resulting from the aging process. When the physician concludes a herniation into the bladder, you know the diagnosis will most likely be stated as a _____ / _____ / _____.
rect/o/cele RĔK-tō-sēl	**7-52** Can you determine the dx of herniation of the rectum into the vagina? _____ / _____ / _____.
nephr/o/ptosis nĕf-rŏp-TŌ-sĭs **nephr/o/pexy** NĔF-rō-pĕks-ē	**7-53** Build medical words meaning prolapse or downward displacement of a kidney: _____ / _____ / _____. surgical fixation of kidney: _____ / _____ / _____.
cyst/o/scope SĬST-ō-skōp **cyst/o/scopy** sĭs-TŎS-kō-pē	**7-54** Cyst/o/scopy is the direct visual examination of the urinary tract by means of a special instrument called a cyst/o/scope that is inserted through the urethra. The endoscope used to perform cyst/o/scopy is specifically called a _____ / _____ / _____. The cyst/o/scope is used to perform the diagnostic procedure called _____ / _____ / _____.
cyst/o/scope SĬST-ō-skōp	**7-55** The cyst/o/scope consists of a hollow tube and optical lighting system for viewing the bladder. Operative devices are inserted through the cyst/o/scope to obtain biopsy specimens of tumors or other growths and for removing polyps or stones. To excise polyps from the urinary bladder, the physician uses the special instrument called a _____ / _____ / _____.
cyst/o **-scope**	**7-56** Besides inserting operative devices through a cyst/o/scope, catheters also are placed through the cyst/o/scope to obtain urine samples and to inject contrast agents into the bladder during radi/o/graphy. Determine the elements in this frame that mean bladder: _____ / _____. instrument for examining: _____.

radi/o **-graphy**	radiation, x-ray; radius (lower arm bone on thumb side): _____ / ____. process of recording: _____.
cyst/ectomy sĭs-TĔK-tō-mē **cyst/o/plasty** SĬS-tō-plăs-tē **cyst/o/scope** SĬST-ō-skōp	**7-57** Construct surgical words meaning excision of the bladder: _____ / _____. surgical repair of the bladder: _____ / ____ / _____. instrument to view the bladder: _____ / ____ / _____.
urethr/o	**7-58** The urethra differs in men and women. In men, it serves a dual purpose of conveying sperm and discharging urine from the bladder. The female urethra performs only the latter function. Regardless of the sex, the combining form for urethra is _____ / ____ .
urethr/itis ū-rē-THRĪ-tĭs **urethr/ectomy** ū-rē-THRĔK-tō-mē **urethr/o/pexy** ū-RĒ-thrō-pĕks-ē **urethr/o/plasty** ū-RĒ-thrō-plăs-tē	**7-59** Form medical words meaning inflammation of the urethra: _____ / _____. excision of the urethra: _____ / _____. surgical fixation of the urethra: _____ / ____ / _____. surgical repair of the urethra: _____ / ____ / _____.
pain, urethra ū-RĒ-thră	**7-60** Urethr/o/dynia is a _____ in the _____.
urethr/algia ū-rē-THRĂL-jē-ă	**7-61** Besides urethr/o/dynia, construct another word meaning pain in the urethra: _____ / _____.
cyst/itis sĭs-TĪ-tĭs **urethr/itis** ū-rē-THRĪ-tĭs **UTI**	**7-62** Cyst/itis and urethr/itis are two common lower urinary tract infections (UTIs) that frequently occur in women. Write the terms that mean inflammation of the bladder: _____ / _____. urethra: _____ / _____. Write the abbreviation for urinary tract infection: _____.

7-63 Urethr/al stricture is a narrowing of the lumen (a tubular space within a structure) caused by scar tissue. Urethr/al stricture commonly results when catheters or surgical instruments are inserted into the urethra. Other causes are untreated gonorrhea and congenital abnormalities. A person with urethr/al stricture has a diminished urinary stream and is prone to develop UTIs because of obstruction of urine flow.

Let us review some of the terminology in this frame by identifying terms that mean

pertaining to the urethra: _____ / _____.

tubular space within a structure: _____.

Write the abbreviation for urinary tract infections: _____.

urethr/al
ū-RĒ-thrăl
lumen
LŪ-měn
UTIs

7-64 Urethr/o/rect/al means pertaining to the

_____ and _____.

urethra, rectum
ū-RĒ-thră, RĔK-tŭm

7-65 Construct a medical word that means inflammation of the urethra and bladder: _____ / ____ / _____ / _____.

urethr/o/cyst/itis
ū-rē-thrō-sĭs-TĪ-tĭs

7-66 Form diagnostic terms that mean

instrument for examining the urethra:

_____ / ____ / _____.

visual examination of the urethra:

_____ / ____ / _____.

urethr/o/scope
ū-RĒ-thrō-skōp

urethr/o/scopy
ū-rē-THRŎS-kō-pē

7-67 Cyst/o/urethr/o/scopy is a visual examination of the urethra and bladder. The instrument used to perform a cyst/o/urethr/o/scopy is a

_____ / ____ / _____ / ____ / _____.

cyst/o/urethr/o/scope
sĭs-tō-ū-RĒ-thrō-skōp

7-68 Identify the element that denotes a noun ending in -algia, -dynia, -pepsia, and -phagia: _____.

-ia

7-69 The element in the suffixes in Frame 7-68 that means condition is _____.

-ia

7-70 Malignant tumors or growths are cancerous, whereas benign tumors are noncancerous. Use the words malignant or benign to complete this frame.

A cancerous tumor is a _____ tumor.

A noncancerous tumor is a _____ tumor.

malignant
mă-LĬG-nănt
benign
bĕ-NĪN

noncancerous	**7-71** Benign tumors are contained within a capsule and do not invade the surrounding tissue. They harm the individual only in that they place pressure on adjacent structures. Benign tumors are (cancerous, non cancerous) _____ growths.
cancerous	**7-72** Malignant tumors spread rather rapidly, are invasive, and are life-threatening. Malignant tumors are (cancerous, noncancerous) _____.
pain, gland	**7-73** The combining form **aden/o** is used in words to denote a *gland*. An aden/o/dynia is a _____ in a _____.
gland **cancer** **tumor**	**7-74** Tumors of the urinary tract may be benign or malignant. An aden/o/carcin/oma is the most common malignant tumor of the kidney. Analyze aden/o/carcin/oma by defining the elements: **aden/o** refers to _____. **carcin/o** refers to _____. -oma refers to _____.
aden/oma ăd-ĕ-NŌ-mă **aden/o/carcin/oma** ăd-ĕ-nō-kăr-sĭn-Ō-mă	**7-75** An aden/oma is a benign glandular tumor composed of the tissue from which it is developing; an aden/o/carcin/oma is a malignant glandular tumor. Determine the words in this frame that mean benign glandular tumor: _____ / _____. malignant glandular tumor: _____ / _____ / _____ / _____.
aden/itis ăd-ĕ-NĪ-tĭs **aden/oma** ăd-ĕ-NŌ-mă **aden/o/pathy** ăd-ĕ-NŎP-ă-thē	**7-76** Form medical words to mean inflammation of a gland: _____ / _____. tumor of a gland: _____ / _____. any disease of a gland: _____ / _____ / _____.
urinary tract infections	**7-77** Urinary tract infections (UTIs) account for most office visits by individuals experiencing urinary tract problems. Define UTIs: _____ _____ _____.
	7-78 Recall that *nephrons* (see Figure 7–2, structure 6) are microscopic filtering units of the kidney designed to filter urea and other waste products effectively from the blood. They also are responsible for maintaining homeostasis (keeping body fluids in balance).

7-79 Urine is collected in the funnel-shaped extensions called the **calyces** (singular, calyx) and empties into the **renal pelvis** and into the ureters, which convey it to the urinary bladder to be stored until the urine is expelled through the urethra during the process of urination, or micturition.

Locate the two structures in Figure 7–1 to see the path of urine as it is expelled through the ureters.

7-80 The combining form **pyel/o** refers to the *renal pelvis*. Pelvis is a word denoting any bowl-shaped structure. Pyel/itis is an

inflammation

_____ of the renal pelvis.

7-81 Construct medical words meaning

pyel/o/pathy
pī-ĕ-LŎP-ă-thē

disease of the renal pelvis: _____ / _____ / _____.

pyel/o/tomy
pī-ĕ-LŎT-ō-mē

incision of the renal pelvis: _____ / _____ / _____.

forming an opening (mouth) into the renal pelvis:

pyel/o/stomy
pī-ĕ-LŎS-tō-mē

_____ / _____ / _____.

Listen and Learn, the audio CD-ROM that accompanies this book, will help you master the pronunciation of selected medical words. Use it to practice pronunciations *of selected terms* from Frames *7–1 to 7–81* for instructions to complete the *Listen and Learn* exercise on the CD-ROM for this section.

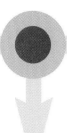

SECTION REVIEW 7 – 3

Using the following table, write the combining form or suffix that matches its definition in the space provided to the left of the definition. There may be more than one word element that matches a definition.

Combining Forms	Suffixes
aden/o	-ectomy
carcin/o	-ectasis
cyst/o	-iasis
enter/o	-itis
pyel/o	-lith
rect/o	-megaly
ureter/o	-oma
urethr/o	-pathy
vesic/o	-plasty
	-rrhaphy
	-scope
	-tomy

1. _____ abnormal condition (produced by something specified)
2. _____ bladder
3. _____ cancer
4. _____ disease
5. _____ enlargement
6. _____ excision, removal
7. _____ dilation, expansion
8. _____ gland
9. _____ incision
10. _____ inflammation
11. _____ instrument for examining
12. _____ intestine (usually small intestine)
13. _____ renal pelvis
14. _____ rectum
15. _____ stone, calculus
16. _____ surgical repair
17. _____ suture
18. _____ tumor
19. _____ ureter
20. _____ urethra

Competency Verification: Check your answers in Appendix B, Answer Key, page 522. If you are not satisfied with your level of comprehension, go back to Frame 7–32 and rework the frames.

Correct Answers _____ × 5 = _____% Score

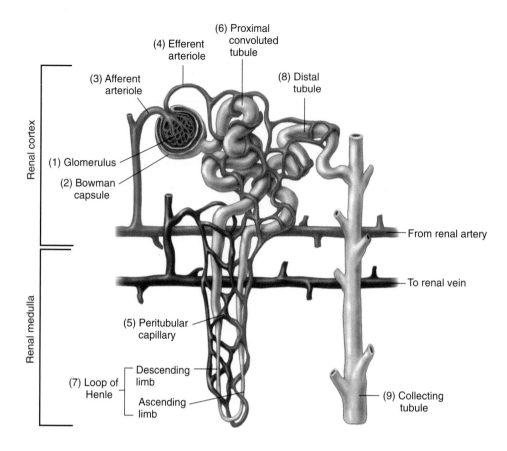

Figure 7-5   Nephron structure.

Nephron Structure

7–82   Label Figure 7–5 as you read the following information. The kidney is composed of an outer layer, called the (1) **renal cortex**, and an inner region, called the (2) **renal medulla.**

7–83   The nephrons, more than 1 million microscopic filtering units in each kidney, are designed to form urine in the process of filtration, reabsorption, and secretion.

Besides numerous other structures, each nephron contains a tiny ball of small, coiled, and intertwined capillaries called the (3) **glomerulus** (plural, glomeruli) and a (4) **collecting tubule.** The collecting tubule conveys the newly formed urine to the renal pelvis for excretion by the kidneys. The nephrons maintain homeostasis in the body by selectively removing waste products from the blood by forming urine, which is expelled from the body. The capsule that surrounds and encloses the glomerulus is (5) **Bowman capsule.**

7–84   An inflammatory disease of the glomerulus known as glomerul/o/nephr/itis is characterized by hyper/tension, olig/uria, electrolyte imbalances, and edema.

hyper/tension hī-pĕr-TĔN-shŭn **olig/uria** ŏl-ĭg-Ū-rē-ă **edema** ĕ-DĒ-mă **glomerul/o/nephr/itis** glō-mĕr-ū-lō-nĕ-FRĬ-tĭs	Identify terms in this frame that are related to high blood pressure: _____ / _____. diminished capacity to pass urine: _____ / _____. swelling (of a body part): _____. inflammation of the glomerulus: _____ / __ / _____ / _____.
glomerul/itis glō-mĕr-ū-LĪ-tĭs **glomerul/o/pathy** glō-mĕr-ū-LŎP-ă-thē	**7-85** Use glomerul/o to form medical words meaning inflammation of a glomerulus: _____ / _____. disease of a glomerulus: _____ / __ / _____.
glomerulus *or* **glomeruli, hardening** glō-MĔR-ū-lŭs, glō-MĔR-ū-lī	**7-86** Glomerul/o/scler/osis literally means an abnormal condition of _____ _____.

Competency Verification: Check your labeling of Figure 7–5 with Appendix B, Answer Key, page 523.

pyel/itis pī-ĕ-LĪ-tĭs	**7-87** The renal pelvis (see Figure 7–1) is a funnel-shaped dilation that drains urine from the kidney into the ureter. An inflammation of the renal pelvis is called _____ / _____.
      KUB	**7-88** To determine urinary tract abnormalities, such as tumors, swollen kidneys, and calculi, the physician may order a radi/o/graph/ic examination called *KUB (kidney, ureter, bladder)*. The radi/o/graph identifies the location, size, shape, and malformation of the kidneys, ureters, and bladder. Stones and calcified areas also may be detected. The diagnostic test of the kidneys, ureters, and bladder may be recorded in the medical chart with the abbreviation _____.
	7-89 Pyel/o/graphy, an important diagnostic tool, provides x-ray images of the renal pelvis and urinary tract after injection of a contrast medium (intra/ven/ous pyel/o/gram). Multiple radiographs of the urinary tract are taken while the contrast medium is excreted, providing detailed information about the structure and function of the kidneys, ureters, bladder, and urethra. Intra/ven/ous pyel/o/graphy (IVP) is used to detect nephr/o/liths and other lesions that may block or irritate the urinary tract.

intra/ven/ous ĭn-tră-VĒ-nŭs **pyel/o/graphy (IVP)** pī-ĕ-LŎG-ră-fē	To confirm a diagnosis of renal stones or other disorders that obstruct or irritate the urinary tract, the physician may order a radiograph that involves intravenous injection of a contrast medium. This type of radiography is known as _____ / _____ / _____ _____ / ____ / _____ (____).
intra/ven/ous ĭn-tră-VĒ-nŭs	**7–90** When a patient has a contrast medium injected within a vein, we are talking about a procedure that is an _____ / _____ / _____ injection.
intra/ven/ous ĭn-tră-VĒ-nŭs **pyel/o/graphy (IVP)** pī-ĕ-LŎG-ră-fē **retro/grade** RĔT-rō-grād **pyel/o/graphy (RP)** pī-ĕ-LŎG-ră-fē	**7–91** The prefix retro- means *backward, behind*. The suffix -grade means *to go*. The term retro/grade is used to describe a specific type of pyel/o/graphy. Retro/grade pyel/o/graphy consists of radiographic images taken after a contrast medium is injected through a urinary catheter directly into the urethra, bladder, and ureters. Pyel/o/graphy in which a contrast medium is injected within a vein is called _____ / _____ / _____ _____ / ____ / _____ (_____). Pyel/o/graphy in which a contrast medium is injected into the urethra is called _____ / _____ _____ / ____ / _____ (_____).
pyel/itis pī-ĕ-LĪ-tĭs **pyel/o/plasty** PĪ-ĕ-lō-plăs-tē **ureter/o/pyel/o/plasty** ū-rē-tĕr-ō-PĪ-ĕl-ō-plăs-tē	**7–92** Build medical terms that mean inflammation of the renal pelvis: _____ / _____. surgical repair of the renal pelvis: _____ / ____ / _____. surgical repair of the ureter and renal pelvis: _____ / _____ / ____ / _____ / _____.
intra/ven/ous ĭn-tră-VĒ-nŭs **pyel/o/gram** PĪ-ĕ-lō-grăm **nephr/o/liths** NĔF-rō-lĭths **ureter/o/liths** ū-RĒ-tĕr-ō-lĭths	**7–93** An intra/ven/ous pyel/o/gram provides visualization of urinary structures. It is used to assess the urinary tract to verify kidney function and identify nephr/o/liths and ureter/o/liths. Determine the words in this frame that mean within a vein: _____ / _____ / _____. record (x-ray) of the renal pelvis: _____ / ____ / _____. stones in the kidney: _____ / ____ / _____. stones in the ureter: _____ / ____ / _____.

nephr/o/scope NĔF-rō-skōp **nephr/o/scopy** nĕ-FRŎ-skŏ-pē	**7-94** The nephr/o/scope, a fiberoptic instrument, is used specifically for visualization of the kidney to disintegrate and remove renal calculi. Use **nephr/o** to construct medical terms meaning instrument for examining the kidney: _____ / _____ / _____. visual examination of the kidney: _____ / _____ / _____.
nephr/o/scopy nĕ-FRŎ-skŏ-pē	**7-95** An incision of the renal pelvis is performed when the physician inserts a nephr/o/scope, usually to assess the inside of the kidney. A visual examination of the kidney is known as _____ / _____ / _____.
pyel/itis pī-ĕ-LĪ-tĭs **pyel/o/nephr/itis** pī-ĕ-lō-nĕ-FRĪ-tĭs	**7-96** Pyel/o/nephr/itis is a bacterial infection of the renal pelvis and kidney caused by bacterial invasion from the middle and lower urinary tract or bloodstream. Bacteria may gain access to the bladder via the urethra and ascend to the kidney. Form medical words meaning inflammation of the renal pelvis: _____ / _____. renal pelvis and kidney : _____ / _____ / _____ / _____.
pyel/o/nephr/itis pī-ĕ-lō-nĕ-FRĪ-tĭs	**7-97** Pyel/o/nephr/itis is an extremely dangerous condition, especially in pregnant women, because it can cause premature labor. A woman who has a bacterial infection of the renal pelvis and kidneys has a condition called _____ / _____ / _____ / _____.
bladder **urethra** ū-RĒ-thră **rectum** RĔK-tŭm **intestine** ĭn-TĔS-tĭn	**7-98** Four common types of hernias (see Figure 7–4) that occur as downward displacements are cyst/o/cele: herniation of the _____. urethr/o/cele: herniation of the _____. rect/o/cele: herniation of the _____. enter/o/cele: herniation of the _____.

	7-99 In the female, the bladder, urethra, or rectum may herniate into the vagina as illustrated in Figure 7–4.
	Practice building medical terms that mean herniation of the
cyst/o/cele SĬS-tō-sēl	bladder: _____ / ____ / _____.
urethr/o/cele ū-RĒ-thrō-sēl	urethra: _____ / ____ / _____.
rect/o/cele RĔK-tō-sēl	rectum: _____ / ____ / _____.
	7-100 The combining form **erythr/o** denotes the color *red*, and **leuk/o** denotes *white*.
white	Leuk/o/rrhea is a discharge that is _____.
red	Erythr/uria is urine that is _____.
	7-101 The combining form for cell is **cyt/o.** The suffix -cyte also means *cell*.
cell	An erythr/o/cyte is a red blood _____.
cell	A leuk/o/cyte is a white blood _____.
	7-102 Ur/o/toxin is a poisonous substance in the
urine Ū-rĭn	_____.
	7-103 From ur/o/toxin, determine the element meaning poisonous:
toxin TŎKS-ĭn	_____.
	7-104 A toxic substance in the body is a substance that resembles or is
poison	caused by _____.
	7-105 Use **ur/o** to form words meaning
ur/o/logy ū-RŎL-ō-jē	study of urine: _____ / ____ / _____.
ur/o/logist ū-RŎL-ō-jĭst	specialist in the study of urine: _____ / ____ / _____.

 Two combining forms that sound alike but have different meanings are **pyel/o** and **py/o.** Here is a useful clarification:

Combining Form	Meaning	Example
pyel/o	renal pelvis	pyel/o/pathy
py/o	pus	py/o/rrhea

pyel/o/plasty
PĪ-ĕ-lō-plăs-tē
pyel/o/gram
PĪ-ĕ-lō-grăm

7-106   Form medical words that mean

surgical repair of the renal pelvis: _____ / ____ / _____.

record (x-ray) of the renal pelvis: _____ / ____ / _____.

py/o/rrhea
pī-ō-RĒ-ă

py/o/nephr/osis
pī-ō-nĕf-RŌ-sĭs

7-107   Use **py/o** *(pus)* to build words meaning

discharge or flow of pus: _____ / ____ / _____.

abnormal condition of pus from the kidney:

_____ / ____ / _____ / _____.

Note: Remember not to use -iasis because the pus is not produced by something specified; the term just denotes that there is pus in the kidneys.

ALERT

py/uria
pī-Ū-rē-ă

7-108   An important diagnostic test that provides early detection of renal problems is the urinalysis. Individual voidings are analyzed for abnormalities, such as foul odors (often seen with infection), blood or pus in the urine, and other physical and chemical properties.

Hemat/uria is a condition of blood in the urine. Form a word meaning pus in the urine: _____ / _____.

an/uria
ăn-Ū-rē-ă

7-109   The prefixes a- and an- are used in words to mean *without* or *not*. The a- usually is used before a consonant. The an- usually is used before a vowel.

Construct a word that literally means without urine: _____ / _____.

hydr/o/nephr/osis
hī-drō-nĕf-RŌ-sĭs

7-110   Hydr/o/nephr/osis, an abnormal dilation of the ren/al pelvis and the calyces of one or both kidneys, is caused by an obstruction of urine production. Although a partial obstruction may not produce symptoms initially, the pressure built up behind the area of obstruction eventually results in symptoms of ren/al dysfunction.

When calculi obstruction causes a cessation of urine flow, it may result in a condition called _____ / ____ / _____ / _____.

hydr/o/nephr/osis
hī-drō-nĕf-RŌ-sĭs

7-111   The presence of ren/al calculi increases the risk for urinary tract infections (UTIs) because the free flow of urine is obstructed. Untreated obstruction of a stone in any of the urinary structures also can result in retention of urine and damage to the kidney.

This condition, known as

_____ / ____ / _____ / _____ eventually results in cessation of urine production.

py/uria pī-Ū-rē-ă **hemat/uria** hĕm-ă-TŪ-rē-ă	**7-112** A person who has hydr/o/nephr/osis may experience pain, hemat/uria, and py/uria. Blood or pus may be present in the urine. Build medical words that mean pus in the urine: _____ / _____. blood in the urine: _____ / _____.
olig/uria ŏl-ĭg-Ū-rē-ă	**7-113** The combining form **olig/o** means *scanty*, or *little*. Combine **olig/o** and -uria to form a word meaning scanty urination: _____ / _____.
olig/uria ŏl-ĭg-Ū-rē-ă	**7-114** A diminished or scanty amount of urine formation is known as _____ / _____.
py/uria pī-Ū-rē-ă	**7-115** Py/uria is the presence of an excessive number of white blood cells in the urine. It is generally a sign of a urinary tract infection. A viral infection of the bladder and urethra may result in the condition called _____ / _____.
poly/uria pŏl-ē-Ū-rē-ă	**7-116** The prefix poly- means *many, much*. Combine poly- and -uria to build a word that means excessive urination: _____ / _____.
poly/cyst/ic pŏl-ē-SĬS-tĭk **ur/emia** ū-RĒ-mē-ă	**7-117** An abnormal condition in which the kidneys are enlarged and contain many cysts is poly/cyst/ic kidney disease (PKD). Kidney failure develops from this disease and progresses to ur/emia and eventually death. Identify the terms in this frame that mean pertaining to many cysts: _____ / _____ / _____. increase in concentration of urea and other nitrogenous wastes in the blood: _____ / _____.
azot/uria ăz-ō-TŪ-rē-ă	**7-118** Azot/emia also means an increase in concentration of urea and other nitrogenous wastes in blood. Use **azot/o** to form a word meaning increase of nitrogenous wastes in urine. _____ / _____.
noct/uria nŏk-TŪ-rē-ă	**7-119** Noct/uria refers to urination at night. If a child has a tendency to urinate at night, the condition is known as _____ / _____.

urination
ū-rǐ-NĀ-shŭn

7-120   Continence indicates self-control and is the ability to control urination and defecation. A person who has urinary continence is able to control urination. A person with urinary in/continence is not able to control

_____.

in/continence
ĭn-KŎN-tĭ-nĕns

7-121   Many patients in nursing homes experience uncontrolled loss of urine from the bladder. These patients have urinary

_____ / _____.

ur/o/logist *or*
nephr/o/logist
ū-RŎL-ō-jĭst,
nĕ-FRŎL-ō-jĭst

7-122   Persons with urinary disorders see the medical specialist called a

_____ / _____ / _____.

hemat/uria
hĕm-ă-TŪ-rē-ă

7-123   Cyst/itis, an inflammatory condition of the urinary bladder, frequently is caused by bacterial infection and is characterized by pain, frequency of urination, and hemat/uria.

If cyst/itis results in traces of blood in the urine, the medical term for this condition is _____ / _____.

cyst/itis
sĭs-TĪ-tĭs

7-124   When a patient has inflammation of the bladder, the condition is diagnosed as _____ / _____.

dys/uria
dĭs-Ū-rē-ă
bacteri/uria
băk-tē-rē-Ū-rē-ă
py/uria
pī-Ū-rē-ă
cyst/itis
sĭs-TĪ-tĭs

7-125   Cyst/itis is more common in women, owing to their shorter urethra and the closeness of the urethr/al orifice to the anus. Symptoms of cyst/itis include dys/uria (painful urination), bacteri/uria (bacteria in the urine), and py/uria (pus in the urine).

Identify the words in this frame that mean

painful urination: _____ / _____.

bacteria in the urine: _____ / _____.

pus in the urine: _____ / _____.

inflammation of the bladder: _____ / _____.

7-126 Pyel/o/nephr/itis, an inflammation of the renal pelvis and the kidney, is a common type of kidney disease and a frequent complication of cystitis.

Build a medical term that means an inflammation of the

nephr/itis
nĕf-RĪ-tĭs

kidney: _____ / _____ .

pyel/o/nephr/itis
pī-ĕ-lō-nĕ-FRĪ-tĭs

renal pelvis and kidney:

_____ / _____ / _____ / _____ .

7-127 Glomerul/o/nephr/itis, a form of nephr/itis in which the lesions involve primarily the glomeruli, may result in protein/uria and hemat/uria.

Determine the medical words in this frame that mean

hemat/uria
hĕm-ă-TŪ-rē-ă
protein/uria
prō-tē-ĭn-Ū-rē-ă
nephr/itis
nĕf-RĪ-tĭs

blood in the urine: _____ / _____ .

protein in the urine: _____ / _____ .

inflammation of the kidney: _____ / _____ .

7-128 A form of nephr/itis that involves the glomeruli is called

glomerul/o/nephr/itis
glō-mĕr-Ū-lō-nĕ-FRĪ-tĭs

_____ / _____ / _____ / _____ .

7-129 Any condition that impairs flow of blood to the kidneys, such as shock, injury, or exposure to toxins, may result in acute renal failure (ARF).

The abbreviation ARF refers to

acute renal failure

_____ _____ _____ .

7-130 Nephr/o/lith/iasis occurs when salts in the urine precipitate (settle out of solution and grow in size). Elimination of the stone(s) may occur spontaneously, but crushing the stone(s) by means of lith/o/tripsy sometimes may be necessary.

Build medical terms that mean

lith/ectomy
lĭ-THĔK-tō-mē
lith/o/tripsy
LĬTH-ō-trĭp-sē

excision of a stone: _____ / _____ .

crushing a stone: _____ / _____ / _____ .

nephr/o/lith/iasis
nĕf-rō-lĭth-Ī-ă-sĭs

abnormal condition (produced by something specified) of kidney stone(s):

_____ / _____ / _____ / _____ .

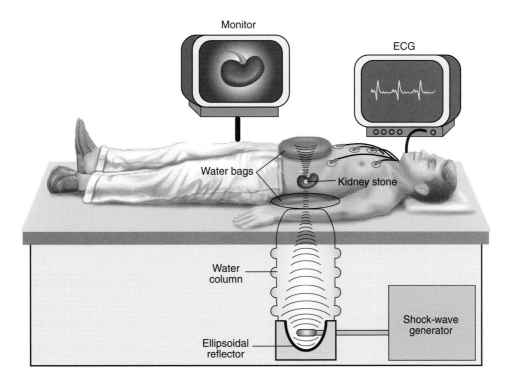

Figure 7-6 Extracorporeal shock-wave lithotripsy.

7-131 *Extracorporeal shock-wave lithotripsy (ESWL)* uses powerful sound wave vibrations to break up calculi in the urinary tract or gallbladder (see Figure 7–6). Ultrasound (US) is used to locate and monitor the stones as they are being destroyed. Complete removal of the stones and their fragments during urination is ensured by administration of an oral dissolution drug.

Identify the abbreviations for

ultrasound: _____.

extracorporeal shock-wave lithotripsy: _____.

US

ESWL

Listen and Learn, the audio CD-ROM that accompanies this book, will help you master the pronunciation of selected medical words. Use it to practice pronunciations *of selected terms* from Frames *7–82 to 7–131* for instructions to complete the *Listen and Learn* exercise on the CD-ROM for this section.

Using the following table, write the combining form, suffix, or prefix that matches its definition in the space provided to the left of the definition. There may be more than one word element that matches a definition.

Combining Forms	Suffixes	Prefixes
cyst/o	-cele	a-
cyt/o	-cyte	an-
erythr/o	-ist	intra-
glomerul/o	-ptosis	poly-
hemat/o		
leuk/o		
nephr/o		
olig/o		
pyel/o		
py/o		
ren/o		
scler/o		
ureter/o		
urethr/o		
ur/o		
vesic/o		

1. _____ bladder

2. _____ blood

3. _____ cell

4. _____ glomerulus

5. _____ hardening; sclera (white of eye)

6. _____ specialist

7. _____ kidney

8. _____ pus

9. _____ red

10. _____ renal pelvis

11. _____ scanty

12. _____ ureter

13. _____ urethra

14. _____ urine

15. _____ white

16. _____ hernia, swelling

17. _____ many, much

18. _____ prolapse, downward displacement

19. _____ in, within

20. _____ without, not

Competency Verification: Check your answers in Appendix B, Answer Key, page 523. If you are not satisfied with your level of comprehension, go back to Frame 7–82 and rework the frames.

Correct Answers _____ × 5 = _____% Score

Abbreviations

This section introduces urinary system–related abbreviations and their meanings. Included are abbreviations contained in the medical record activities that follow.

Abbreviation	Meaning	Abbreviation	Meaning
BUN	blood urea nitrogen	PSA	prostate-specific antigen
BNO	bladder neck obstruction	RP	retrograde pyelography
cysto	cystoscopic examination	TURP	transurethral resection of the prostate
DRE	digital rectal examination	UA	urinalysis
ESWL	extracorporeal shock-wave lithotripsy	US	ultrasonography, ultrasound
IVP	intravenous pyelogram	UTI	urinary tract infection
IVU	intravenous urography	VCUG	voiding cystourethrogram, voiding cystourethrography
KUB	kidney, ureter, bladder		

Pathological, Diagnostic, and Therapeutic Terms

The following are additional terms related to the urinary system. Recognizing and learning these terms will help you understand the connection between a pathological condition, its diagnosis, and the rationale behind the method of treatment selected for a particular disorder.

Pathological

azoturia (ăz-ō-TŪ-rē-ă): increase of nitrogenous substances, especially urea, in urine.

diuresis (dī-ū-RĒ-sĭs): increased formation and secretion of urine.

dysuria (dĭs-Ū-rē-ă): painful or difficult urination, symptomatic of cystitis and other urinary tract conditions.

end-stage renal disease (RĒ-năl): final phase of a kidney disease process; disease has advanced to the point that the kidneys no longer can filter the blood adequately.

enuresis (ĕn-ū-RĒ-sĭs): involuntary discharge of urine after the age by which bladder control should have been established.

In children, voluntary control of urination is usually present by age 5; also called bed-wetting at night or nocturnal enuresis.

hypospadias (hī-pō-SPĀ-dē-ăs): abnormal congenital opening of the male urethra on the undersurface of the penis.

interstitial nephritis (ĭn-tĕr-STĬSH-ăl nĕf-RĪ-tĭs): nephritis associated with pathological changes in the renal interstitial tissue that may be primary or due to a toxic agent, such as a drug or chemical. The end result is that the nephrons are destroyed and renal function is seriously impaired.

renal hypertension (RĒ-năl hī-pĕr-TĔN-shŭn): high blood pressure that results from kidney disease.

uremia (ū-RĒ-mē-ă): elevated level of urea and other nitrogenous waste products in the blood, as occurs in renal failure; also called azotemia.

Wilms tumor (VĬLMZ TOO-mŏr): malignant neoplasm of the kidney occurring in young children, usually before age 5 years. The most frequent early signs are hypertension, a palpable mass, pain, and hematuria.

Diagnostic

blood urea nitrogen (ū-RĒ-ă NĪ-trō-jĕn): laboratory test that measures the amount of urea (nitrogenous waste product) normally excreted by the kidneys into the blood. An increase in the blood urea nitrogen (BUN) level may indicate impaired kidney function.

computed tomography (CT) scan (kŏm-PŪ-tĕd tō-MŎG-ră-fē): radiographic technique that uses a narrow beam of x-rays, which rotates in a full arc around the patient to image the body in cross-sectional slices. A scanner and detector send the images to a computer, which consolidates all of the data it receives from the multiple x-ray views (see Figure 2–5A).

CT scanning is used to diagnose kidney, ureter, and bladder tumors, cysts, inflammation, abscesses, perforation, bleeding, and obstructions. It may be administered with or without a contrast medium.

intravenous pyelogram (ĭn-tră-VĒ-nŭs PĪ-ĕ-lō-grăm): radiographic procedure in which a contrast medium is injected intravenously and serial x-ray films are taken to provide visualization of and important information about the entire urinary tract: kidneys, ureters, bladder, and urethra; also called intravenous urography (IVU) or excretory urogram or IVP.

KUB: term used in a radiographic examination to determine the location, size, shape, and malformation of the kidneys, ureters, and bladder. Stones and calcified areas may be detected.

renal scan (RĒ-năl): imaging procedure that determines renal function and shape. A radioactive substance or radiopharmaceutical that concentrates in the kidney is injected intravenously. The radioactivity is measured as it accumulates in the kidneys and is recorded as an image. This is a nuclear medicine procedure.

retrograde pyelography (RĔT-rō-grād pī-ĕ-LŎG-ră-fē): radiographic procedure in which a contrast medium is introduced through a cystoscope directly into the bladder and ureters, using small-caliber catheters.

Retrograde pyelography (RP) provides detailed visualization of the urinary collecting system and is useful in locating obstruction in the urinary tract. It also may be used as a substitute for an IVP when a patient is allergic to the contrast medium.

urinalysis (ū-rĭ-NĂL-ĭ-sĭs): physical, chemical, and microscopic analysis of urine.

voiding cystourography (sĭs-TŎG-ră-fē): radiography of the bladder and urethra after the introduction of a contrast medium and during the process of voiding urine. The bladder is filled with an opaque contrast medium before the procedure.

Therapeutic

catheterization (kăth-ĕ-tĕr-ĭ-ZĀ-shŭn): insertion of a catheter (hollow flexible tube) into a body cavity or organ to instill a substance or remove fluid. The most common type is to insert a catheter through the urethra into the bladder to withdraw urine.

renal transplantation (RĒ-năl trăns-plăn-TĀ-shŭn): surgical transfer of a complete kidney from a donor to a recipient.

Listen and Learn, the audio CD-ROM that accompanies this book, will help you master the pronunciation of selected medical words. Use it to practice pronunciations of the above-listed medical terms and for instructions to complete the *Listen and Learn* exercise on the CD-ROM for this section.

PATHOLOGICAL, DIAGNOSTIC, AND THERAPEUTIC TERMS REVIEW

Match the medical term(s) below with the definitions in the numbered list.

azoturia   diuresis   interstitial nephritis   urinalysis
blood urea nitrogen dysuria   renal hypertension   voiding cystourography
catheterization   enuresis   retrograde pyelography   Wilms tumor
CT scan   hypospadias   uremia

1. _____ refers to microscopic examination of urine.

2. _____ is a malignant neoplasm in the kidney that occurs in young children.

3. _____ is an increase in nitrogenous compounds in urine.

4. _____ means painful or difficult urination, symptomatic of numerous conditions.

5. _____ means increased formation and secretion of urine.

6. _____ is a radiologic technique in which a contrast medium is introduced through a cystoscope into the bladder and ureters to provide detailed visualization of urinary collecting system.

7. _____ is an abnormal congenital opening of the male urethra on the undersurface of the penis.

8. _____ is nephritis associated with pathological changes in the renal interstitial tissue, which may be primary or due to a toxic agent, such as a drug or chemical.

9. _____ is a test that measures the amount of urea excreted by the kidneys into the blood.

10. _____ means urinary incontinence, including bed-wetting.

11. _____ refers to insertion of a hollow flexible tube into a body cavity or organ to instill a substance or remove fluid.

12. _____ is radiography of the bladder and urethra after the introduction of a contrast medium and during the process of urination.

13. _____ refers to an elevated level of urea and other nitrogenous waste products in the blood.

14. _____ refers to high blood pressure that results from kidney disease.

15. _____ is a diagnostic procedure that uses a narrow beam of x-rays, which rotates in a full arc around the patient to image the body in cross-sectional slices.

Competency Verification: Check your answers in Appendix B, Answer Key, page 523. If you are not satisfied with your level of comprehension, review the pathological, diagnostic, and therapeutic terms, and retake the review.

Correct Answers _____ × 6.67 = _____% Score

Medical Record Activities

The following medical records reflect common real-life clinical scenarios using medical terminology to document patient care. The physician who specializes in the treatment of urinary disorders is a *urologist;* the medical specialty concerned with the diagnosis and treatment of urinary disorders is *urology.* Because some urinary structures in the male perform a dual role, urinary functions and reproductive function (such as the urethra), the urologist also treats male reproductive disorders.

✓ MEDICAL RECORD ACTIVITY 7–1. Cystitis

Terminology

The terms listed in the chart come from the medical record *Cystitis* that follows. Use a medical dictionary such as *Taber's Cyclopedic Medical Dictionary,* the appendices of this book, or other resources to define each term. Then practice reading the pronunciations aloud for each term.

Term	Definition
cholecystectomy kō-lē-sĭs-TĔK-tō-mē	
cholecystitis kō-lē-sĭs-TĪ-tĭs	
choledocholithiasis kō-lĕd-ō-kō-lĭ-THĪ-ă-sĭs	
choledocholithotomy kō-lĕd-ō-kō-lĭth-ŎT-ō-mē	
cholelithiasis kō-lē-lĭ-THĪ-ă-sĭs	
cystitis sĭs-TĪ-tĭs	
cystoscopy sĭs-TŎS-kō-pē	
epigastric ĕp-ĭ-GĂS-trĭk	
hematuria hĕm-ă-TŪ-rē-ă	
nocturia nŏk-TŪ-rē-ă	
polyuria pŏl-ē-Ū-rē-ă	
urinary incontinence Ū-rĭ-nār-ē ĭn-KŎNT-ĭn-ĕns	

Listen and Learn Online! will help you master the pronunciation of selected medical words from this medical record activity. Visit www.fadavis.com/gylys/simplified for instructions in completing the *Listen and Learn Online!* exercise for this section and then to practice pronunciations.

CYSTITIS

Reading

Practice pronunciation of medical terms by reading the following medical report aloud.

This 50-year-old white woman has been complaining of diffuse pelvic pain with urinary bladder spasm since cystoscopy 10 days ago, at which time marked cystitis was noted. She reports nocturia three to four times, urinary frequency, urgency, and epigastric discomfort. The patient has had a history of polyuria, hematuria, and urinary incontinence. There is a history of numerous stones, large and small, in the gallbladder. In 19XX, she was admitted to the hospital with cholecystitis, chronic and acute; cholelithiasis; and choledocholithiasis. Subsequently, cholecystectomy, choledocholithotomy, and incidental appendectomy were performed. My impression is that the urinary incontinence is due to cystitis and is temporary in nature.

Evaluation

Review the medical record above to answer the following questions

1. What was found when the patient had a cystoscopy?

_____

_____

2. What are the symptoms of cystitis?

_____

_____

3. What is the patient's past surgical history?

_____

_____

4. What is the treatment for cystitis?

_____

_____

5. What are the dangers of untreated cystitis?

_____

_____

6. What instrument is used to perform a cystoscopy?

_____

_____

✓ MEDICAL RECORD ACTIVITY 7–2. Benign Prostatic Hypertrophy

Terminology

The terms listed in the chart come from the medical record *Benign Prostatic Hypertrophy* that follows. Use a medical dictionary such as *Taber's Cyclopedic Medical Dictionary,* the appendices of this book, or other resources to define each term. Then practice reading the pronunciations aloud for each term.

Term	Definition
asymptomatic ă-sĭmp-tō-MĂT-ĭk	
auscultation aws-kŭl-TĀ-shŭn	
basal cell carcinoma BĀ-săl SĔL kăr-sĭ-NŌ-mă	
benign prostatic hypertrophy bē-NĬN prŏs-TĂT-ĭk hī-PĔR-trŏ-fē	
bilateral bī-LĂT-ĕr-ăl	
bruits brwēz	
catheterization kăth-ĕ-tĕr-ĭ-ZĀ-shŭn	
colectomy kō-LĔK-tō-mē	
distended dĭs-TĔND-ĕd	
hemorrhoid HĔM-ō-royd	
hydrocele HĪ-drō-sēl	
impotence ĬM-pō-tĕns	
inguinal hernia ĬNG-gwĭ-năl HĔR-nē-ă	
normocephalic nor-mō-sĕ-FĂL-ĭk	
palpable PĂL-pă-bl	

(Continued)

Term	Definition (Continued)
percussion pĕr-KŬSH-ŭn	
pneumothorax nū-mō-THŌ-răks	
transurethral trăns-ū-RĒ-thrăl	

> *Listen and Learn Online!* will help you master the pronunciation of selected medical words from this medical record activity. Visit www.fadavis.com/gylys/simplified for instructions in completing the *Listen and Learn Online!* exercise for this section and then to practice pronunciations.

BENIGN PROSTATIC HYPERTROPHY

Reading

Practice pronunciation of medical terms by reading the following medical report aloud.

PREOPERATIVE ADMISSION: The patient is a 72-year-old white man with no significant voiding symptoms before this admission and recently was found to have colon cancer and is being admitted for colectomy.

HISTORY OF PRESENT ILLNESS: Preoperative catheterization was not possible, and consultation with Dr. Moriarty was obtained.

PAST HISTORY: Negative for transurethral resection of the prostate or any urological trauma or venereal disease. The past history is positive for hemorrhoid symptoms and history of bilateral inguinal hernia repair, history of high cholesterol, history of retinal surgery, spontaneous pneumothorax × 2, and had chest tubes in the past. He also had a basal cell carcinoma.

PHYSICAL EXAMINATION: Head: Normocephalic. **Eyes, Ears, Nose, and Throat:** Within normal limits. **Neck:** No nodes. No bruits over carotids. **Chest:** Clear to auscultation and percussion. **Heart:** Normal heart sounds. No murmur. **Abdomen:** Soft and nontender. No masses are palpable. It is very distended. **Penis:** Normal. There is a right hydrocele. **Rectal:** Examination reveals 35 to 40 g of benign prostatic hypertrophy.

ASSESSMENT: 1. Mild-to-moderate benign prostatic hypertrophy.
2. Status post colon resection for carcinoma of the colon.
3. Right hydrocele, asymptomatic.
4. Impotence.

Evaluation

Review the medical record to answer the following questions.

1. What prompted the consultation with the urologist, Dr. Moriarty?

_____

_____

2. What abnormality did the urologist discover?

_____

_____

3. Did the patient have any previous surgery on his prostate?

_____

_____

4. Where was the patient's hernia?

_____

_____

5. What in the patient's past medical history contributed to his present urological problem?

_____

_____

Chapter Review

Word Elements Summary

The following table summarizes combining forms, suffixes, and prefixes related to the urinary system.

Word Element	Meaning
COMBINING FORMS	
URINARY STRUCTURES	
cyst/o, vesic/o	bladder
glomerul/o	glomerulus
nephr/o, ren/o	kidney
pyel/o	renal pelvis
ureter/o	ureter
urethr/o	urethra
ur/o, urin/o	urine
OTHER	
carcin/o	cancer
enter/o	intestine (usually small intestine)
erythr/o	red
gastr/o	stomach

(Continued)

Word Element	Meaning (Continued)
hemat/o	blood
hepat/o	liver
lith/o	stone, calculus
noct/o	night
olig/o	scanty
py/o	pus
rect/o	rectum
scler/o	hardening; sclera (white of eye)
ven/o	vein
SUFFIXES	
SURGICAL	
-ectomy	excision, removal
-pexy	fixation (of an organ)
-plasty	surgical repair
-rrhaphy	suture
-stomy	forming an opening (mouth)
-tome	instrument to cut
-tomy	incision
-tripsy	crushing
DIAGNOSTIC, SYMPTOMATIC, AND RELATED	
-algia, -dynia	pain
-cele	hernia, swelling
-cyte	cell
-ectasis	dilation, expansion
-edema	swelling
-emesis	vomiting
-gram	record, writing
-graphy	process of recording
-iasis	abnormal condition (produced by something specified)
-itis	inflammation
-lith	stone, calculus

Word Element	Meaning
-logist	specialist in study of
-logy	study of
-megaly	enlargement
-oma	tumor
-osis	abnormal condition; increase (used primarily with blood cells)
-pathy	disease
-pepsia	digestion
-phagia	swallowing, eating
-phobia	fear
-ptosis	prolapse, downward displacement
-rrhea	discharge, flow
-scope	instrument for examining
-scopy	visual examination
-uria	urine

ADJECTIVE

-al, -ic, -ous	pertaining to, relating to

NOUN

-ia	condition
-ist	specialist

PREFIXES

a-, an-	without, not
dys-	bad; painful; difficult
in-	in, not
intra-	in, within
poly-	many, much
supra-	above; excessive; superior

WORD ELEMENTS REVIEW

After you review the Word Elements Summary, complete this activity by writing the meaning of each element in the space provided.

Word Element	Meaning
COMBINING FORMS	
URINARY STRUCTURES	
1. cyst/o, vesic/o	
2. glomerul/o	
3. nephr/o, ren/o	
4. pyel/o	
5. ureter/o	
6. urethr/o	
7. ur/o	
OTHER	
8. aden/o	
9. carcin/o	
10. erythr/o	
11. gastr/o	
12. hemat/o	
13. lith/o	
14. noct/o	
15. olig/o	
16. py/o	
17. rect/o	
18. scler/o	
SUFFIXES	
SURGICAL	
19. -ectomy	
20. -pexy	
21. -plasty	
22. -rrhaphy	
23. -stomy	

Word Element	Meaning
24. -tome	
25. -tomy	
26. -tripsy	
DIAGNOSTIC, SYMPTOMATIC, AND RELATED	
27. -algia, dynia	
28. -cele	
29. -cyte	
30. -ectasis	
31. -edema	
32. -gram	
33. -graphy	
34. -iasis	
35. -itis	
36. -lith	
37. -megaly	
38. -oma	
39. -osis	
40. -pathy	
41. -ptosis	
42. -scope	
43. -scopy	
44. -uria	
PREFIXES	
45. a-, an-	
46. dys-	
47. in-	
48. intra-	
49. poly-	
50. supra-	

Competency Verification: Check your answers in Appendix A, Glossary of Medical Word Elements, page 497. If you are not satisfied with your level of comprehension, review the word elements and retake the review.

Correct Answers _____ × 2 = _____% Score

Chapter 7 Vocabulary Review

Match the medical term(s) with the definitions in the numbered list.

acute renal failure	cystocele	malignant	oliguria
anuria	diuretics	nephrolithotomy	polyuria
benign	edema	nephrons	renal pelvis
bilateral	hematuria	nephroptosis	ureteropyeloplasty
cholelithiasis	IVP	nocturia	urinary incontinence

1. _____ means tending or threatening to produce death; refers to cancerous growths.

2. _____ are microscopic filtering units in the kidney that are responsible for keeping body fluids in balance.

3. _____ refers to formation of gallstones.

4. _____ is a funnel-shaped reservoir that is the basin of the kidney.

5. _____ is an x-ray film of the kidneys after an injection of dye.

6. _____ are drugs that stimulate the flow of urine.

7. _____ means swelling of body tissue.

8. _____ means not cancerous.

9. _____ is an incision into a kidney to remove a stone.

10. _____ is a condition that results from a lack of blood flow to the kidneys.

11. _____ is downward displacement of a kidney.

12. _____ is surgical repair of a ureter and renal pelvis.

13. _____ means pertaining to two sides.

14. _____ means excessive urination at night.

15. _____ refers to inability to hold urine.

16. _____ refers to presence of blood cells in the urine.

17. _____ means excessive discharge of urine.

18. _____ is a diminished amount of urine formation.

19. _____ is absence of urine formation.

20. _____ is herniation of the urinary bladder.

Competency Verification: Check your answers in Appendix B, Answer Key, page 524. If you are not satisfied with your level of comprehension, review the chapter vocabulary and retake the review.

Correct Answers _____ × 5 = _____ % Score

8

Reproductive Systems

OBJECTIVES

Upon completion of this chapter, you will be able to:

■ Describe the main functions of the female and male reproductive systems.

■ Identify the organs of the female and male reproductive systems.

■ Describe pathological, diagnostic, therapeutic, and other terms related to the female and male reproductive systems.

■ Recognize, define, pronounce, and spell terms correctly by completing the audio CD-ROM exercises.

■ Demonstrate your knowledge of this chapter by successfully completing the frames, reviews, and medical report evaluations.

Although the structures of the female and male reproductive systems are different, both have a common purpose. They are specialized to produce and unite *gametes* (reproductive cells) and transport them to sites of fertilization. The reproductive systems of both sexes are designed specifically to perpetuate the species and pass genetic material from generation to generation. In addition, both sexes produce hormones, which are vital in the development and maintenance of sexual characteristics and the regulation of reproductive physiology. In women, the reproductive system includes the ovaries, fallopian tubes, uterus, vagina, clitoris, and vulva (see Figure 8–1). In men, the reproductive system includes the testes, epididymis, vas deferens, seminal vesicles, ejaculatory duct, prostate, and penis. The female and the male reproductive systems are covered in this chapter.

Female Reproductive System

The female reproductive system is composed of internal organs of reproduction and external genitalia. The internal organs are the *ovaries, fallopian tubes* (oviducts, uterine tubes), *uterus,* and *vagina.* The external organs, also called the *genitalia,* are known collectively as the *vulva.* Included in the *vulva* are the *mons pubis, labia majora, labia minora, clitoris,* and *Bartholin glands* (see Figure 8–1). The combined organs of the female reproductive system are designed to: produce and transport *ova* (female sex cells), discharge ova from the body if fertilization does not occur, and nourish and provide a place for the developing fetus throughout pregnancy if fertilization occurs. The female reproductive system also produces the female sex hormones, estrogen and progesterone, which are responsible for the development of secondary sex characteristics, such as breast development and the regulation of the menstrual cycle.

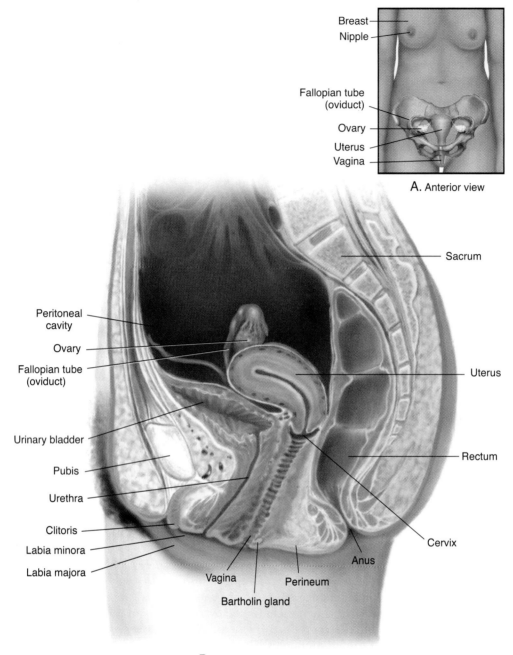

Breast

Nipple

Fallopian tube (oviduct)

Ovary

Uterus

Vagina

A. Anterior view

Peritoneal cavity

Ovary

Fallopian tube (oviduct)

Urinary bladder

Pubis

Urethra

Clitoris

Labia minora

Labia majora

Vagina

Bartholin gland

Perineum

Anus

Cervix

Rectum

Uterus

Sacrum

B. Lateral view

Figure 8-1   Female reproductive system. (A) Anterior view (B) Lateral view.

Word Elements

This section introduces combining forms related to the female reproductive system. Included are key suffixes; prefixes are defined in the right-hand column as needed. Review the following table, and pronounce each word in the word analysis column aloud before you begin to work the frames.

Word Element	Meaning	Word Analysis
COMBINING FORMS		
amni/o	amnion (amniotic sac)	amni/o/centesis (ăm-nē-ō-sĕn-TĒ-sĭs): surgical puncture of the amniotic sac to remove fluid for laboratory analysis *-centesis:* surgical puncture *The sample of amniotic fluid obtained is studied chemically and cytologically to detect genetic abnormalities, biochemical disorders, and maternal-fetal blood incompatibility*
cervic/o	neck; cervix uteri (neck of uterus)	cervic/itis (sĕr-vĭ-SĪ-tĭs): inflammation of the cervix uteri *-itis:* inflammation
colp/o	vagina	colp/o/scopy (kŏl-PŎS-kō-pē): examination of the vagina and cervix with an optical magnifying instrument (colposcope) *-scopy:* visual examination *Colposcopy commonly is performed after a Papanicolaou (Pap) test in the treatment of cervical dysplasia and in obtaining biopsy specimens of the cervix.*
vagin/o		vagin/o/cele (VĂJ-ĭn-ō-sēl): hernia projecting into the vagina; colpocele *-cele:* hernia, swelling
galact/o	milk	galact/o/rrhea (gă-lăk-tō-RĒ-ă): excessive secretion of milk *-rrhea:* discharge, flow
lact/o		lact/o/gen (lăk-tō-JĔN): drug or other substance that enhances the production and secretion of milk *-gen:* forming, producing, origin
gynec/o	woman, female	gynec/o/logist (gī-nĕ-KŎL-ō-jĭst): physician specializing in treating disorders of the female reproductive system *-logist:* specialist in study of
hyster/o	uterus (womb)	hyster/ectomy (hĭs-tĕr-ĔK-tō-mē): excision of the uterus *-ectomy:* excision, removal
uter/o		uter/o/vagin/al (ū-tĕr-ō-VĂJ-ĭ-năl): pertaining to the uterus and vagina *vagin:* vagina *-al:* pertaining to, relating to

(Continued)

Word Element	Meaning	Word Analysis *(Continued)*
mamm/o	breast	mamm/o/gram (MĂM-ō-grăm): radiograph of the breast *-gram:* record, writing
mast/o		mast/o/pexy (MĂS-tō-pĕks-ē): surgical fixation of the breast(s) *-pexy:* fixation (of an organ) *Mastopexy is performed to affix sagging breasts in a more elevated position, often improving their shape.*
men/o	menses, menstruation	men/o/rrhagia (mĕn-ō-RĀ-jē-ă): excessive amount of menstrual flow over a longer duration than a normal menstrual period *-rrhagia:* bursting forth (of)

metr/o	uterus (womb); measure	endo/metr/itis (ĕn-dō-mē-TRĪ-tĭs): inflammatory condition of the endometrium
		   endo-: in, within
		   -itis: inflammation

nat/o	birth	pre/nat/al (prē-NĀ-tl): occurring before birth
		   pre-: before, in front of
		   -al: pertaining to, relating to

oophor/o	ovary	oophor/oma (ō-of-ōr-Ō-mă): ovarian tumor *-oma:* tumor
ovari/o		ovari/o/rrhexis (ō-văr-rē-ō-RĔK-sĭs): rupture of an ovary *-rrhexis:* rupture
perine/o	perineum	perine/o/rrhaphy (pĕr-ĭ-nē-OR-ă-fē): suture of the perineum *-rrhaphy:* suture *Perineorrhaphy is performed to repair a laceration that occurs spontaneously or is made surgically during the delivery of the fetus.*
salping/o	tube (usually fallopian or eustachian [auditory] tubes)	salping/ectomy (săl-pĭn-JĔK-tō-mē): surgical removal of a fallopian tube *-ectomy:* excision, removal
episi/o	vulva	episi/o/tomy (ĕ-pĭs-ē-ĔT-ō-mē): incision of the perineum to enlarge the vaginal opening for delivery *-tomy:* incision
vulv/o		vulv/o/pathy (vŭl-VŎP-ă-thē): any disease of the vulva *-pathy:* disease

Word Element	Meaning	Word Analysis
SUFFIXES		
-arche	beginning	men/arche (mĕn-ĂR-kē): initial menstrual period *men:* menses, menstruation *Menarche usually occurs between age 9 and 17.*
-cyesis	pregnancy	pseudo/cyesis (soo-dō-sī-Ē-sĭs): condition in which a woman believes she is pregnant when she is not; false pregnancy *pseudo-:* false
-gravida	pregnant woman	primi/gravida (prī-mĭ-GRĂV-ĭ-dă): woman during her first pregnancy *primi-:* first
-para	to bear (offspring)	multi/para (mŭl-TĬP-ă-ră): woman who has delivered more than one viable infant *multi-:* many, much
-salpinx	tube (usually fallopian or eustachian [auditory] tubes)	hemat/o/salpinx (hĕm-ă-tō-SĂL-pinks): collection of blood in a fallopian tube *hemat/o:* blood *Hematosalpinx is often associated with a tubal pregnancy; also called hemosalpinx.*
-tocia	childbirth, labor	dys/tocia (dĭs-TŌ-sē-ă): pathological or difficult labor *dys-:* bad; painful; difficult *Dystocia may be caused by an obstruction or constriction of the birth passage or abnormal size, shape, position, or condition of the fetus.*
-version	turning	retro/version (rĕt-rō-VĔR-shŭn): tipping back of an organ *retro-:* backward, behind *Uterine retroversion is measured as first, second, or third degree, depending on the angle of tilt with respect to the vagina.*

Listen and Learn, the audio CD-ROM that accompanies this book, will help you master the pronunciation of selected medical words. Use it to practice pronunciations of the above-listed medical terms and for instructions for completing the *Listen and Learn* exercise on the CD-ROM for this section.

For the following medical terms, first write the suffix and its meaning. Then translate the meaning of the remaining elements starting with the first part of the word. The first word is an example that is completed for you.

Term	Definition
1. primi/gravida	-gravida: pregnant woman; first
2. colp/o/scopy	_____
3. gynec/o/logist	_____
4. perine/o/rrhaphy	_____
5. hyster/ectomy	_____
6. oophor/oma	_____
7. dys/tocia	_____
8. endo/metr/itis	_____
9. mamm/o/gram	_____
10. amni/o/centesis	_____

Competency Verification: Check your answers in Appendix B, Answer Key, page 524. If you are not satisfied with your level of comprehension, review the vocabulary and retake the review.

Correct Answers _____ × 10 = _____ % Score

Internal Structures

8-1 The female reproductive system is composed of internal and external organs of reproduction. The internal reproductive organs are the (1) **ovaries,** (2) **fallopian tubes,** (3) **uterus,** and (4) **vagina.** Label Figures 8–2 and 8–3 as you learn the names of the internal reproductive organs.

tumor
TOO-mŏr

8-2 An oophor/oma is an ovarian _____. Pronounce both initial *o*'s in words with **oophor/o.**

8-3 The main purpose of the ovaries is to produce ovum, the female reproductive cell. This process is called *ovulation.* Another important function of the ovaries is to produce the hormones estrogen and progesterone.

From oophor/oma, construct the combining form for ovary:

_____ / _____.

oophor/o

oophor/o/pathy
ō-ŏf-ŏr-ŎP-ă-thē
oophor/o/plasty
ō-ŎF-ŏr-ō-plăs-tē
oophor/o/pexy
ō-ŏf-ō-rō-PĔK-sē

8–4 Use **oophor/o** to build medical words meaning

disease of the ovaries: _____ / ____ / _____.

surgical repair of an ovary: _____ / ____ / _____.

fixation of a displaced ovary: _____ / ____ / _____.

8–5 The combining form **salping/o** means *tube (usually fallopian or eustachian [auditory] tubes)* and is related to the female reproductive system. The eustachian (auditory) tubes are related to the sense of hearing and are discussed in Chapter 11.

Surgical repair of a fallopian tube (also known as oviduct) is called

salping/o/plasty
săl-PĬNG-gō-plăs-tē

_____ / ____ / _____.

8–6 Approximately once a month, *maturation of the ovum,* or *ovulation,* occurs when the egg leaves the ovary and slowly travels down the fallopian tube to the uterus (see Figure 8–3). If union of the ovum with sperm takes place during this time, fertilization (pregnancy) results.

To form words for the fallopian tube(s), uterine tube(s), or oviduct(s), use the combining form _____ / ____.

salping/o

8–7 If the fertilized egg attaches to the wall of the fallopian tube (instead of the uterus), the tube must be removed to prevent serious bleeding in, or possible death, of the mother.

When a fallopian tube(s) is removed, the surgical procedure is called

salping/ectomy
săl-pĭn-JĔK-tō-mē

_____ / _____.

instrument

8–8 A salping/o/scope is an _____ for viewing the fallopian tube(s).

salping/o/scopy
săl-pĭng-GŎS-kō-pē

8–9 Visual examination of the fallopian tube(s) is called

_____ / ____ / _____.

salping/o/cele
săl-PĬNG-ō-sēl

8–10 Herniation of a fallopian tube(s) is known as

_____ / ____ / _____.

oviducts
Ŏ-vĭ-dŭkts

8–11 Locate the two small tubes leading to each ovary that are called

fallopian tubes, uterine tubes, or _____ (see Figure 8–3).

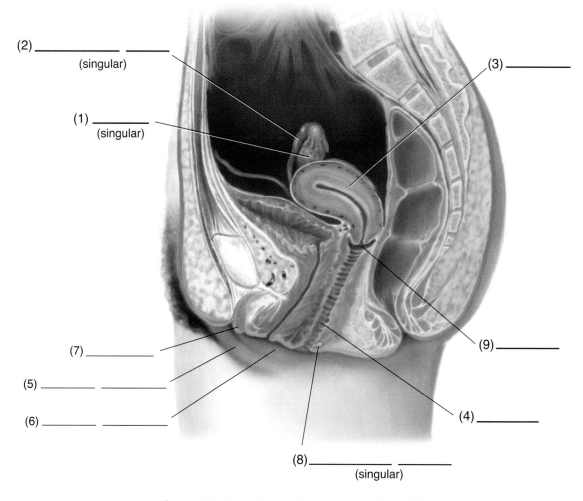

(2) _____ _____
(singular)

(1) _____
(singular)

(3) _____

(7) _____

(5) _____ _____

(6) _____ _____

(8) _____ _____
(singular)

(9) _____

(4) _____

Figure 8-2   Female reproductive system, lateral view.

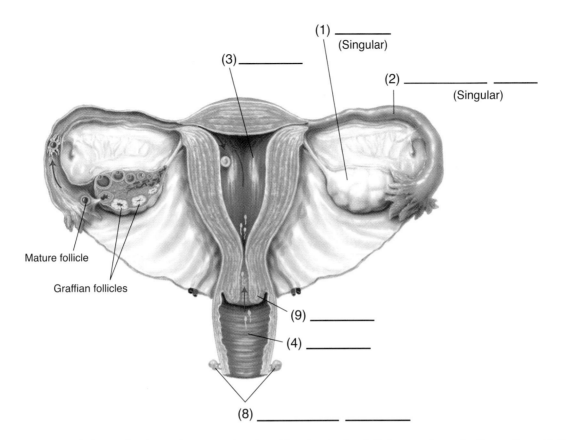

(1) _____ (Singular)

(3) _____

(2) _____ _____ (Singular)

Mature follicle

Graffian follicles

(9) _____

(4) _____

(8) _____ _____

Figure 8-3　Female Reproductive system, anterior view. The developing follicles are shown in the sectioned left ovary; fertilization is shown in the sectioned left fallopian tube. The vagina and uterus are sectioned to show internal structures. The red arrow indicates the movement of the ovum toward the uterus; the blue arrow indicates the movement of the sperm toward the fallopian tube.

hernia *or* **herniation, uterus** HĔR-nē-ă *or* hĕr-nē-Ā-shŭn, Ū-tĕr-ŭs	**8-12**　The uterus, also called the womb, is the organ that contains and nourishes the embryo and fetus from the time the fertilized egg is implanted to the time of birth. The combining form **hyster/o** is used to form words about the uterus as an organ. A hyster/o/cele is a _____ of the _____.
hyster/o/pathy hīs-tĕr-ŎP-ă-thē **hyster/algia,** hĭs-tĕr-ĂL-jē-ā **hyster/o/dynia** hĭs-tĕr-ō-DĬN-ē-ă **hyster/o/spasm** HĬS-tĕr-ō-spăzm	**8-13**　Use **hyster/o** to construct medical words meaning disease of the uterus: _____ / ____ / _____. pain in the uterus: _____ / _____ or _____ / ____ / _____. involuntary contraction, twitching of the uterus: _____ / ____ / _____.

hyster/ectomy hĭs-tĕr-ĔK-tō-mē **hyster/o/tomy** hĭs-tĕr-ŎT-ō-mē	**8-14** Presence of one or more tumors (either benign or malignant) in the uterus may necessitate its removal (see Figure 8–4). Use **hyster/o** to form surgical terms meaning excision of the uterus: _____ / _____. incision of the uterus: _____ / _____ / _____.
dictionary	**8-15** Besides **hyster/o**, the combining forms **metr/o** and **uter/o** also are used to denote the *uterus*. When in doubt about forming medical words with **hyster/o, uter/o,** or **metr/o,** refer to your medical _____.
hyster/o/scopy hĭs-tĕr-ŎS-kō-pē **uter/o/scopy** Ū-tĕr-ŏs-kō-pē	**8-16** The uterus is a muscular, hollow, pear-shaped structure located in the pelvic area between the bladder and rectum (see Figure 8–1). Use **hyster/o** to form a word meaning visual examination of the uterus: _____ / _____ / _____. Use **uter/o** to form another word meaning visual examination of the uterus: _____ / _____ / _____.
hyster/o/ptosis hĭs-tĕr-ŏp-TŌ-sĭs	**8-17** The uterus is supported and held in place by ligaments. Weakening of these ligaments may cause a downward displacement or pro-lapse of the uterus. Combine **hyster/o** and -ptosis to form the word that means a prolapse or downward displacement of the uterus: _____ / _____ / _____.
uterus Ū-tĕr-ŭs **-ine**	**8-18** A dx of uter/ine hemorrhage denotes bleeding from the _____. The element in this frame meaning *pertaining to, relating to* is _____.
hyster/o, uter/o **-pexy**	**8-19** A prolapsed uterus may be caused by heavy physical exertion, pregnancy, or an inherent weakness. The surgical procedure to correct a prolapsed uterus is known as hyster/o/pexy or uter/o/pexy. Write the elements in this frame that mean uterus: _____ / _____, _____ / _____. fixation (of an organ): _____.

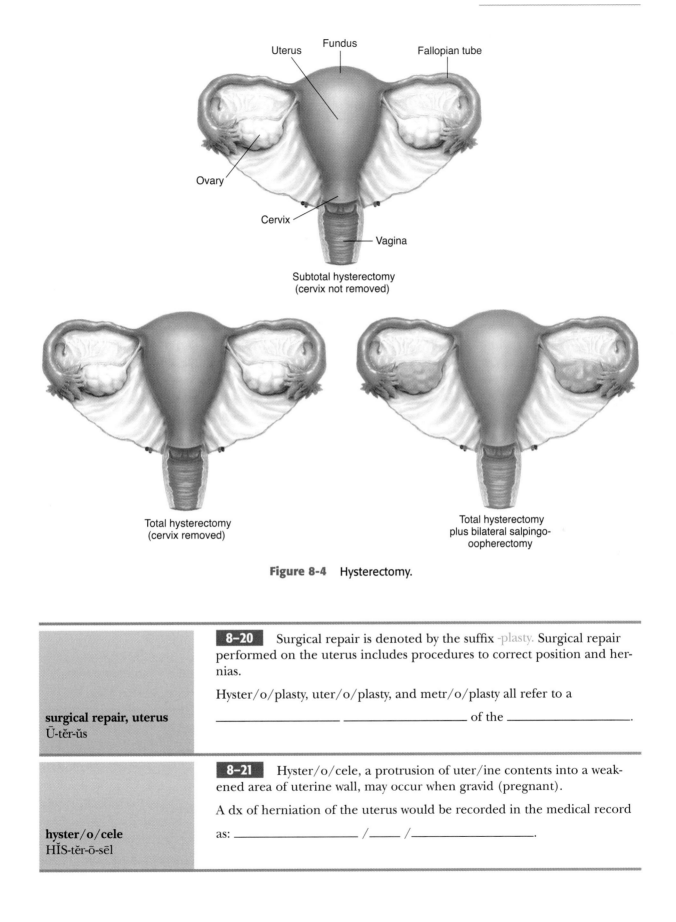

Uterus Fundus Fallopian tube

Ovary

Cervix

Vagina

Subtotal hysterectomy
(cervix not removed)

Total hysterectomy
(cervix removed)

Total hysterectomy
plus bilateral salpingo-
oopherectomy

Figure 8-4 Hysterectomy.

surgical repair, uterus Ū-tĕr-ŭs	**8–20** Surgical repair is denoted by the suffix -plasty. Surgical repair performed on the uterus includes procedures to correct position and hernias. Hyster/o/plasty, uter/o/plasty, and metr/o/plasty all refer to a _____ _____ of the _____.
hyster/o/cele HĬS-tĕr-ō-sēl	**8–21** Hyster/o/cele, a protrusion of uter/ine contents into a weakened area of uterine wall, may occur when gravid (pregnant). A dx of herniation of the uterus would be recorded in the medical record as: _____ / ____ / _____.

estrogen
ĔS-trō-jĕn
progesterone
prō-JĔS-tĕr-ōn

8-22   Two important hormones, estrogen and progesterone, are secreted by the ovaries. These hormones play an important role in the processes of menstruation and pregnancy and in the development of secondary sex characteristics.

When the ovaries are diseased and necessitate removal, the body becomes deficient in hormones known as _____ and

_____.

---

men/o/pause
MĔN-ō-pawz
trans/derm/al
trănz-DĔR-măl

8-23   Men/o/pause, a natural process of the gradual ending of the menstrual cycle, also results in a deficiency of estrogen hormone. Hormone replacement therapy (HRT), given orally or as a trans/derm/al patch, may be used to relieve uncomfortable symptoms of men/o/pause.

Identify the terms in this frame meaning

cessation of the menses: _____ / _____ / _____.

under the skin: _____ / _____ / _____.

---

post/men/o/pause
pōst-MĔN-ō-pawz

8-24   The term *pre/men/o/pause* refers to a time period before men/o/pause. Can you build a word that refers to a time period after men/o/pause? _____ / _____ / _____ / _____.

---

bursting

forth

8-25   The suffixes -rrhage and -rrhagia are used in words to mean *bursting forth (of)*. Hem/o/rrhage denotes a _____ _____ (of) blood.

---

hem/o

8-26   The combining form in hem/o/rrhage that denotes blood is _____ / _____.

---

blood

8-27   The elements **hemat/o, hem/o,** and -emia refer to _____.

---

blood

8-28   Hemat/o/logy is the study of _____.

---

blood

tumor
TOO-mŏr

8-29   A hemat/oma is a localized collection or swelling of blood, usually clotted, in an organ, space, or tissue, caused by a break in the wall of a blood vessel.

Analyze hemat/oma by defining the elements:

hemat/o refers to _____.

-oma refers to a _____.

hemat/o/logist hē-mă-TŎL-ō-jĭst **hemat/o/pathy** hē-mă-TŎP-ăth-ē **hemat/emesis** hēm-ăt-ĔM-ĕ-sĭs	**8-30** Use **hemat/o** to build medical words meaning specialist in the study of blood: _____ / ____ / _____. disease of the blood: _____ / ____ / _____. vomiting blood: _____ / _____.

inflammation, vagina vă-JĪ-nă	**8-31** The vagina is a muscular tube that extends from the cervix (neck of the uterus) to the exterior of the body (see Figure 8–3). In addition to serving as the organ of sexual intercourse and the receptor of semen, the vagina discharges the menstrual flow and acts as a passageway for the delivery of the fetus. The combining forms **colp/o** and **vagin/o** refer to the *vagina*. Colp/itis is an _____ of the _____.

vagin/itis văj-ĭn-Ī-tĭs	**8-32** Form another word besides colp/itis that means inflammation of the vagina: _____ / _____.

colp/algia kŏl-PĂL-jē-ă	**8-33** Colp/o/dynia is pain in the vagina. Use **colp/o** to build another term for pain in the vagina: _____ / _____.

colp/o/spasm KŎL-pō-spăzm **colp/o/ptosis** kŏl-pŏp-TŌ-sĭs **colp/o/pexy** KŎL-pō-pĕk-sē	**8-34** Use **colp/o** to construct medical words meaning spasm or twitching of the vagina: _____ / ____ / _____. prolapse or downward displacement of the vagina: _____ / ____ / _____. fixation of the vagina: _____ / ____ / _____.

vagin/o/plasty vă-JĪ-nō-plăs-tē **vagin/o/scope** VĂJ-ĭn-ō-skōp **vagin/o/tomy** văj-ĭ-NŎT-ō-mē	**8-35** Use **vagin/o** to form medical words meaning surgical repair of the vagina: _____ / ____ / _____. instrument to view the vagina: _____ / ____ / _____. incision of the vagina: _____ / ____ / _____.

suture, vagina SŪ-chŭr, vă-JĪ-nă	**8-36** A prolapsed vagina usually is sutured to the abdominal wall. Colp/o/rrhaphy is a _____ of the _____.
-rrhagia, -rrhage	**8-37** Colp/o/rrhagia is an excessive vaginal discharge or a vaginal hem/o/rrhage. The elements in these words that mean bursting forth (of) are _____ and _____.
hem/o/rrhage HĔM-ĕ-rĭj	**8-38** Form a word meaning bursting forth (of) blood: _____ / ____ / _____.
hernia HĔR-nē-ă **swelling**	**8-39** Recall that -cele designates a _____ or _____.
vagina vă-JĪ-nă	**8-40** A colp/o/cyst/o/cele is a protrusion or herniation of the bladder into the _____.
vagina vă-JĪ-nă **bladder** **hernia, swelling** HĔR-nē-ă	**8-41** Women who have had several vagin/al childbirths may suffer from herniation of the bladder or colp/o/cyst/o/cele. Identify the elements in colp/o/cyst/o/cele: **colp/o** refers to the _____. **cyst/o** refers to the _____. -cele refers to a _____ or _____.
vagin/al VĂJ-ĭn-ăl **hyster/ectomy** hĭs-tĕr-ĔK-tō-mē	**8-42** When the uterus is rcmovcd through the vagina, the surgical procedure is known as a vagin/al hyster/ectomy or a colp/o/hyster/ectomy. Identify the words in this frame that mean pertaining to the vagina: _____ / _____. excision of the uterus: _____ / _____.
muc/ous MŪ-kŭs	**8-43** The vagina is lubricated by mucus. **Muc/o** is the combining form for mucus. Use the adjective ending -ous to form a word that means pertaining to mucus: _____ / _____.

-oid	**8-44** Muc/oid means resembling mucus. The adjective ending element meaning resembling is _____.
resembling fat	**8-45** Lip/oid means _____ _____.
adip/oid ĂD-ĭ-poyd	**8-46** Use **adip/o** to form another term meaning resembling fat: _____ / _____.

 Listen and Learn, the audio CD-ROM that accompanies this book, will help you master the pronunciation of selected medical words. Use it to practice pronunciations *of selected terms* from Frames *8–1 to 8–46* for instructions to complete the *Listen and Learn* exercise on the CD-ROM for this section.

Using the following table, write the combining form and suffix that matches its definition in the space provided to the left of the definition. There may be more than one word element that matches a definition.

Combining Forms		Suffixes	
colp/o	muc/o	-arche	-ptosis
cyst/o	oophor/o	-cele	-rrhage
hemat/o	ovari/o	-logist	-rrhagia
hem/o	salping/o	-logy	-salpinx
hyster/o	uter/o	-oid	-scope
metr/o	vagin/o	-pexy	-tome
		-plasty	-tomy

1. _____ bladder
2. _____ blood
3. _____ bursting forth (of)
4. _____ uterus (womb)
5. _____ hernia, swelling
6. _____ incision
7. _____ instrument to cut
8. _____ instrument for examining
9. _____ tube (usually fallopian or eustachian [auditory] tubes)
10. _____ fixation (of an organ)

11. _____ mucus
12. _____ ovary
13. _____ beginning
14. _____ uterus, womb; (measure)
15. _____ prolapse, downward displacement
16. _____ resembling
17. _____ specialist in study of
18. _____ study of
19. _____ surgical repair
20. _____ vagina

Competency Verification: Check your answers in Appendix B, Answer Key, page 525. If you are not satisfied with your level of comprehension, go back to Frame 8–1 and rework the frames.

Correct Answers _____ × 5 = _____ % Score

Making a set of flash cards from key word elements in this chapter for each section review can help you remember the elements. Make a flash card by writing a word element on one side of a 3 × 5 or 4 × 6 index card. On the other side, write the meaning of the element. Do this for all word elements in the section reviews. Use your flash cards to review each section. You also might use the flash cards to prepare for the chapter review at the end of this chapter.

External Structures

	8-47 The external structures, or genitalia, include the (5) **labia majora** (the outer lips of the vagina), (6) **labia minora** (the smaller, inner lips of the vagina), (7) **clitoris**, and (8) **Bartholin glands.** Label Figures 8–2 and 8–3 to locate the structures of the genitalia.
vulva VŬL-vă	**8-48** The combining form **vulv/o** refers to the *vulva*, the combined external structures of the female reproductive system. Vulv/o/uter/ine refers to the uterus and _____.
clitoris KLĬT-ō-rĭs **Bartholin glands** BĂR-tō-lĭn	**8-49** The external structures, or genitalia, also known as the vulva, include the labia majora, labia minora, _____, and _____ _____.
muc/ous MŪ-kŭs	**8-50** Mucus secretions from the Bartholin glands help keep the vagina moist and lubricated, facilitating intercourse. Use -ous to build a word meaning pertaining to mucus: _____ / _____ (adjective ending).
vulv/itis vŭl-VĪ-tĭs **vulv/o/pathy** vŭl-VŎP-ă-thē	**8-51** Use **vulv/o** to construct words meaning inflammation of the vulva: _____ / _____. disease of the vulva: _____ / _____ / _____.
	8-52 The (9) **cervix** denotes the neck of the uterus and extends into the upper portion of the vagina. Examine the position of the cervix in the lateral and anterior view as you label Figures 8–2 and 8–3.
cervic/itis sĕr-vĭ-SĪ-tĭs	**8-53** The combining form **cervic/o** denotes either the *cervix uteri* or the *neck*. An inflammation of the cervix uteri is called _____ / _____.
vagina vă-JĪ-nă **uteri** Ū-tĕ-rē	**8-54** When **cervic/o** is used in a word, you can determine whether it refers to the *neck* or the *cervix uteri* by reviewing the other parts of the word. colp/o/cervic/al refers to the _____ and cervix _____.
colp/o/scopy kŏl-PŎS-kō-pē	**8-55** A colp/o/scope, an instrument with a magnifying lens, is used to examine vagin/al and cervic/al tissue. Visual examination of vagin/al and cervic/al tissue using a colposcope is called _____ / _____ / _____.

colp/o/scope
KŎL-pō-skōp

8-56 Determine the words in Frame 8–55 that mean instrument for examining the vagina and cervix uteri:

_____ / _____ / _____.

visual examination of the vagina and cervix uteri using a colp/o/scope:

_____ / _____ / _____.

colp/o/scopy
kŏl-PŎS-kō-pē
vagin/al
VĂJ-ĭn-ăl
cervic/al
SĔR-vĭ-kăl

pertaining to the vagina: _____ / _____.

pertaining to the cervix uteri: _____ / _____.

uterus
Ū-tĕr-ŭs

8-57 Cervix uteri refers to the neck of the _____.

Competency Verification: Check your labeling of Figures 8–2 and 8–3 in Appendix B, Answer Key, page 525.

gynec/o/logist
gī-nĕ-KŎL-ō-jĭst

8-58 Gynec/o/logy literally means study of females or women and is the medical specialty for treating female disorders. A specialist in the study of female disorders is called a

_____ / _____ / _____.

gynec/o

8-59 The combining form in the word gynec/o/logy meaning *woman* or *female* is _____ / _____.

gynec/o/pathy
gī-nĕ-KŎP-ă-thē

8-60 Use -pathy to form a word that means disease of a female:

_____ / _____ / _____.

gynec/o/logy
gī-nĕ-KŎL-ō-jē

8-61 GYN is the abbreviation for gynec/o/logy. OB-GYN refers to obstetrics and _____ / _____ / _____.

8-62 Use your medical dictionary to define *obstetrics:*

_____

_____

menses, menstruation
MĔN-sēz,
mĕn-stroo-Ā-shŭn

8-63 The combining form **men/o** denotes the *menses,* also called menstruation, which is the monthly flow of blood and tissue from the uterus.

Men/o/rrhea is a flow of _____ or _____

dys/men/o/rrhea dĭs-mĕn-ō-RĒ-ă	**8-64** Use dys- and men/o/rrhea to develop a word meaning painful or difficult menstrual flow: _____ /_____ /____ /_____.
dys/men/o/rrhea dĭs-mĕn-ō-RĒ-ă	**8-65** Dys/men/o/rrhea is pain associated with menstruation. Primary dys/men/o/rrhea is menstrual pain that results from factors intrinsic to the uterus and the process of menstruation. It is extremely common, occurring at least occasionally in almost all women. If the painful episode is mild and brief, it is considered functional and normal and requires no treatment. The symptomatic term that literally means bad, painful, difficult menstruation is _____ /_____ /____ /_____.
bursting forth **menses** _or_ **menstruation** MĔN-sēz, mĕn-stroo-Ā-shŭn	**8-66** Men/o/rrhagia is excessive bleeding at the time of a menstrual period. Literally it means _____ _____ (of the) _____.
menstruation mĕn-stroo-Ā-shun	**8-67** Men/o/pause terminates the reproductive period of life and is a permanent cessation of menses or _____.
menstruation mĕn-stroo-Ā-shun	**8-68** A/men/o/rrhea is the absence or abnormal stoppage of menstruation. Men/o/rrhea is a flow of the menses or _____.
-pause	**8-69** Identify the element in men/o/pause meaning cessation: _____.
after **before**	**8-70** Post/men/o/paus/al and pre/men/o/paus/al means bleeding that occurs at times other than during the normal menstrual flow. Post- means behind or _____; pre- means in front of or _____.

Breasts

mamm/o, mast/o	**8-71** The breasts, also called mamm/ary glands, are present in both sexes, but they normally function only in females. The biological role of the mammary glands is to secrete milk for the nourishment of the infant, a process called _lactation_. The two combining forms that refer to the breast are _____ /____ and _____ /____.

excision *or* **removal** ĕk-SĬ-zhŭn	**8-72** Mast/ectomy is an _____ of a breast.
mast/ectomy măs-TĔK-tō-mē	**8-73** To prevent the spread of cancer, a malignant breast tumor may be treated with a partial or complete excision. When a breast has to be removed, the patient has a _____ / _____.
	8-74 During puberty, the female's breasts develop as a result of periodic stimulation of the ovarian hormones estrogen and progesterone. Estrogen is responsible for the development of (1) **adipose tissue,** which enlarges the size of the breasts until they reach full maturity around age 16. Breast size is primarily determined by the amount of fat around the (2) **glandular tissue,** but is not a factor in the ability to produce and secrete milk. Label the adipose tissue in Figure 8–5.
	8-75 During pregnancy, high levels of estrogen and progesterone prepare the glands for milk production. Each breast has approximately 20 lobes. Each (3) **lobe** is drained by a (4) **lactiferous duct** that opens on the tip of the raised (5) **nipple.** Circling the nipple is a border of slightly darker skin called the (6) **areola.** Label the structures of the mammary glands in Figure 8–5.
lactation lăk-TĀ-shŭn	**8-76** During pregnancy, the breasts enlarge and remain so until lactation ceases. At menopause, breast tissue begins to atrophy. The ability of mammary glands to secrete milk for the nourishment of the infant is a process called _____.
-graphy **mamm/o**	**8-77** Mamm/o/graphy, an x-ray examination of the breast, is used in the diagnosis of cancer. Determine the element in this frame that means process of recording: _____. breast: _____ / ____.
mamm/o/plasty MĂM-ō-plăs-tē	**8-78** Use **mamm/o** to construct a word meaning surgical reconstruction or surgical repair of a breast: _____ / ____ / _____.
mast/o/plasty MĂS-tō-plăs-tē **mast/o/pexy** MĂS-to-pĕk-sē	**8-79** Correction of pendulous breasts can be performed by a reconstructive procedure in cosmetic surgery to lift the breasts. Use **mast/o** to develop surgical terms meaning surgical repair of the breast: _____ / ____ / _____. fixation of the breast: _____ / ____ / _____.

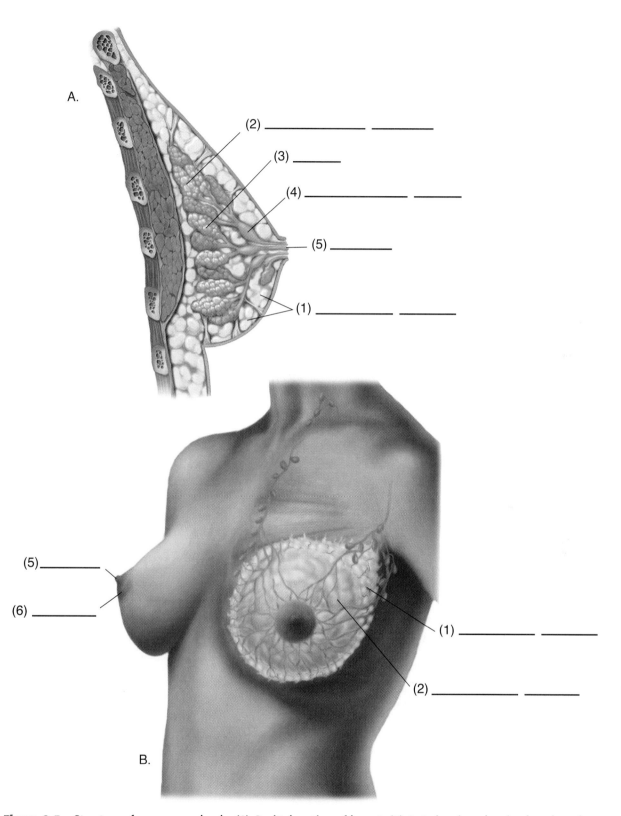

A.

(2) _____ _____

(3) _____

(4) _____ _____

(5) _____

(1) _____ _____

(5) _____

(6) _____

(1) _____ _____

(2) _____ _____

B.

Figure 8-5 Structure of mammary glands. (A) Sagittal section of breast. (B) Anterior view showing lymph nodes and structures of the breast.

mast/o, mamm/o	**8–80** Two combining forms used to designate the breast are _____ / ____ and _____ / ____.
inflammation, breast(s)	**8–81** Breast feeding often causes a blockage of the milk ducts and mast/itis, which is an _____ of the _____.
mast/o/dynia măst-ō-DĬN-ē-ă **mast/algia** măst-ĂL-jē-ă	**8–82** Use **mast/o** to form a word meaning pain in the breast: _____ / ____ / _____ or _____ / _____.

Competency Verification: Check your labeling of Figure 8–5 in Appendix B, Answer Key, page 525.

before **after**	**8–83** The term nat/al means pertaining to birth. Pre/nat/al refers to the time period _____ birth; post/nat/al refers to the time period _____ birth.
neo- **nat/o** **-logy**	**8–84** Identify the elements in neo/nat/o/logy that mean new: _____. birth: _____ / ____. study of: _____.
neo/nat/o/logist nē-ō-nā-TŎL-ō-jĭst	**8–85** Neo/nat/o/logy is the study and treatment of the neonate (newborn infant). A physician who specializes in the care and treatment of the neonate is called a _____ / _____ / ____ / _____.
woman	**8–86** The word *gravida* is used to describe a pregnant woman, as is the suffix -gravida. Primi/gravida is a woman pregnant for the first time; multi/gravida is a woman who has been pregnant more than once. Whenever you see *gravida* in a word, you will know it denotes a pregnant _____.
fourth **second**	**8–87** The word *gravida* also may be followed by numbers to denote the number of pregnancies, as in gravida 1, 2, 3, and 4 (or I, II, III, and IV). Gravida 4 is a woman in her _____ pregnancy. Gravida 2 is a woman in her _____ pregnancy.
gravida 3 GRĂV-ĭ-dă **gravida 5** GRĂV-ĭ-dă	**8–88** A woman in her third pregnancy is a _____. A woman in her fifth pregnancy is a _____.

two, five	**8-89** The word *para* refers to a woman who has given birth to an infant, regardless of whether or not the offspring was alive at birth. It also may be followed by numbers to indicate the number of deliveries, as in para 1, 2, 3, 4 (or I, II, III, or IV). Para 2 means _____ deliveries; para 5 means _____ deliveries.
para 6 PĂR-ă	**8-90** A woman who has delivered three infants would be described as para 3. A woman who has delivered six infants would be described as _____ .
PID	**8-91** Pelvic inflammatory disease (PID) is a collective term for inflammation of the uterus, fallopian tubes, ovaries, and adjacent pelvic structures, usually caused by bacterial infection. The abbreviation for pelvic inflammatory disease is _____ .
path/o/gen PĂTH-ō-jĕn	**8-92** The infection may be confined to a single organ, or it may involve all of the internal female reproductive organs. The disease-producing organisms *(pathogens)* generally enter through the vagina during coitus, induced abortion, childbirth, or the postpartum period. As an ascending infection, the pathogens spread from the vagina and cervix to the upper structures of the female reproductive tract. A term in this frame that means forming, producing, or origin of disease is _____ / ____ / _____ .
sexually transmitted **disease** **pelvic inflammatory** **disease**	**8-93** Two of the most frequent causes of PID are gonorrhea and chlamydia, both of which are sexually transmitted diseases (STDs). Unless treated promptly, PID may result in scarring of the narrow fallopian tubes and of the ovaries causing sterility. The widespread infection of the reproductive structures also can lead to fatal septicemia. The abbreviation STD refers to _____ _____ _____ ; the abbreviation PID refers to _____ _____ _____ .
pelvic inflammatory **disease**	**8-94** Because regions of the uterine tubes have an internal diameter as small as the width of a human hair, the scarring and closure of the tubes caused by PID is one of the major causes of female infertility. Chlamydia and gonorrhea are two of the main causes of PID, which means _____ _____ _____ .
ovary *or* ovaries Ō-vă-rē, Ō-vă-rēz	**8-95** A pelvic infection confined to the uterine tubes is known as salping/itis; a pelvic infection confined to the ovaries is known as oophor/itis. The combining form **oophor/o** refers to the _____ .

oophor/itis ō-ŏf-ō-RĪ-tĭs **oophor/oma** ō-ŏf-ō-RŌ-mă	**8–96** A pelvic infection that involves the ovaries is known as oophor/itis. Use **oophor/o** to build a term meaning inflammation of the ovaries: _____ / _____. tumor of the ovaries: _____ / _____.
pelvic inflammatory disease	**8–97** PID is the abbreviation that means _____ _____ _____.
diagnosis	**8–98** A dx of a cyst or tumor in a fallopian tube may necessitate the surgical procedure known as salping/ectomy. When dx is used in a medical report, it refers to a _____.
salping/ectomy săl-pĭn-JĔK-tō-mē	**8–99** Build a surgical term meaning excision of either one or both fal lopian tubes: _____ / _____.
uterus Ū-tĕr-ŭs	**8–100** A hyster/o/tome is an instrument for incising the _____.
incision, uterus	**8–101** An abdominal incision of the uterus (hyster/o/tomy) is performed to remove the fetus during a cesarean section (CS, C-section). Hyster/o/tomy is an _____ into the _____.
CS, C-section	**8–102** The abbreviations for caesarean section are _____ and _____.

 Listen and Learn, the audio CD-ROM that accompanies this book, will help you master the pronunciation of selected medical words. Use it to practice pronunciations *of selected terms* from Frames *8–47 to 8–102* for instructions to complete the *Listen and Learn* exercise on the CD-ROM for this section.

SECTION REVIEW 8 – 3

Using the following table, write the combining form, suffix, or prefix that matches its definition in the space provided to the left of the definition. There may be more than one word element that matches a definition.

Combining Forms	Suffixes	Prefixes
cervic/o	-algia	dys-
colp/o	-ary	post-
episi/o	-dynia	pre-
gynec/o	-ectomy	
mamm/o	-itis	
mast/o	-logist	
men/o	-ous	
salping/o	-pathy	
vagin/o	-rrhea	
vulv/o	-scope	
	-scopy	
	-tome	

1. _____ after, behind
2. _____ woman, female
3. _____ before, in front of
4. _____ breast
5. _____ disease
6. _____ excision, removal
7. _____ discharge, flow
8. _____ inflammation
9. _____ instrument to cut
10. _____ instrument for examining
11. _____ visual examination

12. _____ menses, menstruation
13. _____ neck; cervix uteri (neck of uterus)
14. _____ pain
15. _____ pertaining to, relating to
16. _____ specialist in study of
17. _____ tube (usually fallopian or eustachian [auditory] tubes)
18. _____ vagina
19. _____ vulva
20. _____ bad; painful; difficult

Competency Verification: Check your answers in Appendix B, Answer Key, page 525. If you are not satisfied with your level of comprehension, go back to Frame 8–47 and rework the frames.

Correct Answers _____ × 5 = _____ % Score

Male Reproductive System

The primary sex organs of the male are called *gonads,* specifically the testes (singular, testis). Gonads produce gametes (sperm) and secrete sex hormones. The remaining accessory reproductive organs are the structures that are essential in caring for and transporting sperm. These structures can be divided into three categories: *sperm transporting ducts, accessory glands,* and *copulatory organ* (see Figure 8–6).

Sperm-transporting ducts include the *epididymis, ductus deferens, ejaculatory duct,* and *urethra.* The accessory glands include the *seminal vesicles, prostate gland,* and *bulbourethral glands.* The copulatory organ, the *penis,* contains erectile tissue. All of these organs and structures are designed to accomplish the male's reproductive role of producing and delivering sperm to the female reproductive tract, where fertilization can occur.

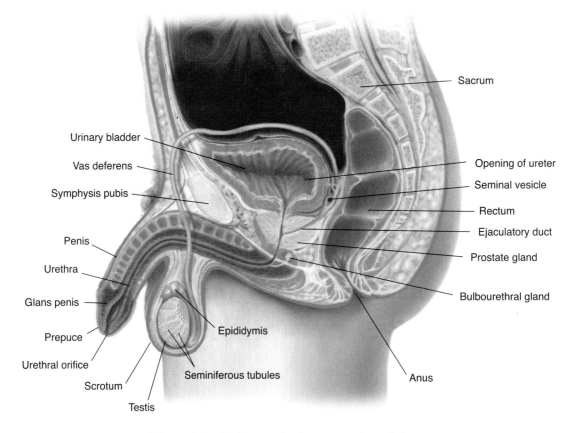

Figure 8-6   Male reproductive system, lateral view.

Word Elements

This section introduces combining forms related to the male reproductive system. Included are key suffixes; prefixes are defined in the right-hand column as needed. Review the following table and pronounce each word in the word analysis column aloud before you begin to work the frames.

Word Element	Meaning	Word Analysis
COMBINING FORMS		
andr/o	male	andr/o/gen (ĂN-drō-jěn): substance producing or stimulating the development of male characteristics (masculinization), such as the hormones testosterone and androsterone *-gen:* forming, producing, origin
balan/o	glans penis	balan/itis (băl-ă-NĪ-tĭs): inflammation of the glans penis *-itis:* inflammation
gonad/o	gonads, sex glands	gonad/o/tropin (gŏn-ă-dō-TRŌ-pĭn): gonad-stimulating hormone that stimulates the function of the testes and ovaries *-tropin:* stimulate
orch/o	testis (plural, testes)	crypt/orch/ism (krĭpt-OR-kĭzm): developmental defect characterized by failure of one or both of the testicles to descend into the scrotum *crypt:* hidden *-ism:* condition *The testicles are retained in the abdomen or inguinal canal. If spontaneous descent does not occur by age 1, hormonal therapy or surgery may be performed.*
orchi/o		orchi/o/pexy (or-kē-ō-PĔK-sē): surgery performed to mobilize an undescended testis, bring it into the scrotum, and attach it so that it will not retract *-pexy:* fixation (of an organ)
orchid/o		orchid/ectomy (or-kĭ-DĔK-tō-mē): excision of one or both testes *-ectomy:* excision, removal
test/o		test/algia (tĕs-TĂL-jē-ă): pain in the testes *-algia:* pain
spermat/o	spermatozoa, sperm cells	spermat/o/cide (SPĔR-mĭ-sīd): chemical substance that kills spermatozoa *-cide:* killing *Spermatocides are effective when used as a contraceptive; also called spermicide.*
sperm/o		a/sperm/ia (ă-SPĔR-mē-ă): failure to form semen or ejaculate *a-:*without, not *-ia:* condition

(Continued)

Word Element	Meaning	Word Analysis *(Continued)*
vas/o	vessel; vas deferens; duct	vas/ectomy (văs-ĔK-tō-mē): removal of all or part of the vas deferens *-ectomy:* excision, removal
varic/o	a dilated vein	varic/o/cele (VĂR-ĭ-kō-sēl): dilated or enlarged vein of the spermatic cord *-cele:* hernia, swelling
vesicul/o	seminal vesicle	vesicul/itis (vĕ-sĭk-ū-LĪ-tĭs): inflammation of the seminal vesicle *-itis:* inflammation

Listen and Learn, the audio CD-ROM that accompanies this book, will help you master the pronunciation of selected medical words. Use it to practice pronunciations of the above-listed medical terms and for instructions for completing the *Listen and Learn* exercise on the CD-ROM for this section.

SECTION REVIEW 8 – 4

For the following medical terms, first write the suffix and its meaning. Then translate the meaning of the remaining elements starting with the first part of the word. The first word is an example that is completed for you.

Term	Meaning
1. vas/ectomy	-ectomy: excision, removal; vessel, vas deferens, duct
2. balan/itis	_____
3. spermat/o/cide	_____
4. gonad/o/tropin	_____
5. orchi/o/pexy	_____
6. a/sperm/ia	_____
7. vesicul/itis	_____
8. orchid/ectomy	_____
9. andr/o/gen	_____
10. crypt/orch/ism	_____

Competency Verification: Check your answers in Appendix B, Answer Key, page 526. If you are not satisfied with your level of comprehension, review the vocabulary and retake the review.

Correct Answers _____ × 10 = _____ % Score

8–103   The (1) **testes** (singular, testis), also called testicles (singular, testicle), are paired oval glands that descend into the (2) **scrotum**. At the onset of puberty, the testes produce the hormone testosterone. Label Figure 8–7 as you learn about the organs of reproduction.

---

disease

testes *or* **testicles**
TĔS-tĭs, TĔS-tĭ-klz

8–104   The combining form **test/o** refers to the *testis*. Test/o/pathy is a
_____ of the
_____ (plural).

---

testis
TĔS-tĭs
testicle
TĔS-tĭ-kl

8–105   The male hormone, testosterone, stimulates and promotes the growth of secondary sex characteristics in the male. This hormone is produced by the testes (plural).

The singular form of testes is _____.

The singular form of testicles is _____.

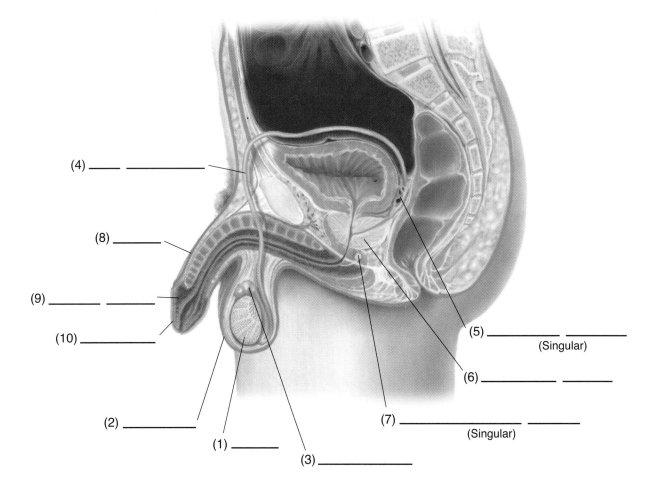

(4) _____ _____

(8) _____

(9) _____ _____

(10) _____

(2) _____

(1) _____

(3) _____

(5) _____ _____
(Singular)

(6) _____ _____

(7) _____ _____
(Singular)

Figure 8-7   Male reproductive system, lateral view.

test/itis tĕs-TĪ-tĭs **test/ectomy** tĕs-TĔK-tō-mē **test/o/pathy** tĕs-TŎP-ă-thē	**8-106** Use **test/o** to form medical words meaning inflammation of a testis: _____ / _____. excision of a testis: _____ / _____. disease of a testis: _____ / _____ / _____.
	8-107 **Spermat/o** is the combining form for *spermatozoa, sperm cells,* the male sex cell produced by the testes.
stone **calculus** KĂL-kū-lŭs	**8-108** A spermat/o/lith is a _____ or _____ in the spermatic duct.

spermat/o/genesis
spĕr-măt-ō-JĔN-ĕ-sĭs

8-109 The suffix -genesis is used in words to mean *forming, producing,* or *origin.* Construct a word meaning producing or forming sperm:

_____ / ____ / _____.

---

spermat/o/cyte
spĕr-MĂT-ō-sīt

8-110 Use **spermat/o** to form a word meaning sperm cell:

_____ / ____ / _____.

---

spermat/oid
SPĔR-mă-toyd

8-111 Build a word that means resembling spermatozoa:

_____ / _____.

---

spermat/uria
spĕr-mă-TŪ-rē-ă

8-112 Spermat/uria is a condition in which there is sperm in the urine. A discharge of semen with urine is also called

_____ / _____.

---

without

8-113 A/spermat/ism is a condition in which there is a lack of male sperm. A/spermat/ism literally means _____ sperm.

---

scanty

8-114 A man who produces a scanty amount of sperm in the semen has a condition called olig/o/sperm/ia.

Olig/o refers to _____.

---

olig/o/sperm/ia
ŏl-ĭ-gō-SPĔR-mē-ă

8-115 When the physician detects an insufficient number of spermatozoa in the semen, the diagnosis is noted in the medical record as

_____ / ____ / _____ / _____.

8-116 A comma-shaped organ, the (3) **epididymis,** stores and propels sperm toward the urethra during ejaculation. The (4) **vas deferens,** also called ductus deferens, is a duct that transports sperm from the testes to the urethra. The sperm is excreted in the semen. Semen, or seminal fluid, is a mixture of secretions from the (5) **seminal vesicles,** (6) **prostate gland,** and (7) **bulbourethral glands,** also known as *Cowper glands.* Label Figure 8–7 as you continue to learn about the male reproductive organs.

---

muc/o

8-117 The ducts of Cowper glands open into the urethra and secrete thick mucus that acts as a lubricant during sexual stimulation.

Write the combining form that refers to mucus: _____ / ____.

---

adjective

8-118 Muc/us is a noun. Muc/ous is a(n) (noun, adjective)

_____.

---

muc/oid
MŪ-koyd

8-119 Use -oid to construct a medical term meaning resembling mucus: _____ / _____.

orchi/o/plasty OR-kē-ō-plăs-tē **orchi/o/rrhaphy** or-kē-OR-ă-fē **orchi/o/pexy** or-kē-ō-PĔK-sē	**8–120** Besides **test/o,** two other combining forms that refer to the *testes* are **orchi/o** and **orchid/o.** Use **orchi/o** to develop medical words meaning surgical repair of the testicle: _____ / ___ / _____. suture of a testicle: _____ / ___ / _____. fixation of a testicle: _____ / ___ / _____.
enlargement	**8–121** The combining form for *prostate gland* is **prostat/o.** The prostate gland secretes a thick fluid that, as part of the semen, helps the sperm to move spontaneously. Prostat/o/megaly is a(n) _____ of the prostate gland.
prostat/o/megaly prŏs-tă-tō-MĔG-ă-lē	**8–122** A common disorder in men older than age 60 in which the prostate becomes enlarged is benign prostatic hypertrophy (BPH) or benign prostatic hyperplasia (see Figure 8–8). BPH is a nonmalignant enlargement that is due to excess growth of prostatic tissue. Construct a medical word to mean enlargement of the prostate gland: _____ / ___ / _____
BPH	**8–123** The abbreviation, used in frame 8–122, for benign growth of cells within the prostate gland is _____.
prostat/ism PRŎS-tă-tĭzm	**8–124** Common symptoms of BPH include urinary obstruction and inability to empty the bladder completely. Combine **prostat** and -ism to form a word that refers to any condition of the prostate that interferes with the flow of urine from the bladder: _____ / _____.
PSA	**8–125** PSA refers to a blood test used to detect prostat/ic cancer and to monitor the patient's response to therapy. The abbreviation for prostate-specific antigen test is _____.
prostat/itis prŏs-tă-TĪ-tĭs **prostat/o/cyst/itis** prŏs-tă-tō-sĭs-TĪ-tĭs	**8–126** Build medical terms meaning inflammation of the prostate gland: _____ / _____. inflammation of the prostate gland and bladder: _____ / ___ / _____ / _____.

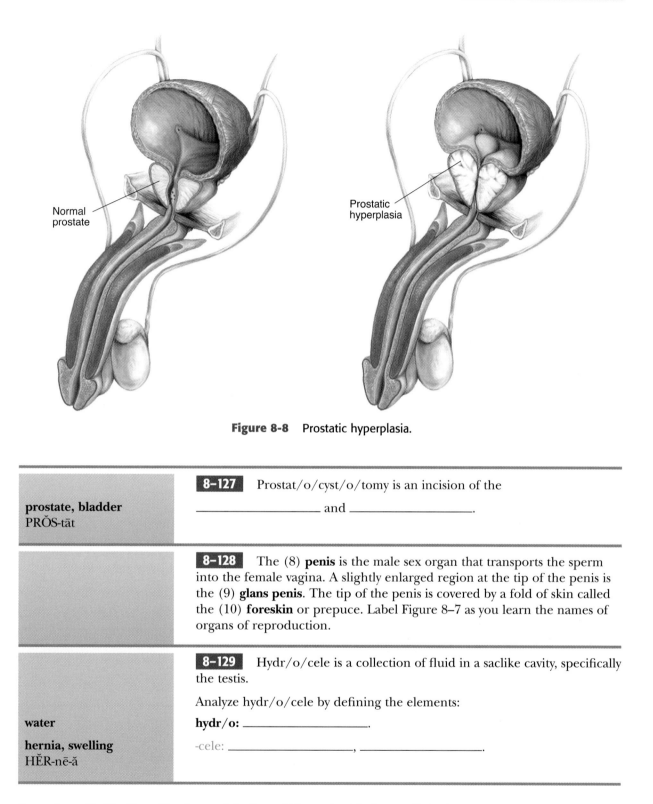

Figure 8-8   Prostatic hyperplasia.

prostate, bladder PRŎS-tāt	**8-127** Prostat/o/cyst/o/tomy is an incision of the _____ and _____.
	8-128 The (8) **penis** is the male sex organ that transports the sperm into the female vagina. A slightly enlarged region at the tip of the penis is the (9) **glans penis**. The tip of the penis is covered by a fold of skin called the (10) **foreskin** or prepuce. Label Figure 8–7 as you learn the names of organs of reproduction.
water **hernia, swelling** HĔR-nē-ă	**8-129** Hydr/o/cele is a collection of fluid in a saclike cavity, specifically the testis. Analyze hydr/o/cele by defining the elements: **hydr/o:** _____. -cele: _____, _____.

Competency Verification: Check your labeling of Figure 8–7 in Appendix B, Answer Key, page XX.

prostat/ectomy prŏs-tă-TĔK-tō-mē	**8-130** Prostate cancer is the third leading cause, after lung and colon cancer, of cancer deaths in men. Surgery may be performed to remove the prostate and adjacent affected tissues. Develop a surgical term meaning excision of the prostate gland: _____ / _____.
cancer	**8-131** Currently PSA is considered the most sensitive tumor marker for prostate _____.
threatening	**8-132** Tumors may be either benign or malignant. Benign tumors are not malignant (cancerous) and not life-threatening. A malignant tumor, however, is cancerous and life-_____.
benign bē-NĪN	**8-133** Tumors also are called neo/plasms (new growths or formations). Similar to tumors, neo/plasms can be either malignant or _____.
cancer/ous KĂN-sĕr-ŭs	**8-134** A benign tumor is non/cancer/ous. A malignant tumor is _____ / _____.
neo/plasm NĒ-ō-plăzm	**8-135** Carcin/omas also are known as malignant neo/plasms. Form a word meaning formation or growth that is new: _____ / _____.
neo/plasm NĒ-ō-plăzm	**8-136** A new growth in any body system or organ is called a _____ / _____.
prostate PRŎS-tăt	**8-137** Prostate cancer also is called carcinoma of the _____.
prostat/itis prŏs-tă-TĪ-tĭs	**8-138** Prostat/itis, an acute or chronic inflammation of the prostate gland, is usually the result of infection. The patient usually complains of burning, urinary frequency, and urgency. Build a symptomatic term meaning inflammation of the prostate gland: _____ / _____
growth	**8-139** The suffixes -plasm and -plasia refer to formation or _____.

dys-

-plasia

8-140 Dys/plasia is an abnormal development of tissue. Identify the element in dys/plasia that means

bad, painful, or difficult: _____.

formation, growth: _____.

---

without, not

formation, growth

8-141 A/plasia means without formation, and it is a condition that is due to failure of an organ to develop or form normally.

Analyze a/plasia by defining the elements:

a- means _____, _____.

-plasia means _____ or _____.

---

hyper-

-plasia

8-142 Hyper/plasia is an excessive increase in the number of cells in a tissue or organ (see Figure 8–8).

Determine the element in hyper/plasia that means

excessive: _____.

formation or growth: _____.

---

vas/o

8-143 Vas/ectomy, a sterilization procedure, involves bi/later/al cutting and tying of the vas deferens to prevent the passage of sperm (see Figure 8–9). This sterilization procedure most commonly is performed at an outpatient surgery center using local an/esthesia.

From the term vas/ectomy, construct the combining form that means vessel, vas deferens, or duct: _____ / _____.

---

an/esthesia
ăn-ĕs-THĒ-zē-ă
bi/later/al
bī-LĂT-ĕr-ăl
vas/ectomy
văs-ĔK-tō-mē

8-144 Identify the terms in Frame 8–143 that mean

without feeling: _____ / _____.

pertaining to two sides: _____ / _____ / _____.

excision of the vas deferens: _____ / _____.

---

prostat/itis
prŏs-tă-TĪ-tĭs

8-145 Vas/ectomy also is performed routinely before removal of the prostate gland to prevent inflammation of the testes and epididymides. Potency is not affected.

An inflammation of the prostate gland is called

_____ / _____.

---

vas/ectomy reversal
văs-ĔK-tō-mē

8-146 Vas/o/vas/o/stomy, also called *vas/ectomy reversal,* is a surgical procedure in which the function of the vas deferens on each side of the testes is restored, having been cut and ligated in a preceding vasectomy (see Figure 8–9).

Another term for vas/o/vas/o/stomy is

_____ / _____ _____.

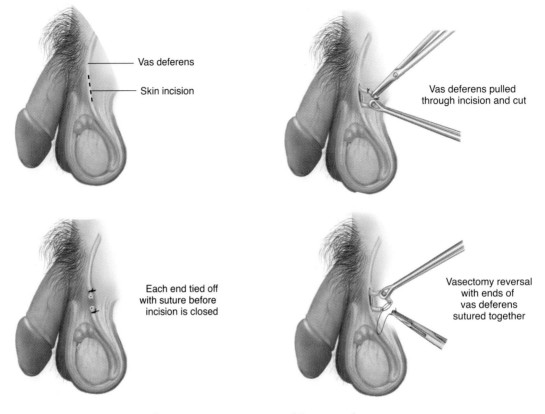

Vas deferens

Skin incision

Vas deferens pulled through incision and cut

Each end tied off with suture before incision is closed

Vasectomy reversal with ends of vas deferens sutured together

Figure 8-9   Vasectomy and its reversal.

---

ur/o/genit/al
ū-rō-JĔN-ĭ-tăl

vas/o/vas/o/stomy
văs-ō-vă-SŎS-tō-mē

8-147   Vas/ectomy reversal may be performed if a man wants to regain his fertility. In most cases, patency (opening up) of the canals is achieved, but in many cases, fertility does not result. This may be due to circulating autoantibodies that disrupt normal sperm activity. The antibodies apparently develop after vas/ectomy because the developing sperm cannot be excreted through the ur/o/genit/al tract.

Identify the term in this frame that means pertaining to urine and the organs of reproduction:

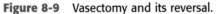

_____ / _____ / _____ / _____.

Identify the surgical term in this frame that is synonymous with *vas/ectomy reversal:* _____ / _____ / _____ / _____ / _____.

Listen and Learn, the audio CD-ROM that accompanies this book, will help you master the pronunciation of selected medical words. Use it to practice pronunciations *of selected terms* from Frames *8–103 to 8–147* for instructions to complete the *Listen and Learn* exercise on the CD-ROM for this section.

Using the following table, write the combining form, suffix, or prefix that matches its definition in the space provided to the left of the definition. There may be more than one word element that matches a definition.

Combining Forms	Suffixes	Prefixes
carcin/o	-cele	dys-
cyst/o	-cyte	hyper-
muc/o	-genesis	neo-
olig/o	-itis	
orchid/o	-megaly	
orchi/o	-pathy	
prostat/o	-pexy	
spermat/o	-rrhaphy	
sperm/o	-tome	
test/o		
vas/o		

1. _____ suture
2. _____ bad; painful; difficult
3. _____ bladder
4. _____ cancer
5. _____ cell
6. _____ disease
7. _____ enlargement
8. _____ hernia, swelling
9. _____ inflammation
10. _____ instrument to cut

11. _____ vessel; vas deferens; duct
12. _____ mucus
13. _____ new
14. _____ forming, producing, origin
15. _____ prostate gland
16. _____ testes
17. _____ scanty
18. _____ spermatozoa, sperm cells
19. _____ fixation (of an organ)
20. _____ excessive, above normal

Competency Verification: Check your answers in Appendix B, Answer Key, page 526. If you are not satisfied with your level of comprehension, go back to Frame 8–103 and rework the frames.

Correct Answers _____ × 5 = _____ % Score

Abbreviations

This section introduces reproductive system–related abbreviations and their meanings. Included are abbreviations contained in the medical record activities that follow.

Abbreviation	Meaning	Abbreviation	Meaning
FEMALE REPRODUCTIVE SYSTEM			
CS	cesarean section	OB-GYN	obstetrics and gynecology
C-section	cesarean section	OCPs	oral contraceptive pills
D&C	dilation (dilatation) and curettage	Pap	Papanicolaou smear
Dx, dx	diagnosis	para 1, 2, 3	unipara, bipara, tripara (number of viable births)
GYN	gynecology	PID	pelvic inflammatory disease
G	gravida (pregnant)	PMP	previous menstrual period
IUD	intrauterine device	TAH	total abdominal hysterectomy
IVF	in vitro fertilization	TSS	toxic shock syndrome
LMP	last menstrual period		
MALE REPRODUCTIVE SYSTEM			
BPH	benign prostatic hyperplasia, benign prostatic hypertrophy	TUR, TURP	transurethral resection of the prostate
GU	genitourinary	XY	male sex chromosomes
SEXUALLY TRANSMITTED DISEASES			
GC	gonorrhea	STD	sexually transmitted disease
HPV	human papillomavirus	VD	venereal disease
HSV	herpes simplex virus		

Pathological, Diagnostic, and Therapeutic Terms

The following are additional terms related to the female and male reproductive systems. Recognizing and learning these terms will help you understand the connection between a pathological condition, its diagnosis, and the rationale behind the method of treatment selected for a particular disorder.

Pathological

Female Reproductive System

candidiasis (kăn-dĭ-DĪ-ă-sĭs): vaginal fungal infection caused by *Candida albicans,* characterized by a curdy or cheeselike discharge and extreme itching.

cervicitis (sĕr-vĭ-SĪ-tĭs): acute or chronic inflammation of the uterine cervix.

The principal causative agent of cervicitis is sexually transmitted diseases, but many infections are nonspecific with unknown pathogenesis.

eclampsia (ē-KLĂMP-sē-ă): gravest form of pregnancy-induced hypertension.

ectopic pregnancy (ĕk-TŎP-ik): implantation of the fertilized ovum outside of the uterine cavity (see Figure 8–10).

Ectopic pregnancy occurs in approximately 1% of pregnancies, mostly in the oviducts (tubal pregnancy). Some types of ectopic pregnancies include ovarian, interstitial, and isthmic.

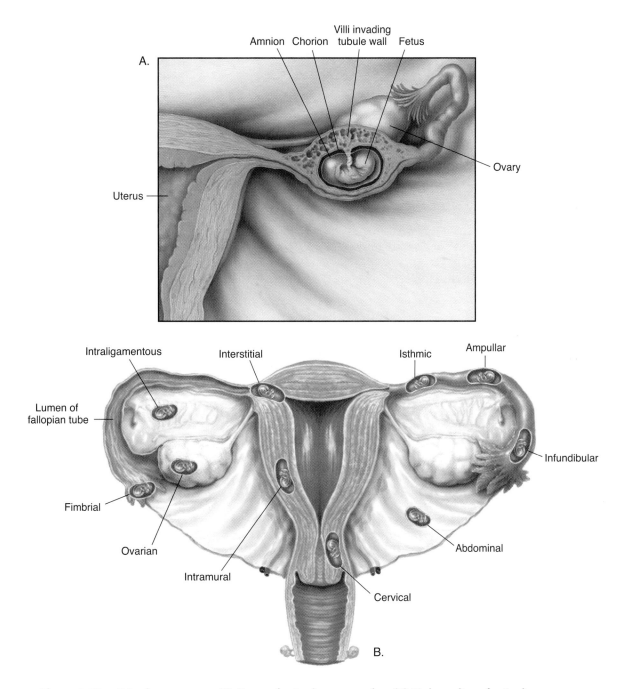

Figure 8-10 Ectopic pregnancy. (A) Types of ectopic pregnancies. (B) Various sites of ectopic pregnancy.

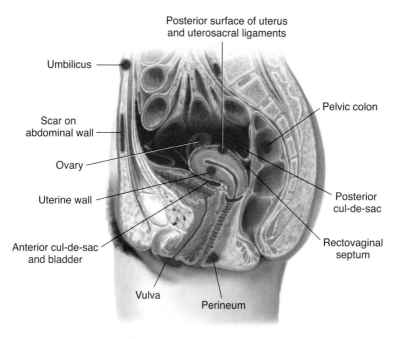

Posterior surface of uterus
and uterosacral ligaments

Umbilicus

Pelvic colon

Scar on
abdominal wall

Ovary

Posterior
cul-de-sac

Uterine wall

Rectovaginal
septum

Anterior cul-de-sac
and bladder

Vulva

Perineum

Figure 8-11 Endometriosis.

endometriosis (ĕn-dō-mē-trē-Ō-sĭs): presence of endometrial tissue outside (ectopic) the uterine cavity such as the pelvis or abdomen (see Figure 8–11).

fibroma (fibroid) of the uterus (fī-BRŌ-mă, FĪ-broyd): benign neoplasm consisting of fibrous encapsulated connective tissue.

leukorrhea (loo-kō-RĒ-ă): white discharge from the vagina.

A greater than usual amount of leukorrhea is normal in pregnancy, and a decrease is to be expected after delivery, during lactation, and after menopause. Leukorrhea is the most common reason women seek gynecological care.

oligomenorrhea (ŏl-ĭ-gō-mĕn-ō-RĒ-ă): scanty or infrequent menstrual flow.

pyosalpinx (pī-ō-SĂL-pĭnks): pus in the fallopian tube.

retroversion (rĕt-rō-VĔR-shŭn): turning, or state of being turned back, especially an entire organ being tipped from its normal position (for example, the uterus).

sterility (stĕr-ĬL-ĭ-tē): inability of a woman to become pregnant or for a man to impregnate a woman.

toxic shock syndrome (TŎK-sĭk SHŎK SĬN-drōm): rare and sometimes fatal disease caused by a toxin or toxins produced by certain strains of the bacterium *Staphylococcus aureus*.

Toxic shock syndrome (TSS) usually occurs in young menstruating women, most of whom were using vaginal tampons for menstrual protection.

Male Reproductive System

anorchism (ăn-ŎR-kĭzm): congenital absence of one or both testes.

balanitis (băl-ă-NĪ-tĭs): inflammation of the skin covering the glans penis.

cryptorchidism (krĭpt-OR-kĭd-ĭzm): failure of testicles to descend into scrotum.

epispadias (ĕp-ĭ-SPĀ-dē-ăs): congenital defect in which the urethra opens on the upper side of the penis, near the glans penis, instead of the tip.

hypospadias (hī-pō-SPĀ-dē-ăs): congenital defect in which the male urethra opens on the undersurface of the penis instead of the tip.

impotence (ĬM-pŏ-tĕns): inability of a man to achieve or maintain a penile erection.

phimosis (fī-MŌ-sĭs): stenosis or narrowness of preputial orifice so that the foreskin cannot be pushed back over the glans penis.

Sexually Transmitted Diseases

A sexually transmitted disease (STD) is any disease that may be acquired as a result of sexual intercourse or other intimate contact with an infected individual and affects the male and female reproductive system. Also called *venereal disease*. The following are some of the common STDs.

chlamydia (klă-MĬD-ē-ă): caused by infection with the bacterium *Chlamydia trachomatis*, the most prevalent and among the most damaging of all STDs.

In women, chlamydial infections cause cervicitis with a mucopurulent discharge and an alarming increase in pelvic infections. In men, chlamydial infections cause urethritis with a whitish discharge from the penis.

genital warts (JĔN-ĭ-tăl wortz): wart(s) in the genitalia caused by human papillomavirus (HPV).

In women, genital warts may be associated with cancer of the cervix.

gonorrhea (gŏn-ō-RĒ-ă): contagious bacterial infection; most often affects the genitourinary tract and occasionally the pharynx or rectum.

Infection results from contact with an infected person or with secretions containing the causative organism Neisseria gonorrhoeae. *In men, symptoms include dysuria and a greenish yellow discharge from the urethra. In women, the chief symptom is a vaginal greenish yellow discharge; can be transmitted to the fetus during delivery.*

herpes genitalis (HĔR-pēz jĕn-ĭ-TĂL-ĭs): infection in females and males of the genital and anorectal skin and mucosa with herpes simplex virus type 2.

This viral infection may be transmitted to the fetus during delivery and may be fatal.

syphilis (SĬF-ĭ-lĭs): infectious, chronic venereal disease characterized by lesions that change to a chancre and may involve any organ or tissue. It usually exhibits cutaneous manifestations.

Relapses of syphilis are frequent; it may exist without symptoms for years and can be transmitted from mother to fetus.

trichomoniasis (trĭk-ō-mō-NĪ-ă-sĭs): infestation with a parasite of genus *Trichomonas;* often causes vaginitis, urethritis, and cystitis.

Diagnostic

Female Reproductive System

amniocentesis (ăm-nē-ō-sĕn-TĒ-sĭs): obstetric procedure of a surgical puncture of the amniotic sac under ultrasound guidance to remove amniotic fluid.

The cells of the fetus, found in the fluid, are cultured and studied chemically and cytologically to detect genetic abnormalities, biochemical disorders, and maternal-fetal blood incompatibility (See Figure 8–12).

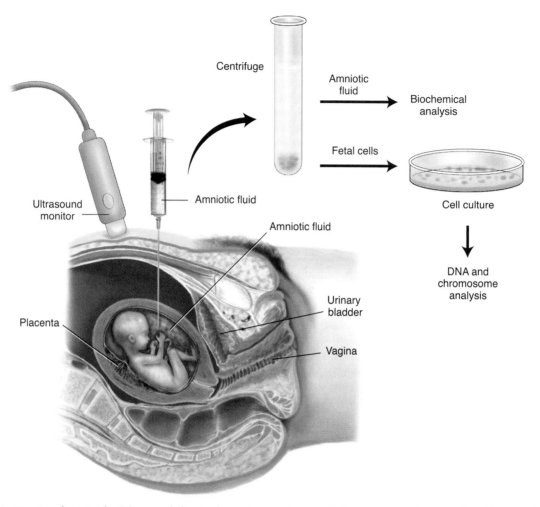

Figure 8-12 Amniocentesis. (A) Transabdominal puncture of the amniotic sac under ultrasound guidance using a needle and a syringe to remove amniotic fluid. (B) Amniotic fluid aspirant for laboratory analysis.

colposcopy (kŏl-PŎS-kō-pē): examination of the vagina and cervix with an optical magnifying instrument (colposcope); this is commonly performed after a Pap test to obtain biopsy specimens of the cervix.

hysterosalpingography (hĭs-tĕr-ō-săl-pĭn-GŎG-ră-fē): radiography of the uterus and oviducts after injection of a contrast medium.

laparoscopy (lăp-ăr-ŎS-kō-pē): visual examination of the abdominal cavity with a laparoscope through one or more small incisions in the abdominal wall, usually at the umbilicus (see Figure 8–13).

Laparoscopy is used for inspection of the ovaries and fallopian tubes, diagnosis of endometriosis, destruction of uterine leiomyomas, myomectomy, and gynecologic sterilization.

mammography (măm-ŎG-ră-fē): radiography of the breast that is used to diagnose benign and malignant tumors.

Papanicolaou (Pap) test (păp-ăh-NĬK-ĕ-lŏw): microscopic analysis of cells taken from the cervix and vagina to detect the presence of carcinoma. Cells are obtained after the insertion of a vaginal speculum and the use of a swab to scrape a small tissue sample from the cervix and vagina.

ultrasonography (ŭl-tră-sŏn-ŎG-ră-fē): imaging technique that uses high-frequency sound waves (ultra-

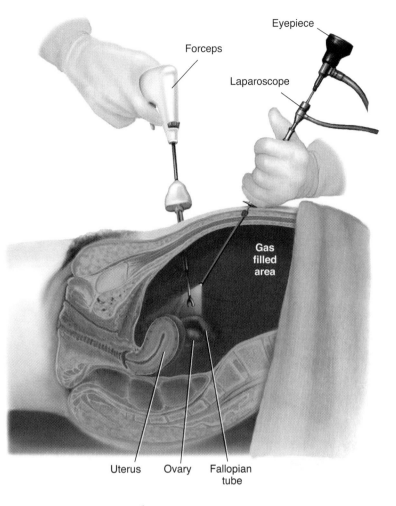

Figure 8-13   Laparoscopy.

sound) that bounce off body tissues and are recorded to produce an image of an internal organ or tissue. Ultrasonic echoes are recorded and interpreted by a computer, which produces a detailed image of the organ or tissue being evaluated.

Pelvic ultrasonography is used to evaluate the female reproductive organs and the fetus during pregnancy; transvaginal ultrasonography places the sound probe in the vagina instead of across the pelvis or abdomen, producing a sharper examination of normal and pathologic structures within the pelvis.

Male Reproductive System

digital rectal examination (dĭj-ĭ-TĂL RĔK-tăl): examination of the prostate gland by finger palpation through the rectum.

Digital rectal examination (DRE) is performed usually during physical examination to detect prostate enlargement.

prostate-specific antigen (PSA) test (ĂN-tĭ-jĕn): blood test to screen for prostate cancer; elevated levels of PSA are associated with prostate cancer and enlargement.

Therapeutic

Female Reproductive System

cerclage (sār-KLŎZH): obstetric procedure in which a nonabsorbable suture is used for holding the cervix closed to prevent spontaneous abortion in a woman who has an incompetent cervix.

dilation and curettage (DĬ-lā-shŭn and kū-rĕ-TĂZH): surgical procedure that expands the cervical canal of the uterus (dilation) so that the surface lining of the uterine wall can be scraped (curettage).

Dilation and curettage (D&C) is performed to stop prolonged or heavy uterine bleeding, diagnose uterine abnormalities, empty uterine contents of conception tissue, and obtain tissue for microscopic examination.

hysterosalpingo-oophorectomy (hĭs-tĕr-ō-săl-pĭng-gō-ō-ŏ-for-ĔK-tō-mē): surgical removal of a fallopian tube and an ovary.

mastectomy (măs-TĔK-tō-mē): complete or partial surgical removal of one or both breasts, most commonly performed to remove a malignant tumor.

A mastectomy may be simple, radical, or modified depending on the extent of the malignancy and the amount of breast tissue excised.

tubal ligation (TŪ-băl lĭ-GĀ-shŭn): sterilization procedure that involves blocking both fallopian tubes by cutting or burning them and tying them off.

Male Reproductive System

circumcision (sĕr-kŭm-SĬ-zhŭn): surgical removal of the foreskin or prepuce of the penis, which usually is performed on the male as an infant.

gonadotropins (gŏn-ă-dō-TRŌ-pĭnz): hormonal preparations used to increase the sperm count in infertility cases.

Listen and Learn, the audio CD-ROM that accompanies this book, will help you master the pronunciation of selected medical words. Use it to practice pronunciations of the above-listed medical terms and for instructions for completing the *Listen and Learn* exercise on the CD-ROM for this section.

PATHOLOGICAL, DIAGNOSTIC, AND THERAPEUTIC TERMS REVIEW

Match the medical term(s) below with the definitions in the numbered list.

anorchism
candidiasis
cerclage
chlamydia
circumcision

cryptorchidism
dilation and curettage (D&C)
endometriosis
gonadotropins
gonorrhea

impotence
leukorrhea
mammography
oligomenorrhea
phimosis

pyosalpinx
sterility
syphilis
toxic shock syndrome
trichomoniasis

1. _____ refers to failure of testicles to descend into scrotum.

2. _____ is pus in the fallopian tube.

3. _____ refers to inability of a woman to become pregnant or for a man to impregnate a woman.

4. _____ refers to congenital absence of one or both testes.

5. _____ is a vaginal fungal infection caused by *Candida albicans* and marked by a curdy discharge and extreme itching.

6. _____ is caused by infection with the bacterium *Chlamydia trachomatis* and occurs in both sexes.

7. _____ is surgical removal of the foreskin or prepuce of the penis.

8. _____ is an obstetric procedure to prevent spontaneous abortion in a woman who has an incompetent cervix.

9. _____ is a discharge from the vagina; common reason for women to seek gynecological care.

10. _____ is a condition in which endometrial tissue is found in various abnormal sites throughout the pelvis or in the abdominal wall.

11. _____ refers to radiography of the breast that is used to diagnose benign and malignant tumors.

12. _____ is a sexually transmitted bacterial infection; most often affects the genitourinary tract and occasionally the pharynx or rectum.

13. _____ is a sexually transmitted venereal disease characterized by lesions that change to a chancre and may involve any organ or tissue; usually exhibits cutaneous manifestations.

14. _____ is a rare and sometimes fatal disease caused by a toxin or toxins produced by certain strains of the bacterium *Staphylococcus aureus;* occurs in menstruating women who use vaginal tampons.

345

15. _____ is an infestation with a parasite of the genus *Trichomonas*, often causing vaginitis, urethritis, and cystitis.

16. _____ refers to widening of the uterine cervix so that the surface lining of the uterus can be scraped.

17. _____ means stenosis of the preputial orifice so that the foreskin does not retract over the glans penis.

18. _____ refers to the inability of a man to achieve a penile erection.

19. _____ refers to scanty or infrequent menstrual flow.

20. _____ are hormonal preparations used to increase the sperm count in infertility cases.

Competency Verification: Check your answers in Appendix B, Answer Key, page 526. If you are not satisfied with your level of comprehension, review the pathological, diagnostic, and therapeutic terms and retake the review.

Correct Answers _____ × 5 = _____ % Score

Medical Record Activities

The following medical records reflect common real-life clinical scenarios using medical terminology to document patient care. The physician who specializes in the treatment of female reproductive disorders is a *gynecologist;* the medical specialty concerned with the diagnoses and treatment of female reproductive disorders is called *gynecology. Obstetrics* is the branch of medicine concerned with pregnancy and childbirth. It involves the care of the mother and fetus throughout pregnancy, childbirth, and postpartum (after birth). An *obstetrician* is a physician who specializes in obstetrics.

The physician who specializes in the treatment of male reproductive and urinary tract disorders is a *urologist.* The medical specialty concerned with the diagnoses and treatment of male reproductive and urinary tract disorders is called *urology.*

✓ MEDICAL RECORD ACTIVITY 8–1. Postmenopausal Bleeding

Terminology

The terms listed in the chart come from the medical record *Postmenopausal Bleeding* that follows. Use a medical dictionary such as *Taber's Cyclopedic Medical Dictionary,* the appendices of this book, or other resources to define each term. Then practice reading the pronunciations aloud for each term.

Term	Definition
axilla ăk-SĬL-ă	
D&C	
gravida 4 GRĂV-ĭ-dă	
laparoscopy lăp-ăr-ŎS-kō-pē (see Figure 8–13)	
lesion LĒ-zhŭn	
mastectomy măs-TĔK-tŏ-mē	
menstrual MĔN-stroo-ăl	
metastases mĕ-TĂS-tă-sēz	
neoplastic NĒ-ō-plăs-tik	
para 4 PĂR-ă	

(Continued)

Term	Definition *(Continued)*
postmenopausal pōst-měn-ō-PAW-zăl	
Premarin PRĔM-ă-rĭn	
preulcerating prē-ŬL-sĕr-āt-ĭng	

> *Listen and Learn Online!* will help you master the pronunciation of selected medical words from this medical record activity. Visit www.fadavis.com/gylys/simplified for instructions in completing the *Listen and Learn Online!* exercise for this section and then to practice pronunciations.

POSTMENOPAUSAL BLEEDING

Reading

Practice pronunciation of medical terms by reading the following medical report aloud.

A 52-year-old gravida 4, para 4, woman had her last menstrual period at age 48. She was in our office last month for an evaluation because of postmenopausal bleeding. She has been taking Premarin and has had vaginal bleeding. The patient is currently admitted for gynecological laparoscopy and diagnostic D&C to rule out the possibility of a neoplastic process.

Last year this patient was admitted to the hospital for a simple mastectomy. The patient had a large preulcerating lesion of the left breast with metastases to the axilla, liver, and bone. Further medical evaluation will be performed next week.

Evaluation

Review the medical record to answer the following questions.

1. How many times has the patient been pregnant? How many children has the patient given birth to?

_____

_____

2. Why is the patient being admitted to the hospital?

_____

_____

3. What is a D&C?

_____

_____

4. What is the patient's past surgical history?

_____

_____

5. At what sites did the patient have malignant growth?

_____

_____

✓ MEDICAL RECORD ACTIVITY 8–2. Bilateral Vasectomy

Terminology

The terms listed in the chart come from the medical record *Bilateral Vasectomy* that follows. Use a medical dictionary such as *Taber's Cyclopedic Medical Dictionary,* the appendices of this book, or other resources to define each term. Then practice reading the pronunciations aloud for each term.

Term	Definition
bilateral bī-LĂT-ĕr-ăl	
cauterized KAW-tĕr-īzd	
Darvocet-N DĂHR-vō-sĕt	
hemostat HĒ-mō-stăt	
prn	
semen SĒ-mĕn	
supine sū-PĪN	
vas VĂS	
vasectomy văs-ĔK-tō-mē (see Figure 8–9)	
Xylocaine ZĪ-lō-kān	

Listen and Learn Online! will help you master the pronunciation of selected medical words from this medical record activity. Visit www.fadavis.com/gylys/simplified for instructions in completing the *Listen and Learn Online!* exercise for this section and then to practice pronunciations.

BILATERAL VASECTOMY

Reading

Practice pronunciation of medical terms by reading the following medical report aloud.

The patient was placed on the table in the supine position and prepped, scrotum shaved, and draped in the usual fashion. The right testicle was grasped and brought to skin level. This area was injected with 1% Xylocaine anesthesia. After a few minutes, a small incision was made, and the right vas was located. A hemostat was used and clamped on the right and left vas. A segment of the right vas was removed, and both ends were cauterized and tied independently with 3–0 silk suture. The skin was closed with 2–0 chromic suture. The same procedure was performed on the left side. There were no complications or bleeding. The patient was discharged to home in care of his wife. Postoperative care instruction sheet was given along with prescription of Darvocet-N, 100 mg, 1 q4h prn, for pain. Patient will be seen for follow-up semen analysis in 6 weeks.

Evaluation

Review the medical record to answer the following questions.

1. What is the end result of a bilateral vasectomy?

_____

_____

2. Was the patient awake during the surgery? What type of anesthesia was used?

_____

_____

3. What was used to prevent bleeding?

_____

_____

4. What type of suture material was used to close the incision?

_____

_____

5. What was the patient given for pain relief at home?

_____

_____

6. Why is it important for the patient to go for a follow-up visit?

_____

_____

Chapter Review

Word Elements Summary

The following table summarizes combining forms, suffixes, and prefixes related to the reproductive system.

Word Element	Meaning
COMBINING FORMS	
FEMALE REPRODUCTIVE SYSTEM	
amni/o	amnion (amniotic sac)
cervic/o	neck; cervix uteri (neck of uterus)
colp/o, vagin/o	vagina
episi/o, vulv/o	vulva
galact/o, lact/o	milk
gynec/o	woman, female
hyster/o, uter/o	uterus (womb)
lapar/o	abdomen
metr/o	uterus (womb); measure
mamm/o, mast/o	breast
men/o	menses, menstruation
nat/o	birth
oophor/o, ovari/o	ovary
perine/o	perineum
salping/o	tube (usually fallopian or eustachian [auditory] tubes)
MALE REPRODUCTIVE SYSTEM	
andr/o	male
balan/o	glans penis
orchid/o, orchi/o, orch/o, test/o	testis (plural, testes)
prostat/o	prostate gland
spermat/o	spermatozoa, sperm cells
vas/o	vessel; vas deferens; duct

(Continued)

Word Element	Meaning *(Continued)*
OTHER COMBINING FORMS	
adip/o, lip/o	fat
carcin/o	cancer
cyst/o	bladder
hemat/o, hem/o	blood
hydr/o	water
muc/o	mucus
olig/o	scanty
SUFFIXES	
SURGICAL	
-ectomy	excision, removal
-pexy	fixation (of an organ)
-plasty	surgical repair
-rrhaphy	suture
-tome	instrument to cut
-tomy	incision
DIAGNOSTIC, SYMPTOMATIC, AND RELATED	
-algia, -dynia	pain
-cele	hernia, swelling
-genesis	forming, producing, origin
-itis	inflammation
-lith	stone, calculus
-logy	study of
-logist	specialist in study of
-megaly	enlargement
-oid	resembling
-oma	tumor
-pathy	disease
-plasia, -plasm	formation, growth
-ptosis	prolapse, downward displacement

Word Element	Meaning
-rrhage, -rrhagia	bursting forth (of)
-rrhea	discharge, flow
-scope	instrument for examining
-spasm	involuntary contraction, twitching
-uria	urine
FEMALE REPRODUCTIVE SYSTEM	
-arche	beginning
-cyesis	pregnancy
-gravida	pregnant woman
-para	to bear (offspring)
-salpinx	tube (usually fallopian or eustachian [auditory] tubes)
-tocia	childbirth, labor
-version	turning
ADJECTIVE	
-al, -ic, -ous	pertaining to, relating to
NOUN	
-ia	condition
-ist	specialist
PREFIXES	
a-, an-	without, not
dys-	bad; painful; difficult
hyper-	excessive, above normal
neo-	new
post-	after, behind
pre-	before, in front of

WORD ELEMENTS REVIEW

After you review the Word Elements Summary, complete this activity by writing the meaning of each element in the space provided.

Word Element	Meaning
COMBINING FORMS	
FEMALE REPRODUCTIVE SYSTEM	
1. amni/o	
2. colp/o, vagin/o	
3. episi/o, vulv/o	
4. galact/o, lact/o	
5. gynec/o	
6. hyster/o, metr/o, uter/o	
7. nat/o	
8. oophor/o, ovari/o	
9. perine/o	
MALE REPRODUCTIVE SYSTEM	
10. vas/o	
11. orchid/o, orchi/o, orch/o, test/o	
12. andr/o	
13. balan/o	
OTHER COMBINING FORMS	
14. adip/o, lip/o	
15. olig/o	
16. hemat/o, hem/o	
17. hydr/o	
18. muc/o	
SUFFIXES	
SURGICAL	
19. -ectomy	
20. -plasty	
21. -pexy	
22. -tomy	

Word Element	Meaning
DIAGNOSTIC, SYMPTOMATIC, AND RELATED	
23. -logist	
24. -genesis	
25. -algia, -dynia	
26. -megaly	
27. -cele	
FEMALE REPRODUCTIVE SYSTEM	
28. -para	
29. -tocia	
30. -version	
31. -cyesis	
32. -salpinx	
33. -gravida	
34. -arche	
NOUN	
35. -ist	
ADJECTIVE	
37. -al, -ic, -ous	
PREFIXES	
38. neo-	
39. dys-	
40. a-, an-	

Competency Verification: Check your answers in Appendix A, Glossary of Medical Word Elements, page 497. If you are not satisfied with your level of comprehension, review the word elements and retake the review.

Correct Answers: _____ × 2.5 = _____ % Score

Chapter 8 Vocabulary Review

Match the medical term(s) below with the definitions in the numbered list.

amenorrhea
aplasia
aspermatism
cervix uteri
dysmenorrhea
epididymis
estrogen

gravida 4
hydrocele
oophoritis
para 4
pelvic inflammatory disease (PID)
postmenopausal
progesterone

prostatic cancer
prostatomegaly
testopathy
testosterone
uterus
vas deferens
vasectomy

1. _____ means enlargement of the prostate gland.

2. _____ refers to disease of the testes.

3. _____ is a male hormone produced by testes.

4. _____ is absence or abnormal stoppage of the menses.

5. _____ is a female hormone(s) produced by the ovaries.

6. _____ is an inflamed condition of the ovaries.

7. _____ is a condition in which there is a lack of male sperm.

8. _____ refers to a woman in her fourth pregnancy.

9. _____ is an organ that nourishes the embryo.

10. _____ is a malignant neoplasm of the prostate.

11. _____ is a tube that temporarily stores sperm.

12. _____ is a collection of fluid in a saclike cavity.

13. _____ is a duct that transports sperm from the testes to the urethra.

14. _____ refers to a woman who has delivered four infants.

15. _____ means neck of the uterus.

16. _____ refers to painful menstruation.

17. _____ means occurring after menopause.

18. _____ is failure or lack of formation or growth.

19. _____ is a procedure to sterilize a man by cutting the vas deferens, which prevents the release of sperm.

20. _____ is collective term for any extensive bacterial infection of the pelvic organs, especially the uterus, uterine tubes, or ovaries.

Competency Verification: Check your answers in Appendix B, Answer Key, page 527. If you are not satisfied with your level of comprehension, review the chapter vocabulary and retake the review.

Correct Answers _____ × 5= _____ % Score

9

Endocrine and Nervous Systems

OBJECTIVES

Upon completion of this chapter, you will be able to:

■ Describe the endocrine system and discuss its primary functions.

■ Describe the nervous system and discuss its primary functions.

■ Describe pathological, diagnostic, therapeutic, and other terms related to the endocrine and nervous systems.

■ Recognize, define, pronounce, and spell terms correctly by completing the audio CD-ROM exercises.

■ Demonstrate your knowledge of this chapter by successfully completing the frames, reviews, and medical report evaluations.

The endocrine and nervous systems work together like interlocking supersystems to control many intricate activities of the body. Together they monitor changes in the body and in the external environment, interpret these changes, and coordinate appropriate responses to reestablish and maintain a relative equilibrium in the internal environment of the body (homeostasis).

Endocrine System

The endocrine system comprises a network of ductless glands (see Figure 9–1), which have a rich blood supply that enables the hormones they produce to enter the bloodstream. Hormone production occurs at one site, but their effects take place at various other sites in the body. The tissues or organs that respond to the effects of a hormone are called *target tissues* or *target organs.*

In contrast to the endocrine system, which slowly discharges hormones into the bloodstream, the nervous system is designed to act instantaneously by transmitting electrical impulses to specific body locations. The nervous system controls all critical body activities and reactions. It is one of the most complicated systems of the body. The nervous system coordinates voluntary (conscious) activities, such as walking, talking, and eating, and involuntary (unconscious) functions, such as reflexes to pain, body changes related to stress, and thought and emotional processes.

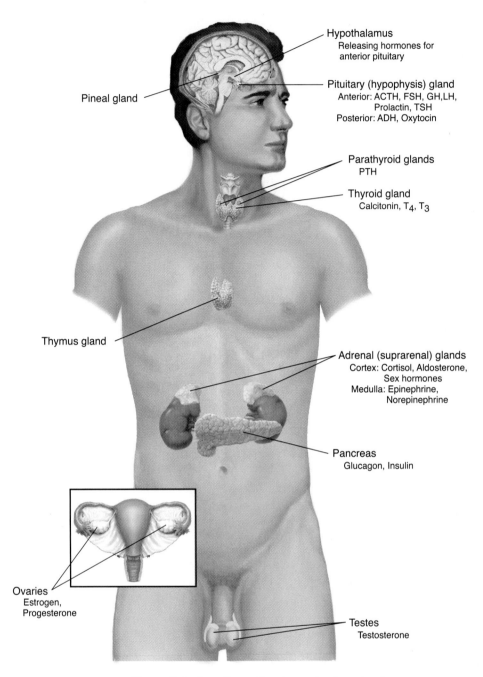

Pineal gland

Hypothalamus
Releasing hormones for
anterior pituitary

Pituitary (hypophysis) gland
Anterior: ACTH, FSH, GH,LH,
Prolactin, TSH
Posterior: ADH, Oxytocin

Parathyroid glands
PTH

Thyroid gland
Calcitonin, T_4, T_3

Thymus gland

Adrenal (suprarenal) glands
Cortex: Cortisol, Aldosterone,
Sex hormones
Medulla: Epinephrine,
Norepinephrine

Pancreas
Glucagon, Insulin

Ovaries
Estrogen,
Progesterone

Testes
Testosterone

Figure 9-1 Locations of major endocrine glands.

Word Elements

This section introduces combining forms related to the endocrine system. Included are key suffixes; prefixes are defined in the right-hand column as needed. Review the following table, and pronounce each word in the word analysis column aloud before you begin to work the frames.

Word Element	Meaning	Word Analysis
COMBINING FORMS		
aden/o	gland	aden/oma (ăd-ĕ-NŌ-mă): tumor composed of glandular tissue *-oma:* tumor

adrenal/o
 	
adren/o
	adrenal glands	adrenal/ectomy (ăd-rē-năl-ĔK-tō-mē): surgical removal of one or both adrenal glands
		   -ectomy: excision, removal
		adren/al (ăd-RĒ-năl): pertaining to the adrenal glands
		   -al: pertaining to, relating to

calc/o	calcium	hypo/calc/emia (hī-pō-kăl-SĒ-mē-ă): deficiency of calcium in the blood
		   hypo-: under, below, deficient
		   -emia: blood condition

gluc/o
 	
glyc/o
	sugar, sweetness	gluc/o/genesis (gloo-kō-JĔN-ĕ-sĭs): formation of glucose
		   -genesis: forming, producing, origin
		hyper/glyc/emia (hī-pĕr-glī-SĒ-mē-ă): greater than normal amount of glucose in the blood
		   hyper-: excessive, above normal
		   -emia: blood condition
		
		Hyperglycemia is associated most frequently with diabetes mellitus.

pancreat/o	pancreas	pancreat/itis (păn-krē-ă-TĪ-tĭs): inflammatory condition of the pancreas *-itis:* inflammation
parathyroid/o	parathyroid glands	parathyroid/ectomy (păr-ă-thī-royd-ĔK-tō-mē): surgical removal of the parathyroid glands *-ectomy:* excision, removal
thym/o	thymus gland	thym/oma (thī-MŌ-mă): tumor of the thymus gland *-oma:* tumor

thyr/o
 	
thyroid/o
	thyroid gland	thyr/o/megaly (thī-rō-MĔG-ă-lē): enlargement of the thyroid gland
		   -megaly: enlargement
		thyroid/ectomy (thī-royd-ĔK-tō-mē): surgical removal of the thyroid gland
		   -ectomy: excision, removal

toxic/o	poison	toxic/o/logist (tŏks-ĭ-KŌL-ō-jĭst): specialist in the study of poisons or toxins *-logist:* specialist in study of

(Continued)

Word Element	Meaning	Word Analysis *(Continued)*
SUFFIXES		
-dipsia	thirst	poly/dipsia (pŏl-ē-DĬP-sē-ă): excessive thirst *poly-:* many, much *Polydipsia is a characteristic symptom of diabetes mellitus.*
-trophy	development, nourishment	hyper/trophy (hī-PĔR-trŏ-fē): increase in the size of an organ *hyper-:* excessive, above normal *Hypertrophy is due to an increase in the size of the cells of an organ rather than an increase in the number of cells, as in carcinoma.*

Listen and Learn, the audio CD-ROM that accompanies this book, will help you master the pronunciation of selected medical words. Use it to practice pronunciations of the above-l isted medical terms and for instructions for completing the *Listen and Learn* exercise on the CD-ROM for this section.

SECTION REVIEW 9 – 1

For the following medical terms, first write the suffix and its meaning. Then translate the meaning of the remaining elements starting with the first part of the word. The first word is an example that is completed for you.

Term	Definition
1. toxic/o/logist	-logist: specialist in study of; poison
2. pancreat/itis	_____
3. thyr/o/megaly	_____
4. hyper/trophy	_____
5. gluc/o/genesis	_____
6. hypo/calc/emia	_____
7. adrenal/ectomy	_____
8. poly/dipsia	_____
9. aden/oma	_____
10. thyroid/ectomy	_____

Competency Verification: Check your answers in Appendix B, Answer Key, page 528. If you are not satisfied with your level of comprehension, review the vocabulary and retake the review.

Correct Answers _____ × 10 = _____ % Score

Hormones

9–1 *Hormones* are chemical substances produced by specialized cells of the body. Because they travel in the blood, hormones reach all body tissues. Only target organs contain receptors that recognize a particular hormone, however. The receptors maintain the tissue's responsiveness to hormonal stimulation.

Review Figure 9–2, which illustrates hormones of the pituitary gland and their target organs. This means the organs shown in Figure 9–2 are directly affected by the amounts of hormones released into the bloodstream by the pituitary gland. For example, an underproduction of growth hormone (GH) in children results in dwarfism.

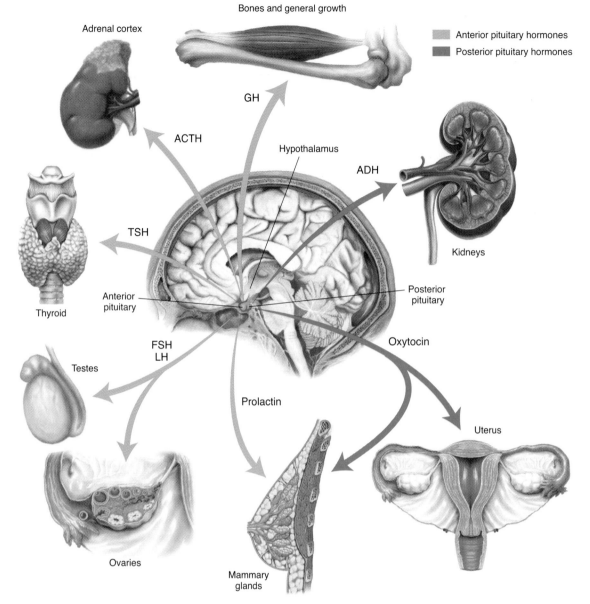

Figure 9-2 Hormones secreted by the anterior and posterior pituitary gland and their target organs.

9-2 Hormone secretion to a target organ is determined by the body's need for the hormone at any given time and is regulated so that there is no overproduction *(hyper/secretion)* or underproduction *(hypo/secretion)*. There are times when the body's regulating mechanism does not operate properly, and hormonal levels become excessive or deficient causing various disorders.

The term in this frame that is synonymous with

overproductions is _____ / _____.

underproduction is _____ / _____.

hyper/secretion
hī-pĕr-sē-KRĒ-shŭn
hypo/secretion
hī-pō-sē-KRĒ-shŭn

9-3   Although all major hormones circulate to virtually all tissues, each hormone exerts specific effects on its target organ. If a hormone has a specific effect on the stomach, that hormone's target organ is the stomach. If the hormone has a specific effect on the heart, the target organ is the

heart

_____.

9-4   Refer to Table 9–1 to complete this frame.

List four common characteristics of hormones.

1. _____

_____

_____

2. _____

_____

_____

3. _____

_____

_____

4. _____

_____

_____

9-5   Dys/function of an endocrine gland may result in either hypo/secretion or hyper/secretion of its hormone. The prefix hyper- means *excessive, above normal;* the prefix hypo- means *under, below, deficient.*

Build medical terms that mean

hyper/secretion
hī-pĕr-sē-KRĒ-shŭn

excessive secretion: _____ / _____.

hypo/secretion
hī-pō-sē-KRĒ-shŭn

deficient secretion: _____ / _____.

Table 9–1. Hormone Characteristics

This table offers four key characteristics of hormones.

- Chemical substances produced by specialized cells of the body
- Released slowly in minute amounts directly into the bloodstream
- Produced primarily by the endocrine glands
- Most are inactivated or excreted by the liver and kidneys

Pituitary Gland

9-6   The (1) **pituitary gland** is one of the most important endocrine glands. Its hormone secretions influence the functions of many organs in the body, as illustrated in Figure 9–2. Located below the brain, it is no larger than a pea.

Label the pituitary gland in Figure 9–3

---

anter/ior
ăn-tē-rē-or
poster/ior
pŏs-TĒ-rē-or

9-7   The pituitary gland consists of two distinct portions—an anter/ior lobe and a poster/ior lobe.

The front lobe is called the _____ / _____ lobe.

The back lobe back is called the _____ / _____ lobe.

---

anter/o

poster/o

9-8   Identify the combining forms meaning

anterior, front: _____ / _____.

back (of body), behind, posterior: _____ / _____.

---

radi/o

9-9   The term anter/o/poster/ior (AP) is used in radi/o/logy to describe the direction or path of an x-ray beam.

From radi/o/logy, determine the combining form for *radiation, x-ray:* _____ / _____.

---

back

9-10   AP is a directional abbreviation meaning passing from the front to the _____ (of the body).

---

poster/ior
pŏs-TĒ-rē-or

9-11   An AP view of the abdomen is a view from the anter/ior to the _____ / _____ part of the abdomen.

AP

PA

9-12   Poster/o/anter/ior (PA) means directed from the back toward the front (of the body).

Identify the abbreviations designating the path of an x-ray beam from the anter/o/poster/ior (part of the body): _____.

posteroanterior (part of the body): _____.

---

above

below

behind

side

9-13   Use the words *above* or *below* to complete directional terms in this frame.

Poster/o/super/ior means located behind and _____ a structure.

Poster/o/infer/ior means located behind and _____ a structure.

Poster/o/later/al means located _____ and at the _____ of a structure.

gland	**9-14** The pituitary gland is also called the *hypophysis.* The anterior lobe of the pituitary gland is called the aden/o/hypophysis; the poster/ior lobe is called the neur/o/hypophysis. The combining form **neur/o** refers to *nerve;* the combining form **aden/o** refers to _____.
anter/ior ăn-TĒ-rē-or **poster/ior** pŏs-TĒ-rē-or **neur/o/hypophysis** nū-rō-hī-PŎF-ĭs-ĭs **aden/o/hypophysis** ăd-ĕ-nō-hī-PŎF-ĭ-sĭs	**9-15** The anter/ior lobe (aden/o/hypophysis) develops from an upgrowth of the pharynx and is glandular in nature; the poster/ior lobe (neur/o/hypophysis) develops from a downgrowth from the base of the brain and consists of nervous tissue. Although both lobes secrete various hormones that regulate body functions, the two hormones secreted by the neur/o/hypophysis are produced in the hypothalamus. The neur/o/hypophysis merely acts as a storage site until the hormones are released. (See Table 9–2) Identify the words in this frame that mean in front of: _____ / _____. behind, back (of body): _____ / _____. hypophysis composed of nervous tissue: _____ / _____ / _____. hypophysis composed of glandular tissue: _____ / _____ / _____.
neur/o/hypophysis nū-rō-hī-PŎF-ĭs-ĭs	**9-16** The poster/ior lobe of the pituitary gland, composed primarily of nervous tissue, is called _____ / _____ / _____.
aden/o/hypophysis ăd-ē-nō-hī-PŎF-ĭ-sĭs	**9-17** The anter/ior lobe of the pituitary gland, composed primarily of glandular tissue, is called _____ / _____ / _____.
	9-18 Table 9–2 outlines pituitary hormones, along with their target organs and functions and selected associated disorders. Refer to Table 9–2 to complete Frames 9–18 through 9–23. The two hormones released by the neur/o/hypophysis are _____ _____ and _____.
	9-19 Define the following abbreviations: GH: _____ TSH: _____

ADH:

_____

LH:

_____

9-20 Briefly state the important function of ADH in the kidneys.

_____

_____

9-21 Briefly state two functions of GH.

_____

_____

_____

_____

9-22 The hormone that causes contraction of the uterus during childbirth is _____.

9-23 Write the abbreviation of the hormone that initiates sperm production in men: _____.

9-24 Overproduction of GH in children produces an exceptionally large person, a condition known as *gigant/ism*. Underproduction of GH in children is likely to produce an exceptionally small person, a condition called *dwarf/ism*.

An abnormally short or undersized person is known as a

_____; an abnormally tall or oversized person is known as a

_____.

dwarf

giant

9-25 Acr/o/megaly, a chronic metabolic condition, is characterized by a gradual marked enlargement and thickening of the bones of the face and jaw. This condition, which afflicts middle-aged and older persons, is caused by overproduction of growth hormone and is treated by radiation, pharmacologic agents, or surgery, often involving partial resection of the pituitary gland.

A term that literally means enlargement of the extremities is

_____ / ____ / _____.

acr/o/megaly

ăk-rō-MĔG-ă-lē

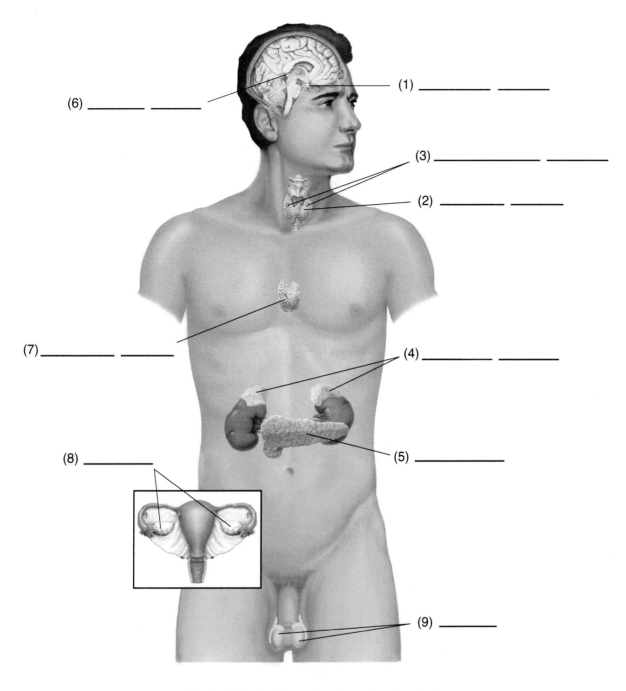

(6) _____ _____

(1) _____ _____

(3) _____ _____

(2) _____ _____

(7) _____ _____

(4) _____ _____

(5) _____

(8) _____

(9) _____

Figure 9-3 Locations of major endocrine glands.

Table 9–2. Pituitary Hormones

This table outlines pituitary hormones, along with their target organs and functions and selected associated disorders.

Hormone	Target Organ and Functions	Disorders
POSTERIOR PITUITARY HORMONES (NEUROHYPOPHYSIS)		
Antidiuretic hormone (ADH)	Kidney—increases water reabsorption (water returns to the blood)	Hyposecretion causes diabetes insipidus Hypersecretion causes syndrome of inappropriate antidiuretic hormone (SIADH)
Oxytocin	Uterus—stimulates uterine contractions; initiates labor Breast—promotes milk secretion from the mammary glands	Unknown
ANTERIOR PITUITARY HORMONES (ADENOHYPOPHYSIS)		
Adrenocorticotropic hormone (ACTH)	Adrenal cortex—promotes secretions of some hormones by adrenal cortex, especially cortisol	Hyposecretion is rare Hypersecretion causes Cushing disease
Follicle-stimulating hormone (FSH)	Ovaries—in females, stimulates egg production; increases secretion of estrogen Testes—in males, stimulates sperm production	Hyposecretion causes failure of sexual maturation Hypersecretion has no known important effects
Growth hormone (GH) or somatotropin	Bone, cartilage, liver, muscle, and other tissues—stimulates somatic growth; increases use of fats for energy	Hyposecretion in children causes pituitary dwarfism Hypersecretion in children causes gigantism; hypersecretion in adults causes acromegaly
Luteinizing hormone (LH)	Ovaries—in females, promotes ovulation; stimulates production of estrogen and progesterone Testes—in males, promotes secretion of testosterone	Hyposecretion causes failure of sexual maturation Hypersecretion has no known important effects
Prolactin	Breast—in conjunction with other hormones, promotes lactation	Hyposecretion in nursing mothers causes poor lactation Hypersecretion in nursing mothers causes galactorrhea
Thyroid-stimulating hormone (TSH)	Thyroid gland—stimulates secretion of thyroid hormone	Hyposecretion in infants causes cretinism; hyposecretion in adults causes myxedema Hypersecretion causes Graves disease, exophthalmos (see Figure 9–4)

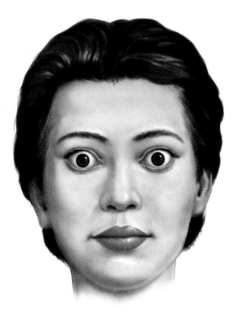

Figure 9-4   Exophthalmos caused by Graves disease.

Thyroid Gland

	9–26 The (2) **thyroid gland** is located on the front and sides of the trachea just below the larynx. Its two lobes are separated by a strip of tissue called the isthmus. Label the thyroid gland in Figure 9–3.
thyroid/ectomy thī-royd-ĔK-tō-mē	**9–27** The combining forms for the *thyroid gland* are **thyr/o** and **thyroid/o**. Use **thyroid/o** to form a word meaning excision of the thyroid gland: _____ / _____.
thyr/o/megaly thī-rō-MĔG-ă-lē **thyr/o/pathy** thī-RŎP-ă-thē **thyr/o/tomy** thī-RŎT-ō-mē	**9–28** Use **thyr/o** to construct words meaning enlargement of the thyroid gland: _____ / ____ / _____. disease of the thyroid gland: _____ / ____ / _____. incision of the thyroid gland: _____ / ____ / _____.
	9–29 Table 9–3 outlines thyroid hormones, along with their functions and selected associated disorders. Refer to the table to complete Frames 9–29 through 9–31. The thyroid gland produces two hormones that regulate the body's metabolism (rate at which food is converted into heat and energy). These hormones are called _____ and _____.

9-30 In conjunction with PTH, calcium levels in the blood are regulated by secretion of the hormone called _____.

9-31 When does calcitonin exert its most important effects in the body?

_____

_____

_____

9-32 Hyper/thyroid/ism is caused by excessive secretion of the thyroid gland, which increases the body's metabolism and intensifies the demand for food.

Analyze hyper/thyroid/ism by defining the elements:

excessive, above normal

Hyper- means _____, _____ _____.

thyroid gland
THĪ-royd

thyroid/o means _____ _____.

condition

-ism means _____.

9-33 Hyper/thyroid/ism involves enlargement of the thyroid gland associated with hypersecretion of thyroxine. It is characterized by ex/ophthalm/os (bulging of the eyes), which develops because of edema in the tissues of the eye sockets and swelling of the extrinsic eye muscles. Hyper/thyroid/ism also is called Graves disease, *ex/ophthalm/ic goiter*, *thyr/o/toxic/osis*, and *tox/ic goiter* (see Figures 9–4 and 9–5).

Identify the terms in this frame that mean

ex/ophthalm/os or
ĕks-ŏf-THĂL-mŏs
ex/ophthalm/ic
ĕks-ŏf-THĂL-mĭc

bulging of the eyes: _____ / _____ / _____.

abnormal condition of thyroid gland poisoning:

thyr/o/toxic/osis
thī-rō-tŏks-ĭ-KŌ-sĭs

_____ / ____ / _____ / _____.

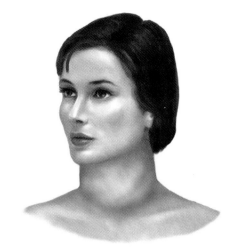

Figure 9-5   Enlargement of the thyroid gland in goiter.

Table 9–3. Thyroid Hormones

This table outlines thyroid hormones, along with their functions and selected associated disorders.

Hormone	Functions	Disorders
Calcitonin	In conjunction with parathyroid hormone (PTH), calcitonin helps to regulate calcium levels in the blood Decreases elevated calcium levels to maintain homeostasis	Calcitonin exerts its most important effects in childhood when the bones are growing and changing dramatically in mass, size, and shape
Thyroxine (T_4) and triiodothyronine (T_3)	Increases energy production from all food types Increases rate of protein synthesis	Hyposecretion in infants causes cretinism; hyposecretion in adults causes myxedema Hypersecretion causes Graves disease, exophthalmos (see Figure 9–4)

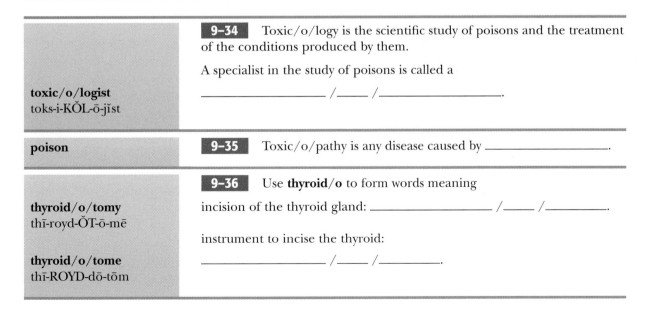

toxic/o/logist
toks-i-KŎL-ō-jĭst

9–34   Toxic/o/logy is the scientific study of poisons and the treatment of the conditions produced by them.

A specialist in the study of poisons is called a

_____ / ____ / _____.

poison

9–35   Toxic/o/pathy is any disease caused by _____.

thyroid/o/tomy
thī-royd-ŎT-ō-mē

thyroid/o/tome
thī-ROYD-dō-tōm

9–36   Use **thyroid/o** to form words meaning

incision of the thyroid gland: _____ / ____ / _____.

instrument to incise the thyroid:

_____ / ____ / _____.

blood	**9-37** The combining form for *calcium* is **calc/o.** The term calc/emia indicates an abnormal presence of calcium in the _____.
hyper/calc/emia hī-pĕr-kăl-SĒ-mē-ă	**9-38** Hypo/calc/emia is a condition of abnormally low blood calcium. A person with excessively high blood calcium has a condition called: _____ / _____ / _____.

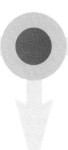

SECTION REVIEW 9 – 2

Using the following table, write the combining form, suffix, or prefix that matches its definition in the space provided to the left of the definition. There may be more than one word element that matches a definition.

Combining Forms	Suffixes	Prefixes
acr/o	-emia	dys-
aden/o	-logist	hyper-
anter/o	-megaly	hypo-
calc/o	-osis	poly-
neur/o	-pathy	
poster/o	-tome	
radi/o	-tomy	
thyr/o		
thyroid/o		
toxic/o		

1. _____ abnormal condition; increase (used primarily with blood cells)

2. _____ excessive, above normal

3. _____ back (of body), behind, posterior

4. _____ bad; painful; difficult

5. _____ blood condition

6. _____ calcium

7. _____ disease

8. _____ enlargement

9. _____ extremity

10. _____ anterior, front

11. _____ gland

12. _____ incision

13. _____ instrument to cut

14. _____ nerve

15. _____ poison

16. _____ radiation, x-ray; radius (lower arm bone on thumb side)

17. _____ specialist in study of

18. _____ many, much

19. _____ thyroid gland

20. _____ under, below, deficient

Competency Verification: Check your answers in Appendix B, Answer Key, page 528. If you are not satisfied with your level of comprehension, go back to Frame 9–1 and rework the frames.

Correct Answers _____ × 5 = _____% Score

Making a set of flash cards from key word elements in this chapter for each section review can help you remember the elements. Make a flash card by writing a word element on one side of a 3 × 5 or 4 × 6 index card. On the other side, write the meaning of the element. Do this for all word elements in the section reviews. Use your flash cards to review each section. You also might use the flash cards to prepare for the chapter review at the end of this chapter.

Parathyroid Glands

	9–39 The (3) **parathyroid glands** are located on the posterior surface of the thyroid gland. The parathyroid glands are so called because they are located around the thyroid gland. Label the parathyroid glands in Figure 9–3.
para/thyr/oid glands păr-ă-THĪ-royd	**9–40** Usually there are two pairs of para/thyr/oid glands associated with each of the thyroid's lobes, but the exact number varies. Nevertheless, as many as eight glands have been reported. The para/thyr/oid glands were detected accidentally. Surgeons observed that most patients who had either a partial or total thyroid/ectomy recovered uneventfully, whereas some experienced uncontrolled muscle spasms and severe pain and subsequently died. It was only after several such unexpected deaths that the parathyroid glands were discovered and their hormonal function, quite different from that of the thyroid gland hormones, became obvious. When we discuss the two pairs of glands located in the posterior aspect of the thyroid glands, we are talking about the _____ / _____ / _____ _____.
para-	**9–41** Identify the element in the previous frame that means located near, beside; beyond: _____.
PTH	**9–42** The hormone produced by the parathyroid glands is called para/thormone or para/thyroid hormone (PTH). The abbreviation for para/thormone or para/thyr/oid hormone is _____.
	9–43 Table 9–4 outlines parathyroid hormones along with their target organs and functions and selected associated disorders. Refer to the table to complete this frame. The major function of PTH is to regulate levels of _____ and _____.

Table 9–4. Parathyroid Hormone

This table outlines the parathyroid hormone, along with its target organs, functions, and selected associated disorders.

Hormone	Target Organ and Functions	Disorder
Parathyroid hormone (PTH)	Bones—increases reabsorption of calcium and phosphate from bone to blood Kidneys—increases calcium absorption and phosphate excretion Small intestine—increases absorption of calcium and phosphate	Hyposecretion causes tetany Hypersecretion causes osteitis fibrosa cystica

	9-44 *Oste/itis fibrosa cystica* is an inflammatory degenerative condition in which normal bone is replaced by cysts and fibrous tissue. It usually is associated with hyper/para/thyroid/ism.
	The term in this frame that means abnormal endocrine condition characterized by hypersecretion of PTH is
hyper/para/thyroid/ism hī-pĕr-păr-ă-THĪ-roy-dĭzm	_____ / _____ / _____ / _____.

	9-45 Calc/emia refers to calcium in the blood.
	Use hypo- and hyper- to form words meaning
	excessive calcium in the blood:
hyper/calc/emia hī-pĕr-kăl-SĒ-mē-ă **hypo/calc/emia** hī-pō-kăl-SĒ-mē-ă	_____ / _____ / _____. deficiency of calcium in the blood: _____ / _____ / _____.

Adrenal Glands

	9-46 The (4) **adrenal glands,** also known as the supra/ren/al glands, are paired structures located super/ior to the kidneys. Label Figure 9-3 as you continue to learn about the endocrine system.

	9-47 Indicate the words in Frame 9-46 that mean above or superior to a kidney:
supra/ren/al soo-pră-RĒ-năl **super/ior**	_____ / _____ / _____. pertaining to upper or above: _____ / _____.

	9-48 **Adren/o** and **adrenal/o** are combining forms for the adrenal glands.
enlargement, adrenal	Adren/o/megaly is an _____ of the _____ glands.
	Use **adrenal/o** to form a word meaning an excision of an adrenal gland:
adrenal/ectomy ăd-rē-năl-ĔK-tō-mē	_____ / _____.

	9-49 Each adrenal gland is structurally and functionally differentiated into two sections—the outer adrenal cortex, which comprises the bulk of the gland, and the inner portion, the adrenal medulla. The hormones produced by each part have different functions.
kidneys	The adrenal glands are perched atop the _____

	9-50 Table 9-5 outlines adrenal hormones, along with their target organs and functions and selected associated disorders. Review the table to learn about hormones and their effects on target organs.

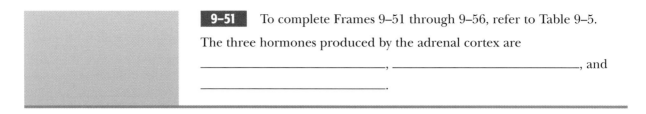

9–51 To complete Frames 9–51 through 9–56, refer to Table 9–5.

The three hormones produced by the adrenal cortex are

_____, _____, and

_____.

Table 9–5. Adrenal Hormones

This table outlines the adrenal hormones, along with their target organs, functions, and selected associated disorders.

Hormone	Target Organ and Functions	Disorders
ADRENAL CORTEX HORMONES		
Glucocorticoids (mainly cortisol)	Body cells—promote gluconeogenesis; regulate metabolism of carbohydrates, proteins, and fats; help depress inflammatory and immune responses	Hyposecretion causes Addison disease Hypersecretion causes Cushing syndrome (see Figure 9–6)
Mineralocorticoids (mainly aldosterone)	Kidneys—increase blood levels of sodium and decrease blood levels of potassium	Hyposecretion causes Addison disease Hypersecretion causes aldosteronism
Sex hormones (any of the androgens, estrogens, or related steroid hormones) produced by the ovaries, testes, and adrenal cortices	In females, possibly responsible for female libido and source of estrogen after menopause; otherwise, effects in adults are insignificant	Hypersecretion of adrenal androgen in females leads to virilism (development of male characteristics) Hypersecretion of adrenal estrogen and progestin secretion in males leads to feminization (development of feminine characteristics) Hyposecretion has no known significant effects
Epinephrine (adrenaline) and norepinephrine	Sympathetic nervous system target organs—hormone effects mimic sympathetic nervous system activation (sympathomimetic); increase metabolic rate and heart rate; raises blood pressure by promoting vasoconstriction	Hyposecretion has no known significant effects Hypersecretion causes prolonged "fight-or-flight" reaction; hypertension

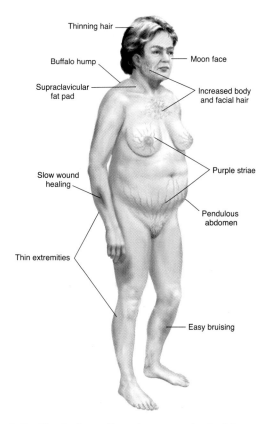

Thinning hair

Buffalo hump

Supraclavicular
fat pad

Moon face

Increased body
and facial hair

Slow wound
healing

Purple striae

Pendulous
abdomen

Thin extremities

Easy bruising

Figure 9-6   Physical manifestations seen in Cushing syndrome.

9-52   Identify at least two hormone(s) produced by the adrenal cortex that maintain(s) secondary sex characteristics: _____ and

_____ .

9-53   Epinephrine helps the body to cope with dangerous situations. Nerves transmit the message of fear to the glands, which react by rushing adrenaline to all parts of the system. Epinephrine is also called

_____ .

9-54   When a person is experiencing a stressful situation, the adrenal medulla produces adrenaline. This hormone is also called

_____ .

9-55   The hormones produced by the adrenal medulla that increase blood pressure are _____ and _____ .

9-56   The main glucocorticoid hormone secreted by the adrenal cortex is _____ .

Pancreas (Islets of Langerhans)

9-57 The (5) **pancreas** is located posterior to the stomach. The hormone-producing cells of the pancreas are called *islets of Langerhans.* The islets produce two distinct hormones: Alpha cells produce *glucagons,* and beta cells produce *insulin.* Both hormones play an important role in the proper metabolism of sugars and starches in the body. Label the pancreas in Figure 9–3.

pancreat/oma
păn-krē-ă-TŌ-mă

pancreat/o/lith
păn-krē-ĂT-ō-lĭth

pancreat/o/lith/iasis
păn-krē-ă-tō-lĭ-THĪ-ă-sĭs

pancreat/o/pathy
păn-krē-ă-TŎP-ă-thē

9-58 Use **pancreat/o** (*pancreas*) to build medical words meaning

tumor of the pancreas: _____ / _____.

calculus or stone in the pancreas:

_____ / ____ / _____.

abnormal condition of a pancreatic stone:

_____ / ____ / _____ / _____.

disease of the pancreas:

_____ / ____ / _____.

pancreas
PĂN-krē-ăs

9-59 The suffix -lysis is used in words to mean separation, destruction, loosening. Pancreat/o/lysis is a destruction of the _____.

9-60 Refer to Table 9–6 to complete Frames 9–60 through 9–62. The two hormones produced by the pancreas are _____ and _____.

9-61 Determine the pancreat/ic hormone that does the following
lowers blood sugar: _____.
increases blood sugar: _____.

9-62 How does insulin lower blood sugar?

_____

_____

Table 9–6. Pancreatic Hormones

This table outlines the pancreatic hormones, along with their target organs, functions, and selected associated disorders.

Hormone	Target Organ and Functions	Disorders
Glucagon	Liver and blood—increases blood glucose level by accelerating conversion of glycogen into glucose in liver (glycogenolysis) and conversion of other nutrients into glucose in the liver (gluconeogenesis) and releasing glucose into blood; converts glycogen to glucose	Persistently low blood sugar levels (hypoglycemia) may be caused by deficiency in glucagon
Insulin	Tissue cells—lowers blood glucose level by accelerating glucose transport into cells; converts glucose to glycogen	Hyposecretion of insulin causes diabetes mellitus Hypersecretion of insulin causes hyperinsulinism

glyc/o/gen
GLĪ-kō-jĕn

9–63   Gluc/ose is the chief source of energy for living organisms. **Gluc/o** and **glyc/o** are combining forms that mean sugar, sweetness.

The suffix -gen refers to *forming, producing, origin.*

Combine **glyc/o** and -gen to form a word meaning forming or producing sugar: _____ / _____ / _____.

gluc/o/genesis
gloo-kō-JĔN-ĕ-sĭs
glyc/o/genesis
glī-kō-JĔN-ĕ-sĭs

9–64   Use -genesis to form words that mean forming, producing, or origin of sugar: _____ / _____ / _____ and

_____ / _____ / _____.

gluc/o/meter
gloo- KŎM-tĕr

9–65   The gluc/o/meter is used to calculate blood glucose from one drop of blood. The instrument used by patients with diabetes to monitor their blood glucose levels is known as a

_____ / _____ / _____.

-emia

hyper-

hypo-

glyc

9–66   Hyper/glyc/emia is an excessive amount of glucose or sugar in the blood. A deficiency of glucose (sugar) in the blood is hypo/glyc/emia.

Identify the elements in this frame that mean

blood condition: _____.

excessive, above normal: _____.

under, below, deficient: _____.

sugar, sweetness: _____.

hypo/glyc/emia
hī-pō-glī-SĒ-mē-ă

9–67   A less than normal amount of gluc/ose in the blood, usually caused by excessive secretion of insulin by the pancreas, administration of too much insulin, or dietary deficiency, is called hypo/glyc/emia. Treatment is administration of glucose by mouth if the person is conscious or an intravenous (IV) solution if the person is unconscious.

A deficiency of blood glucose is called

_____ / _____ / _____.

-gen, -genesis

9–68   In the terms glyc/o/gen and glyc/o/genesis, write the elements that mean forming, producing, or origin:

_____ , _____ .

insulin
ĬN-sū-lĭn

9–69   *Diabetes mellitus* commonly results in hyper/glyc/emia. This condition occurs if the pancreas does not produce sufficient amounts of insulin or if the cells of the body become resistant to insulin and do not use insulin properly. Insulin, an essential hormone for conversion of sugar, starches, and other food into energy, is required for normal daily living.

If hypo/glyc/emia occurs, the diabetic person can reduce the amount of gluc/ose in the blood by injecting himself or herself with the hormone called _____ .

type 1 diabetes
dī-ă-BĒ-tēz

9–70   Diabetes is a general term that, when used alone, refers to *diabetes mellitus*, a disease that occurs in two primary forms: *type 1 diabetes,* also called insulin-dependent diabetes mellitus (IDDM) and *type 2 diabetes,* also called non-insulin-dependent diabetes mellitus (NIDDM).

Insulin-dependent diabetes mellitus (IDDM) is usually referred to as

_____ ____ _____ .

hypo/glyc/emia
hī-pō-glī-SĒ-mē-ă

9–71   People with diabetes who use too much insulin have abnormally low blood sugar. The medical term for this condition is

_____ / _____ / _____ .

hypo/glyc/emia
hī-pō-glī-SĒ-mē-ă

9–72   Hyper/glyc/emia increases susceptibility to infection and often results in a diabetic coma. The opposite of hyper/glyc/emia is

_____ / _____ / _____ .

9-73   The suffix -dipsia denotes a condition of thirst.

Poly/dipsia, poly/uria, and poly/phagia are three cardinal signs of diabetes mellitus. Write the words used in this frame that mean

excessive thirst: _____ /_____.

excessive urination: _____ /_____.

excessive eating: _____ /_____.

poly/dipsia
pŏl-ē-DĬP-sē-ă
poly/uria
pŏl-ē-Ū-rē-ă
poly/phagia
pŏl-ē-FĀ-jē-ă

9-74   When a person drinks too much water, he or she may experience a condition of excessive urine production (urination). The medical term for this condition is _____ /_____.

poly/uria
pŏl-ē-Ū-rē-ă

Pineal and Thymus Glands

9-75   The (6) **pineal gland** and (7) **thymus gland** are classified as endocrine glands, but little is known about their endocrine function. Label these structures in Figure 9–3.

9-76   **Thym/o** is the combining form for the thymus gland.

Build medical words meaning

excision of the thymus gland: _____ /_____.

tumor of the thymus gland: _____ /_____.

disease of the thymus gland: _____ /_____ /_____.

destruction of the thymus gland:

_____ /_____ /_____.

thym/ectomy
thī–MĔK-tō–mē
thym/oma
thī–MŌ–mă
thym/o/pathy
thī-MŎP-ă-thē

thym/o/lysis
thī-MŎL-ĭ-sĭs

Ovaries and Testes

9-77   The (8) **ovaries** are a pair of small, almond-shaped glands positioned in the upper pelvic cavity, one on each side of the uterus. The (9) **testes** are paired oval glands surrounded by the scrotal sac. The functions of the ovaries and testes are covered in Chapter 8. Label the ovaries and testes in Figure 9–3.

9-78   Recall the combining forms for

ovaries: _____ /_____ or _____ /_____.

testes: _____ /_____, _____ /_____, or

_____ /_____.

oophor/o, ovari/o

orchid/o, orchi/o,

orch/o

oophor/o/pathy ō-ŏf-or-ŎP-ă-thē **oophor/o/tomy** ō-ŏf-or-ŎT-ō-mē	**9–79** Use **oophor/o** to construct medical words meaning disease of an ovary: _____ / ___ / _____. incision of an ovary: _____ / ___ / _____.
orchid/o/pexy OR-kĭd-ō-pĕk-sē	**9–80** Use **orchid/o** to form a word meaning surgical fixation of a testis: _____ / ___ / _____.

Competency Verification: Check your labeling of Figure 9–3 in Appendix B, Answer Key, page 528.

Listen and Learn, the audio CD-ROM that accompanies this book, will help you master the pronunciation of selected medical words. Use it to practice pronunciations *of selected terms* from Frames *9–1 to 9–80* and for instructions to complete the *Listen and Learn* exercise on the CD-ROM for this section.

Using the following table, write the combining form, suffix, or prefix that matches its definition in the space provided to the left of the definition. There may be more than one word element that matches a definition.

Combining Forms	Suffixes	Prefixes
adrenal/o	-dipsia	hypo-
adren/o	-gen	para-
gluc/o	-genesis	poly-
glyc/o	-iasis	supra-
orch/o	-lith	
orchi/o	-lysis	
orchid/o	-pathy	
pancreat/o	-pexy	
thym/o	-phagia	
toxic/o	-rrhea	
	-uria	

1. _____ abnormal condition (produced by something specified)
2. _____ above; excessive; superior
3. _____ adrenal glands
4. _____ disease
5. _____ fixation (of an organ)
6. _____ discharge, flow
7. _____ many, much
8. _____ near, beside; beyond
9. _____ pancreas
10. _____ forming, producing, origin

11. _____ separation; destruction; loosening
12. _____ stone, calculus
13. _____ sugar, sweetness
14. _____ swallowing, eating
15. _____ testis (plural, testes)
16. _____ thirst
17. _____ thymus gland
18. _____ under, below, deficient
19. _____ urine
20. _____ poison

Competency Verification: Check your answers in Appendix B, Answer Key, page 528. If you are not satisfied with your level of comprehension, go back to Frame 9–39 and rework the frames.

Correct Answers _____ × 5 = _____% Score

Nervous System

The nervous system is an extensive, intricate network of structures that activates, coordinates, and controls the functions of all other body systems and can be grouped into two main divisions: the central nervous system (CNS) and the peripheral nervous system (PNS). The CNS consists of the brain and spinal cord and is the control center of the body. The PNS consists of the peripheral nerves, which include the cranial nerves (emerging from the base of the skull) and the spinal nerves (emerging from the spinal cord). The PNS connects the CNS to remote body parts to relay and receive messages, and its autonomic nerves regulate involuntary functions of the internal organs.

Despite the complex organization of the nervous system, it consists of only two principal types of cells, *neurons* and *neuroglia*. *Neurons* are the basic structural and functional units of the nervous system (see Figure 9–7). They are specialized to respond to physical and chemical stimuli, conduct electrochemical impulses, and release specific chemical regulators. Through these activities, neurons perform such functions as the perception of sensory stimuli, learning, memory, and control of muscles and glands. *Neuroglia* do not carry impulses, but perform the functions of support and protection. Many neuroglial or *glial* cells form a supporting network by twining around nerve cells or lining certain structures in the brain and spinal cord. Others bind nervous tissue to supporting structures and attach the neurons to their blood vessels. Certain small *glial cells* are phagocytic. In other words, they protect the CNS from disease by engulfing invading microbes and clearing away debris. *Neuroglia* are of clinical interest because they are a common source of tumors (gliomas) of the nervous system.

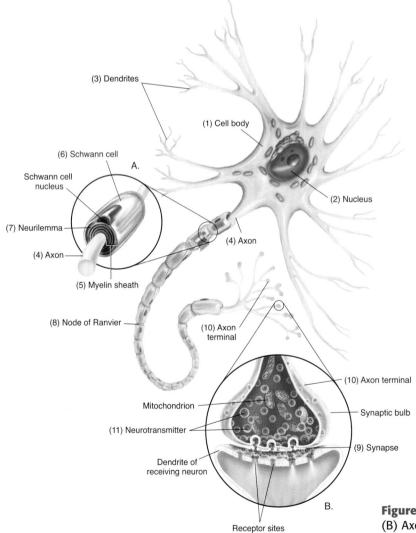

Figure 9-7   Neuron. (A) Schwann cell (B) Axon terminal synapse

Word Elements

This section introduces combining forms related to the nervous system. Included are key suffixes; prefixes are defined in the right-hand column as needed. Review the following table and pronounce each word in the word analysis column aloud before you begin to work the frames.

Word Element	Meaning	Word Analysis
COMBINING FORMS		
cerebr/o	cerebrum	cerebr/o/spin/al (sĕr-ĕ-brō-SPĪ-năl): pertaining to the brain and spinal cord *-al:* pertaining to, relating to *spin:* spine
encephal/o	brain	encephal/itis (ĕn-sĕf-ă-LĪ-tĭs): inflammatory condition of the brain *-itis:* inflammation
gli/o	glue; neuroglial tissue	gli/oma (glī-Ō-mă): tumor composed of neuroglia tissue (supportive tissue of nervous system) *-oma:* tumor
mening/o	meninges (membranes covering brain and spinal cord)	mening/o/cele (mĕn-ĬN-gō-sēl): saclike protrusion of the meninges through the skull or vertebral column *-cele:* hernia, swelling *Meningocele is a congenital (occurs at birth) defect and can be repaired by surgery.*
meningi/o		meningi/oma (mĕn-ĭn-jē-Ō-mă): tumor composed of the meninges *-oma:* tumor
myel/o	bone marrow; spinal cord	myel/algia (mī-ĕl-ĂL-jē-ă): pain of the spinal cord or its membranes *-algia:* pain
neur/o	nerve	neur/o/lysis (nū-RŎL-ĭs-ĭs): destruction of a nerve *-lysis:* separation; destruction; loosening

(Continued)

Word Element	Meaning	Word Analysis *(Continued)*
SUFFIXES		
-paresis	partial paralysis	hemi/paresis (hĕm-ē-păr-Ē-sĭs): paralysis of one half of the body (right half or left half) *hemi-:* one half
-phasia	speech	a/phasia (ă-FĀ-zē-ă): absence of speech *a-:* without, not *Aphasia is an abnormal neurologic condition in which language function is defective or absent because of an injury to certain areas of the cerebral cortex.*
-plegia	paralysis	quadri/plegia (kwŏd-rĭ-PLĒ-jē-ă): paralysis of all four extremities *quadri-:* four

Listen and Learn, the audio CD-ROM that accompanies this book, will help you master the pronunciation of selected medical words. Use it to practice pronunciations of the above-listed medical terms and for instructions for completing the *Listen and Learn* exercise on the CD-ROM for this section.

SECTION REVIEW 9–4

For the following medical terms, first write the suffix and its meaning. Then translate the meaning of the remaining elements starting with the first part of the word. The first word is an example that is completed for you.

Term	Meaning
1. meningi/oma	-oma: tumor; meninges
2. neur/o/lysis	_____
3. hemi/paresis	_____
4. myel/algia	_____
5. cerebr/o/spin/al	_____
6. a/phasia	_____
7. mening/o/cele	_____
8. encephal/itis	_____
9. gli/oma	_____
10. quadri/plegia	_____

Competency Verification: Check your answers in Appendix B, Answer Key, page 529. If you are not satisfied with your level of comprehension, review the vocabulary and retake the review.

Correct Answers _____ × 10 = _____% Score

---

myel/o

neur/o

encephal/o

9–81 The nervous system consists of the brain, spinal cord, and peripheral nerves. Together with the endocrine system, the nervous system coordinates and controls many body activities.

Identify the combining forms related to the nervous system.

bone marrow, spinal cord: _____ /_____.

nerve: _____ /_____.

brain: _____ /_____.

---

encephal/itis
ĕn-sĕf-ă-LĪ-tĭs
encephal/oma
ĕn-sĕf-ă-LŌ-mă

9–82 *Encephal/itis,* an inflammatory condition of the brain, usually is caused by a virus infection transmitted by the bite of an infected mosquito. It also may be the result of lead or other poisoning or of hem/o/rrhage.

Use **encephal/o** to build words meaning

inflammation of the brain: _____ /_____.

tumor of the brain: _____ /_____.

387

myel/itis mī-ĕ-LĪ-tĭs **myel/o/malacia** mī-ĕ-lō-mă-LĀ-shē-ă **myel/oma** mī-ĕ-LŌ-mă	**9-83** Use **myel/o** (bone marrow, spinal cord) to form medical words meaning inflammation of the spinal cord: _____ / _____. softening of the spinal cord: _____ / _____ / _____. tumor of the bone marrow: _____ / _____.
cell	**9-84** The combining form **thromb/o** refers to a *blood clot.* A thromb/o/cyte is a blood-clotting _____.
thromb/o/cyte THRŎM-bō-sīt	**9-85** A thromb/o/cyte (platelet) promotes the formation of clots and prevents bleeding. Another name for platelet is _____ / _____ / _____.
clot	**9-86** Thromb/o/lysis is the destruction or loosening of a blood _____.
thromb/o/genesis thrŏm-bō-JĔN-ĕ-sĭs	**9-87** Use -genesis to form a word meaning producing, forming, or origin of a blood clot: _____ / _____ / _____.
hem/o/rrhage HĔM-ĕ-rĭj **cerebr/o/vascul/ar** sĕr-ĕ-brō-VĂS-kū-lăr **thrombus** THRŎM-bŭs	**9-88** Cerebr/o/vascul/ar accident (CVA), or stroke, is a disruption of normal blood supply (ischemia) to the brain. It is characterized by occlusion by an embolus, thrombus, or hem/o/rrhage. The resulting neur/o/logic/al symptoms vary according to the site and degree of occlusion. Write the terms in this frame that mean bursting forth (of) blood: _____ / _____ / _____. pertaining to the cerebrum and blood vessels: _____ / _____ / _____ / _____. blood clot: _____.
aneurysm/ectomy ăn-ū-rĭz-MĔK-tō-mē	**9-89** CVA caused by hem/o/rrhage from a cerebral artery is often fatal. This usually results from high blood pressure, atherosclerosis, or the bursting of an arterial *aneurysm* (localized dilation of the blood vessel wall). The combining form **aneurysm/o** means *a widening or a widened blood vessel.* Use **aneurysm/o** to construct a medical word that means excision of an aneurysm: _____ / _____.

cerebr/o/scler/osis sĕr-ē-brō-sklĕ-RŌ-sĭs	**9–90**　Combine **cerebr/o** + scler + osis to form a word meaning an abnormal condition of hardening of the cerebrum: _____ / ____ / _____ / _____.
cerebr/oid SĔR-ē-broyd	**9–91**　Construct a medical term meaning resembling the cerebrum: _____ / _____.
mening/itis mĕn-ĭn-JĪ-tĭs **mening/o/cele** mĕn-ĬN-gō-sēl **meningi/oma** mĕn-ĭn-jē-Ō-mă	**9–92**　The *meninges* are three layers of membranes that surround and protect the brain and spinal cord: the *dura matter,* the *arachnoid,* and the *pia matter.* Both **mening/o** and **meningi/o** refer to the *meninges.* Use **mening/o** to construct a word meaning inflammation of the meninges: _____ / _____. Use **mening/o** to build a word meaning hernia or swelling of the meninges: _____ / ____ / _____. Use **meningi/o** to construct a word meaning tumor of the meninges: _____ / _____.
mening/o/cele mĕn-ĬN-gō-sēl	**9–93**　The outer layer, the *dura mater,* is a tough, fibrous membrane that covers the entire length of the spinal cord and contains channels for blood to enter brain tissue. The middle layer, the *arachnoid,* runs across the space known as the sub/dur/al space, which contains cerebr/o/spin/al fluid. The innermost layer, the *pia mater,* is a thin membrane containing many blood vessels that nourish the spinal cord. Herniation of the meninges may occur through a defect in the skull or spinal cord. When herniation of the meninges occurs, the condition is called _____ / ____ / _____.
epi- **dur** **-al**	**9–94**　The space between the *pia mater* and the bones of the spinal cord is called the *epi/dur/al space* and contains blood vessels and some fat. It is the space into which anesthetics may be injected to dull pain, or contrast material may be injected for certain diagnostic procedures. Identify the elements in this frame meaning above, on: _____. dura mater; hard: _____. pertaining to, relating to: _____.

-rrhagia **-rrhage**	**9-95** Hem/o/rrhage occurs when there is a loss of large amounts of blood in a short period. Hem/o/rrhage may be arterial, venous, or capillary. The two suffixes that mean bursting forth (of) are _____ and _____ .
neur/o/glia nū-RŎG-lē-ă	**9-96** As discussed earlier, the entire nervous system is composed of two principal types of cells, *neurons* and *neuroglia*. The supporting cells in the CNS collectively are called neur/o/glia. A term that literally means nerve glue is _____ / ____ / _____ .
inflammation, nerves	**9-97** Neur/itis is an _____ of _____ .
neur/algia nū-RĂL-jē-ă	**9-98** Another term besides neur/o/dynia that means pain in a nerve is _____ / _____ .
inflammation **nerves**	**9-99** Neur/o/myel/itis is an _____ of _____ and spinal cord.
neur/o/cyte NŪ-rō-sīt	**9-100** A neur/o/cyte, commonly called a neuron, is a nerve cell. A term that literally means nerve cell is _____ / ____ / _____ .

Listen and Learn, the audio CD-ROM that accompanies this book, will help you master the pronunciation of selected medical words. Use it to practice pronunciations of *selected terms from frames 9–81 to 9–100* and for instructions to complete the *Listen and Learn* exercise on the CD-ROM for this section.

SECTION REVIEW 9 – 5

Using the following table, write the combining form, suffix, or prefix that matches its definition in the space provided to the left of the definition. There may be more than one word element that matches a definition.

Combining Forms	Suffixes	Prefixes
cerebr/o	-glia	a-
encephal/o	-malacia	dys-
gli/o	-osis	
mening/o	-phasia	
meningi/o	-rrhage	
myel/o	-rrhagia	
neur/o		
scler/o		
thromb/o		
vascul/o		

1. _____ abnormal condition; increase (used primarily with blood cells)
2. _____ bad; painful; difficult
3. _____ blood clot
4. _____ vessel
5. _____ brain
6. _____ bursting forth (of)
7. _____ glue; neuroglial tissue
8. _____ hardening; sclera (white of eye)
9. _____ meninges (membranes covering brain and spinal cord)
10. _____ nerve
11. _____ cerebrum
12. _____ softening
13. _____ speech
14. _____ bone marrow; spinal cord
15. _____ without, not

Competency Verification: Check your answers in Appendix B, Answer Key, page 529. If you are not satisfied with your level of comprehension, go back to Frame 9–81 and rework the frames.

Correct Answers _____ × 6.67 = _____% Score

Abbreviations

This section introduces endocrine and nervous systems–related abbreviations and their meanings. Included are abbreviations contained in the medical record activities that follow.

Abbreviation	Meaning	Abbreviation	Meaning
ENDOCRINE SYSTEM			
ADH	antidiuretic hormone	LH	luteinizing hormone
BS	blood sugar	NIDDM	non-insulin-dependent diabetes mellitus
DM	diabetes mellitus	PGH	pituitary growth hormone
GH	growth hormone	PTH	parathyroid hormone
ICSH	interstitial cell–stimulating hormone	RAIU	radioactive iodine uptake
IDDM	insulin-dependent diabetes mellitus	TSH	thyroid-stimulating hormone
NERVOUS SYSTEM			
CNS	central nervous system	EEG	electroencephalogram
CSF	cerebrospinal fluid	EMG	electromyogram
CVA	cerebrovascular accident	LP	lumbar puncture
CVD	cerebrovascular disease		
ABBREVIATIONS RELATED TO RADIOGRAPHIC PROCEDURES			
po	orally	CT	computed tomography
AP	anteroposterior	PET	positron emission tomography
PA	posteroanterior	MRI	magnetic resonance imaging
IV	intravenously		

Pathological, Diagnostic, and Therapeutic Terms

The following are additional terms related to the endocrine and nervous systems. Recognizing and learning these terms will help you understand the connection between a pathological condition, its diagnosis, and the rationale behind the method of treatment selected for a particular disorder.

Pathological

Endocrine System

Addison disease (Ă-dĭ-sŭn): relatively uncommon chronic disorder caused by deficiency of cortical hormones; results when the adrenal cortex is damaged or atrophied. Atrophy of the adrenal glands is usually the result of an autoimmune process in which circulating adrenal antibodies slowly destroy the gland.

Cushing syndrome (KOOSH-ing): cluster of symptoms caused by excessive amounts of cortisol or adrenocorticotropin hormone (ACTH) circulating in the blood

Most cases of Cushing syndrome are caused by administration of glucocorticoids in the treatment of immune disorders, such as asthma, rheumatoid arthritis, and lupus erythematosus.

diabetes (dī-ă-BĒ-tēz): general term that when used alone refers to diabetes mellitus, a disease that occurs in two primary forms, type 1 and type 2 diabetes, which are defined below.

diabetes mellitus (dī-ă-BĒ-tēz MĚ-lĭ-tŭs): chronic metabolic disorder marked by *hyperglycemia* and occurs in two primary forms, *type 1 diabetes* and *type 2 diabetes*.

When body cells are deprived of glucose, their principal energy fuel, they begin to metabolize fats and proteins, depositing unusually high levels of wastes in the blood causing a condition called ketosis. Hyperglycemia and ketosis are responsible for the host of troubling and commonly life-threatening symptoms of diabetes mellitus.

type 1 diabetes: diabetes that is abrupt in onset and usually is diagnosed in children and young adults. It is due to the failure of the pancreas to produce insulin, making this type of disease difficult to regulate; also called *insulin-dependent diabetes mellitus (IDDM)*.
Treatment includes insulin injections to maintain a normal level of glucose in the blood.

type 2 diabetes: diabetes that is gradual onset and is the most common form. It is usually diagnosed in adults older than age 40 and results from the body's deficiency in producing enough insulin, or the body's cells are resistant to insulin action; also called *non-insulin-dependent diabetes mellitus (NIDDM)*.
Management of this disease is less problematic than that of type 1. Treatment includes diet, weight loss, and exercise. It also may include insulin or oral antidiabetic agents, which activate the release of pancreatic insulin and improve the body's sensitivity to insulin.

exophthalmos (ĕks-ŏf-THĂL-mŏs): abnormal protrusion of eyeball(s); may be due to thyrotoxicosis, tumor of the orbit, orbital cellulitis, leukemia, or aneurysm.

Graves disease (GRĀVZ): multisystem autoimmune disorder that involves growth of the thyroid associated with hypersecretion of thyroxine.

Graves disease is characterized by an enlarged thyroid gland and exophthalmos (bulging of the eyes), which develops because of edema in the tissues of the eye sockets and swelling of the extrinsic eye muscles; also called exopthalmic goiter, thyrotoxicosis, or toxic goiter.

insulinoma (ĭn-sū-lĭn-Ō-mā): tumor of the islets of Langerhans; pancreatic tumor.

myxedema (mĭks-ĕ-DĒ-mă): advanced hypothyroidism in adults resulting from hypofunction of the thyroid gland; affects body fluids, causing edema and increasing blood volume, increasing blood pressure.

panhypopituitarism (păn-hī-pō-pǐ-TŪ-ǐ-tăr-ĭzm): total pituitary impairment that brings about a progressive and general loss of hormonal activity.

pheochromocytoma (fē-ō-krō-mō-sī-TŌ-mă): small chromaffin cell tumor, usually located in the adrenal medulla.

pituitarism (pǐ-TŪ-ǐ-tăr-ĭzm): any disorder of the pituitary gland and its function.

Nervous System

Alzheimer disease (ĂLTS-hī-měr): chronic, organic mental disorder; a form of presenile dementia caused by atrophy of frontal and occipital lobes.

> *Onset is usually between age 40 and 60. Involves progressive irreversible loss of memory, deterioration of intellectual functions, apathy, speech and gait disturbances, and disorientation. Course may take from a few months to 4 or 5 years to progress to complete loss of intellectual function.*

cerebrovascular accident (sěr-ě-brō-VĂS-kū-lăr): brain tissue damage caused by a disorder within the blood vessels; usually due to the formation of a clot or a ruptured blood vessel; the resulting functional deficit depends on the area of the brain affected; also called apoplexy, cerebral infarction, stroke, or CVA.

epilepsy (ĔP-ǐ-lěp-sē): disorder affecting the central nervous system, characterized by recurrent seizures.

Huntington chorea (HŬN-tǐng-tŭn kō-RĒ-ă): hereditary nervous disorder caused by the progressive loss of brain cells, leading to bizarre, involuntary, dancelike movements.

hydrocephalus (hī-drō-SĚF-ă-lŭs): cranial enlargement caused by accumulation of fluid within the ventricles of the brain.

multiple sclerosis (MŬL-tǐ-pl sklě-RŌ-sǐs): progressive degenerative disease of the CNS characterized by inflammation, hardening, and loss of myelin throughout the spinal cord and brain, which produces weakness and other muscular symptoms.

neuroblastoma (nū-rō-blăs-TŌ-mă): malignant tumor composed principally of cells resembling neuroblasts; occurs chiefly in infants and children.

palsy (PAWL-zē): partial or complete loss of motor function; paralysis.
> **Bell:** facial paralysis caused by dysfunction of a facial nerve of unknown etiology.
> *With Bell palsy, the person may not be able to close an eye or control salivation on the affected side. The condition often results in grotesque facial disfigurement and facial spasms, but complete recovery is possible.*
> **cerebral** (sěr-ě-brō): bilateral, symmetrical, nonprogressive motor dysfunction and partial paralysis usually caused by damage to the cerebrum during gestation or birth trauma but can be hereditary.

Parkinson disease (PĂR-kǐn-sŭn): progressive, degenerative neurological disorder affecting the portion of the brain responsible for controlling movement.

> *The unnecessary skeletal muscle movements often interfere with voluntary movement, causing the hand to shake, which is called tremor, the most common symptom of Parkinson disease.*

poliomyelitis (pō-lē-ō-mī-ěl-Ī-tǐs): inflammation of the gray matter of the spinal cord caused by a virus, often resulting in spinal and muscle deformity and paralysis.

sciatica (sī-ĂT-ǐ-kă): severe pain in the leg along the course of the sciatic nerve, which travels from the hip to the foot.

seizure (SĒ-zhūr): convulsion or other clinically detectable event caused by a sudden discharge of electrical activity in the brain that may be classified as partial or generalized; characteristic symptom of epilepsy.

shingles (SHĬNG-lz): eruption of acute, inflammatory, herpetic vesicles on the trunk of the body along a peripheral nerve caused by herpes zoster virus.

spina bifida (SPĪ-nă BĬF-ĭ-dă): congenital neural tube defect characterized by incomplete closure of the spinal canal through which the spinal cord and meninges may or may not protrude. It usually occurs in the lumbosacral area and has several forms.

    spina bifida occulta (SPĪ-nă BĬF-ĭ-dă ŏ-KŬL-tă): most common and least severe form of this defect without protrusion of the spinal cord or meninges.

    spina bifida cystica (SPĪ-nă BĬF-ĭ-dă SĬS-tĭk-ă): more severe type of this defect; involves protrusion of the meninges (meningocele), spinal cord (myelocele), or both (meningomyelocele). The severity of the neurological dysfunction depends directly on the degree of nerve involvement

transient ischemic attack (TRĂN-zhĕnt ĭs-KĒ-mĭk): temporary interference with blood supply to the brain, lasting a few minutes to a few hours.

Diagnostic

Endocrine System

computed tomography (CT) scan (kŏm-PŪ-tĕd tō-MŎG-ră-fē): radiographic technique that uses a narrow beam of x-rays, which rotates in a full arc around the patient to image the body in cross-sectional slices. A scanner and detector send the images to a computer, which consolidates all of the data it receives from the multiple x-ray views (see Figure 2–5A).

CT scans of endocrine organs are used to assist in the diagnosis of various pathologies; also may involve the use of a contrast medium.

magnetic resonance imaging (măg-NĔT-ĭc RĔZ-ĕn-ăns ĬM-ĭj-ĭng): radiographic technique that uses electro-magnetic energy to produce multiplanar cross-sectional images of the body (see Figure 2–5B).

Magnetic resonance imaging (MRI) is used to identify abnormalities of pituitary, pancreatic, adrenal, and thyroid glands.

radioactive iodine uptake (RAIU) test: imaging procedure that measures levels of radioactivity in the thyroid after administration of radioactive iodine either orally (po) or intravenously (IV).

RAIU is used to determine thyroid function by monitoring the thyroid's ability to take up (uptake) iodine from the blood.

Nervous System

cerebrospinal fluid analysis (sĕr-ĕ-brō-SPĪ-năl FLOO-ĭd): cerebrospinal fluid obtained from a lumbar puncture is evaluated for the presence of blood, bacteria, malignant cells, and the amount of protein and glucose present.

computed tomography (CT) scan (kŏm-PŪ-tĕd tō-MŎG-ră-fē): radiographic technique that uses a narrow beam of x-rays, which rotates in a full arc around the patient to image the body in cross-sectional slices. A scanner and detector send the images to a computer, which consolidates all of the data it receives from the multiple x-ray views (see Figure 2–5A).

CT brain scan provides a computerized cross-sectional view of the brain. Contrast medium also may be injected intravenously. CT scans help in differentiating intracranial pathologies such as tumors, cysts, edema, hemorrhage, blood clots, and cerebral aneurysms.

magnetic resonance imaging (măg-NĔT-ĭc RĔZ-ĕn-ăns ĬM-ĭj-ĭng): radiographic technique that uses electromagnetic energy to produce multiplanar cross-sectional images of the body (see Figure 2–5B).

MRI of the brain produces cross-sectional, frontal, and sagittal plane views of the brain. It is regarded as superior to computed tomography for most CNS abnormalities, particularly those of the brainstem and spinal cord. A contrast medium is not required but may be used to enhance internal structure visualization.

positron emission tomography (PŎZ-ĭ-trŏn ē-MĬSH-ŭn tō-MŎG-ră-fē): radiographic technique that combines computed tomography with the use of radiopharmaceuticals. PET produces a cross-sectional (transverse) image of the dispersement of radioactivity (through emission of positrons) in a section of the body to reveal the areas where the radiopharmaceutical is being metabolized and where there is a deficiency in metabolism; also called *PET scan* (see Figure 2–5D).

Positron emission tomography (PET) aids in the diagnosis of neurologic disorders such as brain tumors, epilepsy, stroke, Alzheimer disease, and abdominal and pulmonary disorders.

Therapeutic

craniotomy (krā-nē-ŎT-ō-mē): surgical procedure to create an opening in the skull to gain access to the brain during neurosurgical procedures.

A craniotomy also is performed to relieve intracranial pressure, to control bleeding, or to remove a tumor.

hormone replacement therapy: oral administration or injection of synthetic hormones to replace a hormone deficiency, such as of estrogen, testosterone, or thyroid hormone.

thalamotomy (thăl-ă-MŎT-ō-mē): partial destruction of the thalamus to treat psychosis or intractable pain.

Listen and Learn, the audio CD-ROM that accompanies this book, will help you master the pronunciation of selected medical words. Use it to practice pronunciations of the above-listed medical terms and for instructions for completing the *Listen and Learn* exercise on the CD-ROM for this section.

PATHOLOGICAL, DIAGNOSTIC, AND THERAPEUTIC TERMS REVIEW

Match the medical term(s) below with the definitions in the numbered list.

Alzheimer disease	exophthalmos	MRI	pheochromocytoma	shingles
Bell palsy	Graves disease	myxedema	pituitarism	spina bifida
CVA	Huntington chorea	neuroblastoma	poliomyelitis	thalamotomy
CT scan	hydrocephalus	panhypopituitarism	PET	type 1 diabetes
Cushing syndrome	insulinoma	Parkinson disease	sciatica	type 2 diabetes
epilepsy				

1. _____ is facial paralysis caused by a functional disorder of the seventh cranial nerve and any or all of its branches.

2. _____ refers to brain tissue damage caused by a disorder within the blood vessels; usually due to the formation of a clot or a ruptured blood vessel; also called *apoplexy* or *stroke*.

3. _____ is a central nervous system disorder characterized by recurrent seizures.

4. _____ is abnormal protrusion of eyeball that may be due to thyrotoxicosis.

5. _____ means hyperthyroidism, also called toxic goiter; involves growth of the thyroid associated with hypersecretion of thyroxine; characterized by exophthalmos.

6. _____ is a tumor of the pancreas.

7. _____ means advanced hypothyroidism in adults, resulting from hypofunction of the thyroid gland, causing edema and increasing blood pressure.

8. _____ is a small chromaffin cell tumor, usually located in the adrenal medulla.

9. _____ is a progressive degenerative neurological disorder affecting the portion of the brain responsible for controlling movement, causing hand tremors.

10. _____ refers to inflammation of the gray matter of the spinal cord caused by a virus, often resulting in spinal and muscle deformity and paralysis.

11. _____ refers to severe pain in the leg along the course of the sciatic nerve, which travels from the hip to the foot.

12. _____ is a congenital defect characterized by incomplete closure of the spinal canal through which the spinal cord and meninges may or may not protrude; it usually occurs in the lumbosacral area and has several forms.

13. _____ is cranial enlargement caused by accumulation of fluid within the ventricles of the brain.

14. _____ is a malignant tumor composed principally of cells resembling neuroblasts; occurs chiefly in infants and children.

15. _____ is a brain disorder marked by deterioration of mental capacity (dementia), beginning in middle age, and leading to total disability and death.

16. _____ is a radiographic technique that uses electromagnetic energy to produce cross-sectional, frontal, and sagittal plane views of the brain.

17. _____ is a disease caused by complete absence of insulin secretion; also called *insulin-dependent diabetes mellitus*.

18. _____ refers to eruption of acute, inflammatory, herpetic vesicles on the trunk of the body along a peripheral nerve caused by herpes zoster virus.

19. _____ refers to any disorder of the pituitary gland and its function,

20. _____ refers to total pituitary impairment that brings about a progressive and general loss of hormonal activity.

21. _____ is a hereditary nervous disorder caused by the progressive loss of brain cells that leads to bizarre, involuntary, dancelike movements.

22. _____ results from hypersecretion of the adrenal cortex in which there is excessive production of glucocorticoids.

23. _____ is a radiographic technique that uses a narrow beam of x-rays, which rotates in a full arc around the patient to image the body in cross-sectional slices; scanner and detector send the images to a computer, which consolidates all of the data it receives from the multiple x-ray views.

24. _____ refers to partial destruction of the thalamus to treat psychosis or intractable pain.

25. _____ produces cross-sectional image of the dispersement of radioactivity in a section of the body to reveal the areas where the radiopharmaceutical is being metabolized and where there is a deficiency in metabolism.

Competency Verification: Check your answers in Appendix B, Answer Key, page 529. If you are not satisfied with your level of comprehension, review the pathological, diagnostic, and therapeutic terms and retake the review.

Correct Answers _____ × 4 = _____ % Score

Medical Record Activities

The following medical records reflect common real-life clinical scenarios using medical terminology to document patient care. The physician who specializes in the treatment of endocrine disorders is an *endocrinologist;* the medical specialty concerned in the diagnoses and treatment of endocrine disorders is called *endocrinology.* The physician who specializes in the treatment of neurological disorders is a *neurologist;* the medical specialty concerned in the diagnoses and treatment of neurological disorders is called *neurology.*

✓ MEDICAL RECORD ACTIVITY 9–1. Diabetes Mellitus

Terminology

The terms listed in the chart come from the medical record *Diabetes Mellitus* that follows. Use a medical dictionary such as *Taber's Cyclopedic Medical Dictionary,* the appendices of this book, or other resources to define each term. Then practice reading the pronunciations aloud for each term.

Term	Definition
acidosis ăs-ĭ-DŌ-sĭs	
ADA	
BS	
diabetes mellitus dī-ă-BĒ-tēz MĔ-lĭ-tŭs	
electrolytes ē-LĔK-trō-lītz	
glycemic glī-SĒ-mĭk	
glycosuria glĭ-kō-SŪ-rē-ă	
Humulin L HŪ-mū-lĭn	
Humulin R HŪ-mū-lĭn	
insulin-dependent diabetes mellitus ĬN-sū-lĭn dē-PĔN-dĕnt dī-ă-BĒ-tēz MĔ-lĭ-tŭs	
ketones KĒ-tōnz	
metabolically mĕt-ĕ-BŎL-ĭk-ă-lĭ	
polydipsia pŏl-ē-DĬP-sē-ă	
polyuria pŏl-ē-Ū-rē-ă	
WNL	

Listen and Learn Online! will help you master the pronunciation of selected medical words from this medical record activity. Visit www.fadavis.com/gylys/simplified for instructions in completing the *Listen and Learn Online!* exercise for this section and then to practice pronunciations.

DIABETES MELLITUS

Reading

Practice pronunciation of medical terms by reading the following medical report aloud.

ADMITTING DIAGNOSIS: Diabetes mellitus, new onset.

DISCHARGE DIAGNOSIS: Insulin-dependent diabetes mellitus, new onset.

HISTORY OF PRESENT ILLNESS: This patient is a 15-year-old white boy who presented in the office complaining of increased appetite, polydipsia, and polyuria and was found to have elevated blood sugar of 400 and glycosuria. He was sent to the hospital for further evaluation and treatment.

HOSPITAL COURSE: On admission, laboratory tests showed electrolytes WNL, and ketones were negative. Urinalysis showed a trace of sugar, BS was 380, and there was no evidence of acidosis. Metabolically the patient was stable. Patient was started on split-mixed insulin dosing. The patient and his family received full diabetic instruction during his hospitalization and seemed to understand this well. The patient picked up on all of this information quickly, asked appropriate questions, and appeared to be coping well with his new condition. By the 5th day, his polyuria and polydipsia resolved. When the patient was able to draw up and give his own insulin and perform his own fingersticks, he was discharged.

DISCHARGE INSTRUCTIONS: The patient was discharged to home with parents, on a mixture of Humulin L 12 units and Humulin R 6 units each morning, with Humulin L 5 units and Humulin R 6 units each afternoon. He will continue with fingerstick BS four times daily at home until seen in the office for follow-up. I warned him of all glycemic symptoms to watch for, and he is to call the office with any problems that may occur. He is to follow an ADA 2000-calorie diet.

DISCHARGE CONDITION: The patient's overall condition was much improved, and at the time of discharge BS levels were stabilized and he was doing well.

Evaluation

Review the medical record to answer the following questions.

1. What symptoms of DM did the patient experience before his office visit?

_____

_____

2. What confirmed the patient's new diagnosis of DM?

_____

_____

3. What conditions had to be met before the patient could be discharged from the hospital?

_____

_____

4. How many times a day does the patient have to take insulin?

_____

_____

5. Why does the patient have to perform fingersticks four times a day?

_____

_____

6. What is an ADA 2000-calorie diet? Why is it important?

_____

_____

✓ MEDICAL RECORD ACTIVITY 9–2. Cerebrovascular Accident

Terminology

The terms listed in the chart come from the medical record *Cerebrovascular Accident* that follows. Use a medical dictionary such as *Taber's Cyclopedic Medical Dictionary*, the appendices of this book, or other resources to define each term. Then practice reading the pronunciations aloud for each term.

Term	Definition
adenocarcinoma ăd-ĕ-nō-kăr-sĭn-Ō-mă	
anorexia ăn-ō-RĔK-sē-ă	
aphasia ă-FĀ-zē-ă	
biliary BĬL-ē-ār-ē	
cardiovascular kăr-dē-ō-VĂS-kū-lăr	
cholecystojejunostomy kō-lē-sĭs-tō-jĕ-jū-NŎS-tō-mē	
CVA	
deglutition dē-gloo-TĬSH-ŭn	
diplopia dĭp-LŌ-pē-ă	
Dx	
jaundice JAWN-dĭs	
jejunojejunostomy jē-jū-nō-jĕ-jū-NŎS-tō-mē	
metastasis mĕ-TĂS-tă-sis	
pruritus proo-RĪ-tŭs	
vertigo VĔR-tĭ-gō	

Listen and Learn Online! will help you master the pronunciation of selected medical words from this medical record activity. Visit www.fadavis.com/gylys/simplified for instructions in completing the *Listen and Learn Online!* exercise for this section and then to practice pronunciations.

CEREBROVASCULAR ACCIDENT

Reading

Practice pronunciation of medical terms by reading the following medical report aloud.

The patient is a moderately obese white woman who was admitted to Riverside Hospital because of a sudden episode of CVA. She recalls an episode of vertigo 3 days ago. The patient is being nursed at home by her daughter because of terminal adenocarcinoma of the head of the pancreas with metastasis to the liver, which was diagnosed in December. About 5 hours before the CVA, the patient fell to the floor with paralysis of the right arm and right leg and aphasia. She has not noticed any difficulty with deglutition. Apparently with the onset of the CVA attack she also experienced diplopia. She denies any difficulty with her cardiovascular system in the past. The patient was in the hospital 5 years ago because of generalized biliary-type disease with jaundice, pruritus, weight loss, and anorexia. Subsequently, she was seen in consultation, and cholecystojejunostomy and jejunojejunostomy was performed.

Dx: (1) CVA, probably secondary to metastatic lesion of the brain or cerebrovascular disease; (2) evidence of the previously described deterioration secondary to carcinoma of the pancreas with metastases of the liver.

Evaluation

Review the medical record to answer the following questions.

1. Did the patient have a history of cardiovascular problems before her CVA?

   _____

   _____

2. What symptoms did the patient experience just before her CVA?

   _____

   _____

3. What is the primary site of this patient's cancer?

   _____

   _____

4. What is cerebrovascular disease?

   _____

   _____

5. What is the probable cause of the patient's CVA?

   _____

   _____

Chapter Review

Word Elements Summary

The following table summarizes combining forms, suffixes, and prefixes related to the endocrine and nervous systems.

Word Element	Meaning
COMBINING FORMS	
aden/o	gland
adren/o, adrenal/o	adrenal glands
anter/o	anterior, front
calc/o	calcium
cerebr/o	cerebrum
encephal/o	brain
gli/o	glue; neuroglial tissue
gluc/o, glyc/o	sugar, sweetness
mening/o, meningi/o	meninges (membranes covering brain and spinal cord)
myel/o	bone marrow; spinal cord
neur/o	nerve
pancreat/o	pancreas
thym/o	thymus gland
thyroid/o	thyroid gland
vascul/o	blood vessel
OTHER COMBINING FORMS	
acr/o	extremities
carcin/o	cancer
cyst/o	bladder
cyt/o	cell
dermat/o	skin
enter/o	intestine (usually small intestine)
gastr/o	stomach
hem/o	blood

(Continued)

Word Element	Meaning *(Continued)*
hepat/o	liver
hidr/o	sweat
nephr/o, ren/o	kidney
orchid/o, orchi/o, orch/o	testis (plural, testes)
poster/o	back (of body), behind, posterior
scler/o	hardening; sclera (white of eye)
spin/o	spine
thromb/o	blood clot
toxic/o	poison

SUFFIXES

SURGICAL

-ectomy	excision, removal
-lysis	separation; destruction; loosening
-pexy	fixation (of an organ)
-tome	instrument to cut
-tomy	incision

DIAGNOSTIC, SYMPTOMATIC, AND RELATED

-algia, -dynia	pain
-dipsia	thirst
-emia	blood condition
-gen, -genesis	forming, producing, origin
-glia	glue; neuroglial tissue
-iasis	abnormal condition (produced by something specified)
-ism	condition
-itis	inflammation
-lith	stone, calculus
-logist	specialist in study of
-logy	study of

Word Element	Meaning
-megaly	enlargement
-malacia	softening
-oid	resembling
-oma	tumor
-osis	abnormal condition; increase (used primarily with blood cells)
-pathy	disease
-penia	decrease, deficiency
-phagia	swallowing, eating
-phasia	speech
-plegia	paralysis
-rrhagia	bursting forth (of)
-rrhea	discharge, flow
-uria	urine
PREFIXES	
a-	without, not
dys-	bad; painful; difficult
endo-	within
hyper-	excessive, above normal
hypo-	under, below, deficient
para-	near, beside; beyond

WORD ELEMENTS REVIEW

After you review the word elements summary, complete this activity by writing the meaning of each element in the space provided.

Word Element	Meaning
COMBINING FORMS	
1. aden/o	
2. adren/o, adrenal/o	
3. calc/o	
4. cerebr/o	
5. encephal/o	
6. gli/o	
7. gluc/o, glyc/o	
8. mening/o, meningi/o	
9. myel/o	
10. neur/o	
11. pancreat/o	
12. thym/o	
13. thyroid/o	
OTHER COMBINING FORMS	
14. hem/o	
15. hepat/o	
16. hidr/o	
17. toxic/o	
SUFFIXES	
SURGICAL	
18. -ectomy	
19. -lysis	
20. -pexy	
21. -tome	
22. -tomy	

Word Element	Meaning
DIAGNOSTIC, SYMPTOMATIC, AND RELATED	
23. -dipsia	
24. -emia	
25. -gen, -genesis	
26. -glia	
27. -iasis	
28. -ism	
29. -itis	
30. -lith	
31. -logist	
32. -logy	
33. -megaly	
34. -malacia	
35. -oid	
36. -oma	
37. -osis	
38. -pathy	
39. -penia	
40. -phagia	
41. -phasia	
42. -plegia	
43. -rrhagia	
44. -rrhea	
45. -uria	
PREFIXES	
46. a-	
47. endo-	
48. hyper-	
49. hypo-	
50. para-	

Competency Verification: Check your answers in Appendix A, Glossary of Medical Word Elements, page 497. If you are not satisfied with your level of comprehension, review the word elements and retake the review.

Correct Answers _____ × 2= _____% Score

Chapter 9 Vocabulary Review

Match the medical term(s) below with the definitions in the numbered list.

acromegaly   deglutition   hyperglycemia   neurohypophysis   polydipsia
adenohypophysis   diabetes mellitus insulin   neuromalacia   polyphagia
adrenalectomy   glycogenesis   jaundice   pancreatolith   pruritus
adrenaline   hormone   meningocele   pancreatolysis   thyrotoxicosis
cerebral palsy   hypercalcemia   metastasis   pancreatopathy   vertigo

1. _____ means enlargement of the extremities.

2. _____ means destruction of the pancreatic substance by pancreatic enzymes.

3. _____ is the anterior lobe of the pituitary, composed of glandular tissue.

4. _____ refers to partial paralysis and lack of muscular coordination caused by damage to the cerebrum before or during the birth process.

5. _____ refers to excessive amounts of calcium in the blood.

6. _____ is a pancreatic hormone that decreases blood sugar level.

7. _____ is the posterior lobe of the pituitary, composed primarily of nerve tissue.

8. _____ means disease of the pancreas.

9. _____ refers to excessive consumption of food.

10. _____ is a chronic metabolic disorder marked by *hyperglycemia;* occurs in two primary forms.

11. _____ means increase of blood sugar, as in diabetes.

12. _____ is a calculus or stone in the pancreas.

13. _____ refers to excessive thirst.

14. _____ is a toxic condition due to hyperactivity of the thyroid gland; exophthalmic goiter.

15. _____ means excision of an adrenal gland.

16. _____ is a hormone secreted by the adrenal medulla that causes some of the physiological expressions of fear and anxiety; epinephrine.

17. _____ means production or formation of sugar.

18. _____ refers to protrusion of the membranes of the brain or spinal cord through a defect in the skull or spinal column.

19. _____ means softening of nerve tissue.

20. _____ refers to severe itching.

21. _____ refers to the act of swallowing.

22. _____ is an illusion of movement.

23. _____ is yellowish discoloration of the skin and eyes.

24. _____ refers to spread of a malignant tumor beyond its primary site to a secondary organ or location.

25. _____ is a chemical substance produced by specialized cells of the body and released slowly into the bloodstream.

Competency Verification: Check your answers in Appendix B, Answer Key, page 530. If you are not satisfied with your level of comprehension, review the chapter vocabulary and retake the review.

Correct Answers _____ × 5= _____% Score

10

Musculoskeletal System

OBJECTIVES

Upon completion of this chapter, you will be able to:

■ Describe the musculoskeletal system and discuss its primary functions.

■ Describe pathological, diagnostic, therapeutic, and other terms related to the musculoskeletal system.

■ Recognize, define, pronounce, and spell terms correctly by completing the audio CD-ROM exercises.

■ Demonstrate your knowledge of this chapter by successfully completing the frames, reviews, and medical report evaluations.

Skeletal System

The musculoskeletal system is composed of bones, joints, and muscles. The skeletal system of a human adult consists of 206 individual bones, but only the major bones are covered in this chapter. For anatomical purposes, the human skeleton is divided into the axial skeleton (distinguished with bone color in Figure 10–1) and the appendicular skeleton (distinguished with blue color in Figure 10–1). The axial skeleton protects internal organs and provides central support for the body, and the appendicular skeleton enables the body to move. The ability to walk, run, or catch a ball is possible due to the movable joints of the limbs.

The main function of bones is to form a skeleton to support and protect the body and serve as storage areas for mineral salts, especially calcium and phosphorus. Joints are the places where two bones articulate, or connect. Because bones cannot move without the help of muscles, contraction must be provided by muscular tissue.

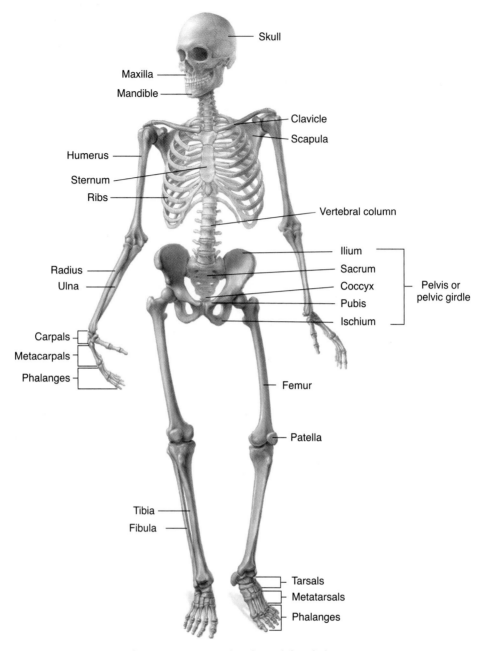

Figure 10-1   Anterior view of the skeleton.

Word Elements

This section introduces combining forms related to the skeletal system. Included are key suffixes; prefixes are defined in the right-hand column as needed. Review the following table, and pronounce each word in the word analysis column aloud before you begin to work the frames.

Word Element	Meaning	Word Analysis
COMBINING FORMS		
SPECIFIC BONES OF UPPER EXTREMITIES		
carp/o	carpus (wrist bones)	carp/o/ptosis (kăr-pŏp-TŌ-sĭs): wrist drop *-ptosis:* prolapse, downward displacement
cost/o	ribs	sub/cost/al (sŭb-KŎS-tăl): beneath the ribs *sub-:* under, below *-al:* pertaining to, relating to
crani/o	cranium (skull)	crani/o/tomy (krā-nē-ŎT-ō-mē): incision through the cranium, usually to gain access to the brain during neurosurgical procedures *-tomy:* incision *Craniotomy is performed to relieve intracranial pressure, to control bleeding, or to remove a tumor.*
humer/o	humerus (upper arm bone)	humer/al (HŪ-měr-ăl): pertaining to the humerus *-al:* pertaining to, relating to
metacarp/o	metacarpus (hand bones)	metacarp/ectomy (mĕt-ă-kăr-PĔK-tō-mē): excision or resection of one or more metacarpal bones *-ectomy:* excision, removal
phalang/o	phalanges (bones of fingers and toes)	phalang/itis (făl-ăn-JĪ-tĭs): inflammation of one or more phalanges *-itis:* inflammation
spondyl/o (used to form words about the condition of the structure)	vertebrae (backbone)	spondyl/itis (spŏn-dĭl-Ī-tĭs): inflammation of any of the vertebrae, usually characterized by stiffness and pain *-itis:* inflammation *Spondylitis may result from a traumatic injury to the spine, infection, or rheumatoid disease; also called ankylosing spondylitits.*
vertebr/o (used to form words that describe the structure)		vertebr/al (VĔR-tě-brăl): pertaining to a vertebra or the vertebral column *-al:* pertaining to, relating to
stern/o	sternum (breastbone)	stern/o/cost/al (stěr-nō-KŎS-tăl): pertaining to the sternum and ribs *cost:* ribs *-al:* pertaining to, relating to
SPECIFIC BONES OF LOWER EXTREMITIES		
calcane/o	calcaneum (heel bone)	calcane/o/dynia (kăl-kăn-ē-ō-DĬN-ē-ă): painful condition of the heel *-dynia:* pain

(Continued)

Word Element	Meaning	Word Analysis *(Continued)*
femor/o	femur (thigh bone)	femor/al (FĔM-or-ăl): pertaining to the femur *-al:* pertaining to, relating to
fibul/o	fibula (smaller, outer bone of lower leg)	fibul/ar (FĬB-ū-lăr): pertaining to the fibula *-ar:* pertaining to, relating to
patell/o	patella (kneecap)	patell/ectomy (păt-ĕ-LĔK-tō-mē): excision of the patella *-ectomy:* excision, removal
pelv/i	pelvis	pelv/i/metry (pĕl-VĬM-ĕ-trē): measurement of the pelvic dimensions or proportions *-metry:* act of measuring *Pelvimetry helps determine whether or not it will be possible to deliver a fetus through the normal route.*
pelv/o		pelv/is (PĔL-vĭs): pertaining to the pelvis *-is:* noun ending *A woman's pelvis is usually less massive but wider and more circular than a man's pelvis.*
tibi/o	tibia (larger inner bone of lower leg)	tibi/al (TĬB-ē-ăl): pertaining to the tibia (shin bone) *-al:* pertaining to, relating to

OTHER RELATED STRUCTURES

Word Element	Meaning	Word Analysis
ankyl/o	stiffness; bent, crooked	ankyl/osis (ăng-kĭ-LŌ-sĭs): immobility of a joint *-osis:* abnormal condition; increase (used primarily with blood cells) *Ankylosis may be congenital, or it may be due to disease, trauma, surgery, or contractures resulting from immobility.*
arthr/o	joint	arthr/itis (ăr-THRĪ-tĭs): inflammation of a joint, often accompanied by pain, swelling, stiffness, and deformity *-itis:* inflammation
cervic/o	neck; cervix uteri (neck of uterus)	cervic/al (SĔR-vĭ-kăl): pertaining to or in region of the neck; pertaining to constricted area of necklike structure, such as neck of a tooth or the cervix uteri *-al:* pertaining to, relating to
chondr/o	cartilage	cost/o/chondr/itis (kŏs-tō-kŏn DRĪ-tĭs): inflammation of the costal cartilage of the anterior chest wall *-itis:* inflammation *Costochondritis is characterized by pain and tenderness that may radiate from the initial site of inflammation.*
lamin/o	lamina (part of vertebral arch)	lamin/ectomy (lăm-ĭ-NĔK-tō-mē): excision of the bony arches of one or more vertebrae *-ectomy:* excision, removal
myel/o	bone marrow; spinal cord	myel/o/cele (MĪ-ĕ-lō-sēl): sacklike protrusion of spinal cord through congenital defect in vertebral column *-cele:* hernia, swelling

Word Element	Meaning	Word Analysis
orth/o	straight	orth/o/ped/ics (or-thō-PĒ-dĭks): branch of medicine concerned with the prevention and correction of musculoskeletal system disorders *ped:* foot, child *-ics:* pertaining to, relating to
oste/o	bone	oste/itis (ŏs-tē-Ī-tĭs): inflammation of bone *-itis:* inflammation
radi/o	radiation, x-ray; radius (lower arm bone, thumb side)	radi/o/graph (RĀ-dē-ō-grăf): x-ray image *-graph:* instrument for recording

SUFFIXES

Word Element	Meaning	Word Analysis
-clasia	to break	arthr/o/clasia (ăr-thrō-KLĀ-zē-ă): forcible breaking of a joint *arthr/o:* joint
-cyte	cell	oste/o/cyte (ŎS-tē-ō-sīt): bone cell *oste/o:* bone
-desis	binding, fixation (of a bone or joint)	arthr/o/desis (ăr-thrō-DĒ-sĭs): stiffening of a joint by operative means *arthr/o:* joint
-malacia	softening	oste/o/malacia (ŏs-tē-ō-mă-LĀ-shē-ă): gradual softening and bending of the bones *oste/o:* bone *Osteomalacia is due to vitamin D deficiency that results in a shortage or loss of calcium salts, causing bones to become increasingly soft, flexible, brittle, and deformed.*
-physis	growth	dia/physis (dī-ĂF-ĭ-sĭs): shaft or middle region of a long bone *dia-:* through, across
-porosis	porous	oste/o/porosis (ŏs-tē-ō-por-Ō-sĭs): disorder characterized by abnormal loss of bone density and deterioration of bone tissue, with an increased fracture risk *oste/o:* bone

 Listen and Learn, the audio CD-ROM that accompanies this book, will help you master the pronunciation of selected medical words. Use it to practice pronunciations of the above-listed medical terms and for instructions to complete the *Listen and Learn* exercise on the CD-ROM for this section.

SECTION REVIEW 10–1

For the following medical terms, first write the suffix and its meaning. Then translate the meaning of the remaining elements starting with the first part of the word. The first word is an example that is completed for you.

Term	Meaning
1. dia/physis	-physis: growth; through, across
2. sub/cost/al	_____
3. oste/o/malacia	_____
4. lamin/ectomy	_____
5. pelv/i/metry	_____
6. myel/o/cele	_____
7. oste/o/porosis	_____
8. ankyl/osis	_____
9. carp/o/ptosis	_____
10. crani/o/tomy	_____

Competency Verification: Check your answers in Appendix B, Answer Key, page 531. If you are not satisfied with your level of comprehension, review the vocabulary and retake the review.

Correct Answers _____ × 10 = _____% Score

Structure and Function of Bones

oste/o	**10-1** To understand the skeletal system, it is important to know the types and names of major bones, their functions, and where they are located. Regardless of the size or shape of a bone, the combining form used to designate bone is _____ /_____.
	10-2 There are four principal types of bones—*long bones, short bones, flat bones,* and *irregular bones*. The *long bones* of the extremities are the strongest bones of the arms and legs. The cube-shaped *short bones* include the bones of the ankles, wrists, and toes. *Flat bones* are the broad bones found in the skull, shoulder, and ribs. *Irregular bones* have varied shapes and sizes and are often clustered, such as the bones of the vertebrae and certain bones of the ears and face.

irregular bones

long bones

short bones

flat bones

Identify the four types of bones described below.

Certain bones of the ears and the bones of the vertebrae:

_____ _____.

The strongest bones of the arms and legs:

_____ _____.

Cube-shaped bones of the wrists, ankles, and toes:

_____ _____.

The broad bones in the shoulders and ribs:

_____ _____.

10-3   Typically, long bones are found in the extremities of the body. The main elongated portion of such a bone, the (1) **diaphysis,** is composed of several tissue layers: the thin fibrous outer membrane, the (2) **periosteum;** the thick layer of hard (3) **compact bone;** and the inner (4) **medullary cavity**. Label the parts of the long bone in Figure 10–2.

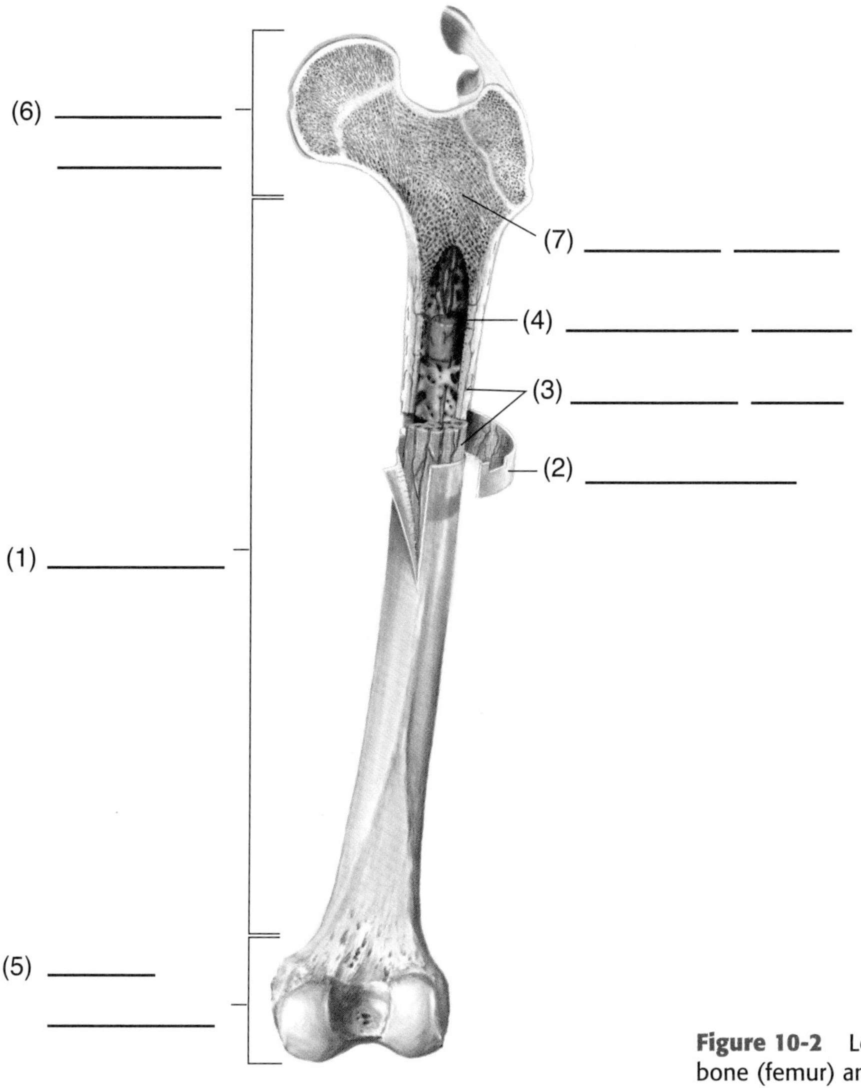

(6) _____
   _____

(7) _____ _____

(4) _____ _____

(3) _____ _____

(2) _____

(1) _____

(5) _____
   _____

Figure 10-2 Longitudinal section of a long bone (femur) and interior bone structure.

10-4 The two ends of bones, the (5) **distal epiphysis** and (6) **proximal epiphysis,** have a bulbous shape to provide space for muscle and ligament attachments near the joints. Label these structures in Figure 10–2.

10-5 There are two kinds of bone tissue, based on porosity, and most bones have both types. Compact (dense) bone tissue is the hard, outer layer; spongy (cancellous) bone tissue is the porous, highly vascular inner portion. Compact bone tissue is covered by periosteum that serves for attachment of muscles, provides protection, and gives durable strength to the bone. The (7) **spongy bone** tissue makes the bone lighter and provides a space for bone marrow where blood cells are produced. Label the spongy bone in Figure 10–2, and note the position and structure of compact and spongy bone.

10-6 In Figure 10–2, observe how the diaphysis forms a cylinder that surrounds the medullary cavity. In adults, the medullary cavity contains fat yellow marrow, so named because of the large amounts of fat it contains.

10-7 The peri/oste/um, as illustrated in Figure 10–2, covers the entire surface of the bone. Its blood vessels supply nutrients, and its nerves signal pain. In growing bones, the inner layer contains the bone-forming cells known as *oste/o/blasts*. Because blood vessels and oste/o/blasts are located here, the peri/oste/um provides a means for bone repair and general bone nutrition. Bones that lose peri/oste/um through injury or disease usually scale or die. As discussed earlier, the peri/oste/um also provides a point of attachment for muscles.

Identify the terms in this frame that mean

embryonic cell (that develops into) bone:

_____ / _____ / _____.

structure around bone: _____ / _____ / _____.

oste/o/blasts
ŎS-tē-ō-blăstz
peri/oste/um
pĕr-ē-ŎS-tē-ŭm

10-8 Oste/o/genesis is the formation or development of bones.

Identify the elements in this frame that mean

forming, producing, origin: _____.

bone: _____ / _____.

When we are talking about bone cells, the medical term to use is

_____ / _____ / _____.

-genesis

oste/o

oste/o/cytes
ŎS-tē-ō-sītz

10-9 In an adult, the production of red blood cells *(erythr/o/poiesis)* occurs in red bone marrow. Red bone marrow is also responsible for the formation of white blood cells *(leuk/o/poiesis)* and platelets.

Identify the terms in this frame that mean

leuk/o/poiesis
loo-kō-poy-Ē-sĭs

formation or production of white blood cells:

_____ / ____ / _____.

erythr/o/poiesis
ĕ-rĭth-rō-poy-Ē-sĭs

formation or production of red blood cells:

_____ / ____ / _____.

10–10   Cartilage, which is more elastic than bone, composes parts of the skeleton. It is found chiefly in the joints, thorax, trachea, and nose.

Use **chondr/o** _(cartilage)_ to form words meaning

chondr/itis
kŏn-DRĪ-tĭs

inflammation of cartilage: _____ / _____.

chondr/oma
kŏn-DRŌ-mă

tumor composed of cartilage: _____ / _____.

producing or forming cartilage:

chondr/o/genesis
kŏn-drō-JĔN-ĕ-sĭs

_____ / ____ / _____.

10–11   Use -cyte to build a word meaning cartilage cell:

chondr/o/cyte
KŎN-drō-sīt

_____ / ____ / _____.

Competency Verification: Check your labeling of Figure 10–2 with Appendix B, Answer Key, page 531.

10–12   Oste/algia refers to pain in a bone. Form another term meaning pain in a bone:

oste/o/dynia
ŏs-tē-ō-DĬN-ē-ă

_____ / ____ / _____.

10–13   Bone is living tissue composed of oste/o/cytes, blood vessels, and nerves.

Determine the medical term for bone cells:

oste/o/cytes
ŎS-tē-ō-sītz

_____ / ____ / _____.

10–14   Practice developing medical words that mean

oste/itis
ŏs-tē-Ī-tĭs

inflammation of bone: _____ / _____.

oste/o/pathy
ŏs-tē-ŎP-ă-thē

disease of bone: _____ / ____ / _____.

oste/o/tomy
ŏs-tē-ŎT-ō-mē

incision of bone: _____ / ____ / _____.

oste/o/rrhaphy
ŏs-tē-OR-ă-fē

suture of bone (wiring of bone fragments):

_____ / ____ / _____.

oste/o/scler/osis
ŏs-tē-ō-sklĕ-RŌ-sĭs

abnormal condition of bone hardening:

_____ / ____ / _____ / _____.

dist/o	**10-15** *Dist/al* is a directional word meaning farthest from the point of attachment to the trunk, or far from the beginning of a structure. From dist/al, construct the combining form that means far or farthest: _____ / ____.
proxim/o	**10-16** Proxim/al is a directional word meaning near the point of attachment to the trunk, or near the beginning of a structure. From proxim/al, construct the combining form that means near or nearest: _____ / ____.
farthest **nearest**	**10-17** Use the words farthest or nearest to complete this frame. The dist/al epiphysis is located _____ from the trunk. The proxim/al epiphysis is located _____ the trunk.
oste/o/malacia ŏs-tē-ō-mă-LĀ-shē-ă **oste/o/genesis** ŏs-tē-ō-JĔN-ĕ-sĭs	**10-18** Milk is a good source of vitamin D. A deficiency of this vitamin results in a softening and weakening of the skeleton causing pain and bowing of the bones. Construct medical terms meaning softening of bones: _____ / ____ / _____. producing or forming bone: _____ / ____ / _____.
oste/o/malacia ŏs-tē-ō-mă-LĀ-shē-ă	**10-19** Oste/o/malacia is the result of an inadequate amount of phosphorus and calcium available in the blood for mineralization of the bones. It may be caused by a diet lacking these minerals, deficiency in vitamin D, or a metabolic disorder causing malabsorption of minerals. The medical term meaning softening of bones is _____ / ____ / _____.
oste/o/malacia ŏs-tē-ō-mă-LĀ-shē-ă	**10-20** A form of oste/o/malacia known as rickets is seen in infants and children in many underdeveloped countries as a result of vitamin D deficiency. Symptoms of rickets include soft pliable bones causing deformities such as bowlegs and knock-knees. Rickets is another name for _____ / ____ / _____.
oste/o/malacia ŏs-tē-ō-mă-LĀ-shē-ă	**10-21** Rickets is marked by an abnormality in the shapes of bones and is a form of _____ / ____ / _____.
rickets RĬK-ĕts	**10-22** Calcium provides bone strength that is needed for its supportive functions. Many children in underdeveloped countries have rickets because of inadequate milk supply. When oste/o/malacia occurs in children, it is called _____.

calc/emia kăl-SĒ-mē-ă	**10-23** Combine **calc/o** and -emia to form a word meaning calcium in the blood: _____ / _____ .
under, below, deficient	**10-24** Recall that hypo- means _____ , _____ , _____ .
hyper/calc/emia hī-pĕr-kăl-SĒ-mē-ă	**10-25** Hypo/calc/emia is a deficiency of calcium in the blood; the term _____ / _____ / _____ is an excessive amount of calcium in the blood.
radi/o/logist rā-dē-ŎL-ō-jĭst	**10-26** Radi/o/logy, initially widely called roentgen/o/logy, was developed after the discovery of an unknown ray in 1895 by Wilhelm Roentgen, who called his discovery a roentgen (x-ray). Occasionally you still may see words with **roentgen/o,** but **radi/o** is the preferred term used in the context of medical imaging today. Radi/o/logy is the branch of medicine concerned with radioactive substances. A physician who specializes in the study of x-rays is called a _____ / ____ / _____ .
radi/o/therapy rā-dē-ō-THĔR-ă-pē	**10-27** Radiation is used for diagnostic and therapeutic purposes. Radiation therapy, also called radi/o/therapy, is the treatment of diseases using either an external source of high-energy rays or internally implanted radioactive substances. These rays and substances are effective in damaging cancer cells and halting their growth. Treatment of disease using radiation is called _____ / ____ / _____ .
radi/o/logist rā-dē-ŎL-ō-jĭst	**10-28** Combine **radi/o** + -logist to build a word that means a physician specialist who studies, or interprets, x-rays: _____ / ____ / _____ .
muscle **bone marrow, spinal cord**	**10-29** Although **my/o** and **myel/o** sound alike, they have different meanings. **My/o** refers to _____ ; **myel/o** refers to _____ or _____ .
	10-30 Find three words that contain **myel/o** in your medical dictionary and write brief definitions in the spaces provided. **Term** **Meaning** _____ _____ _____ _____ _____ _____

myel/o	**10–31** A myel/o/gram is a radi/o/graph of the spinal cord after injection of a contrast medium. The combining form for bone marrow and spinal cord is _____ /_____.
myel/o/genesis mī-ĕ-lō-JĔN-ĕ-sĭs	**10–32** Use -genesis to build a word meaning formation of bone marrow: _____ /_____ /_____.
myel/o/malacia mī-ĕl-ō-mă-LĀ-shē-ă **myel/o/gram** MĪ-ĕl-ō-grăm	**10–33** Develop medical words meaning softening of the spinal cord: _____ /_____ /_____. record of the spinal cord: _____ /_____ /_____.
myel/o/gram MĪ-ĕl-ō-grăm	**10–34** A myel/o/gram, a radiograph of the spinal canal after injection of a contrast medium, is used to identify and study spinal lesions caused by trauma or disease. To identify any distortions of the spinal cord, the physician may order a radiograph called a _____ /_____ /_____.

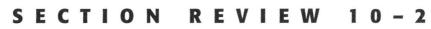

SECTION REVIEW 10 – 2

Using the following table, write the combining form, suffix, or prefix that matches its definition in the space provided to the left of the definition. There may be more than one word element that matches a definition.

Combining Forms	Suffixes		Prefixes
calc/o	-algia	-graphy	hyper-
chondr/o	-cele	-itis	hypo-
dist/o	-cyte	-logist	peri-
my/o	-dynia	-malacia	
myel/o	-emia	-oma	
oste/o	-genesis	-rrhaphy	
proxim/o	-gram	-tomy	
radi/o			
scler/o			

1. _____ excessive, above normal
2. _____ around
3. _____ blood condition
4. _____ bone
5. _____ cartilage
6. _____ calcium
7. _____ cell
8. _____ far, farthest
9. _____ hardening; sclera (white of eye)
10. _____ hernia, swelling
11. _____ incision
12. _____ inflammation
13. _____ near, nearest

14. _____ muscle
15. _____ pain
16. _____ process of recording
17. _____ forming, producing, origin
18. _____ record, writing
19. _____ softening
20. _____ specialist in study of
21. _____ bone marrow; spinal cord
22. _____ suture
23. _____ tumor
24. _____ under, below, deficient
25. _____ radiation, x-ray; radius (lower arm bone on thumb side)

Competency Verification: Check your answers in Appendix B, Answer Key, page 531. If you are not satisfied with your level of comprehension, go back to Frame 10–1 and rework the frames.

Correct Answers _____ × 4 = _____% Score

Making a set of flash cards from key word elements in this chapter for each section review can help you remember the elements. Make a flash card by writing a word element on one side of a 3 × 5 or 4 × 6 index card. On the other side, write the meaning of the element. Do this for all word elements in the section reviews. Use your flash cards to review each section. You also might use the flash cards to prepare for the chapter review at the end of this chapter.

Joints

synarthroses sĭn-ăhr-THRŌ-sēz **diarthroses** dī-ăhr-THRŌ-sēz **amphiarthroses** ăm-fē-ăr-THRŌ-sēz	**10–35** To allow for body movements, bones must have points where they meet *(articulate)*. These articulating points form joints that have various degrees of mobility. Some are freely movable *(diarthroses)*, others are only slightly movable *(amphiarthroses)*, and the remaining are totally immovable *(synarthroses)*. All three types are necessary for smooth, coordinated body movements. Use the above information to identify and pronounce the following types of joints. Totally immovable joints: _____. Freely movable joints: _____. Slightly movable joints: _____.
arthr/o/pathy ăr-THRŎP-ă-thē **arthr/itis** ăr-THRĪ-tĭs **arthr/o/centesis** ăr-thrō-sĕn-TĒ-sĭs	**10–36** Use **arthr/o** *(joint)* to develop medical words meaning disease of a joint: _____ / _____ / _____. inflammation of a joint: _____ / _____. surgical puncture of a joint: _____ / _____ / _____.
joints	**10–37** Just as a piece of machinery is lubricated by oil, joints are lubricated by synovial fluid, which is secreted within the synovial membranes. Synovial fluid allows free movement of the _____.
arthr/o/centesis ăr-thrō-sĕn-TĒ-sĭs	**10–38** To aspirate or remove accumulated fluid from a joint, a surgical puncture of a joint is performed. This surgical procedure is called _____ / _____ / _____.
arthr/o/dynia ăr-thrō-DĬN-ē-ă	**10–39** A person with arthr/itis suffers not only from an inflammation of the joints, but also from arthr/algia. Construct another medical word meaning pain in a joint: _____ / _____ / _____.
arthr/itis ăr-THRĪ-tĭs **oste/o/arthr/itis** ŏs-tē-ō-ăr-THRĪ-tĭs	**10–40** Although there are various forms of arthr/itis, all of them result in an inflammation of the joints that usually is accompanied by pain and swelling. Form medical words meaning inflammation of joints: _____ / _____. inflammation of bones and joints: _____ / _____ / _____ / _____.

oste/o/arthr/o/pathy
ŏs-tē-ō-ăr-THRŎP-ă-thē

10–41   A disease of the bones and joints is called

_____ / _____ / _____ / _____ / _____.

oste/o/arthr/osis
ŏs-tē-ō-ăr-THRŌ-sĭs

10–42   Select element(s) from oste/o/arthr/o/pathy to build a word meaning an abnormal condition of the bones and joints.

_____ / _____ / _____ / _____.

Combining Forms Related to Specific Bones

10–43   The word roots/combining forms of bones are derived from the specific names of the bones. Learn the combining forms for the bones as you label them in Figure 10–3.

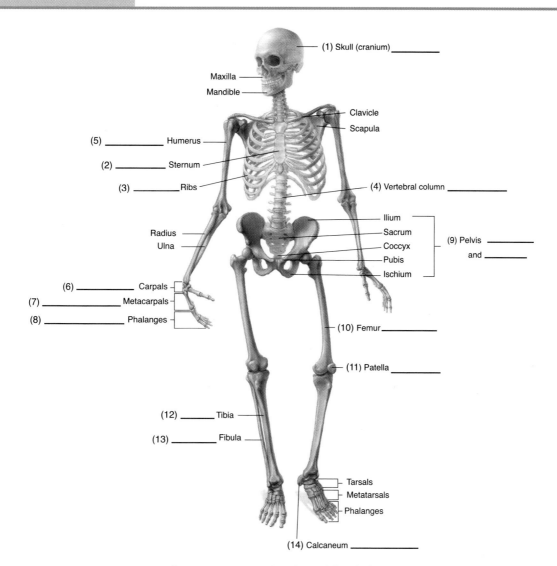

Figure 10-3   Anterior view of the skeleton.

(1) **crani/o** refers to the *cranium (skull)*.

(2) **stern/o** refers to the *sternum (breastbone)*.

(3) **cost/o** refers to the *ribs*, which are attached to the sternum.

(4) **vertebr/o** refers to the *vertebrae (backbone)*. The vertebral column also is called the spinal column and is composed of 26 bones called vertebr/ae (singular, vertebra).

(5) **humer/o** refers to the *humerus (upper arm bone)*. The humerus articulates with the scapula at the shoulder and with the radius and ulna at the elbow.

(6) **carp/o** refers to the *carpus (wrist bones)*. There are eight wrist bones.

(7) **metacarp/o** refers to the *metacarpus (hand bones)*. The metacarpals (plural) radiate from the wristlike spokes and form the palm of the hand.

(8) **phalang/o** refers to the *phalanges (bones of fingers and toes)*.

(9) **pelv/i** and **pelv/o** refer to the *pelvis*. The *pelvis*, also called the *pelvic girdle*, is composed of three pairs of fused bones (the ilium, pubis, and ischium), the sacrum, and the coccyx. The pelvis provides attachment for the legs and supports the soft organs of the abdominal cavity (see Figure 10–1).

(10) **femor/o** refers to the *femur (thigh bone)*. The femur is the longest and strongest bone in the body. It articulates with the hip bone and the bones of the lower leg.

(11) **patell/o** refers to the *patella (kneecap)*. The patella articulates with the femur, but essentially is a floating bone. The main function of this bone is to protect the knee joint, but its exposed position makes it vulnerable to dislocation and fracture.

(12) **tibi/o** refers to the *tibia (larger inner bone of lower leg)*. The tibia is the weight-bearing bone of the lower leg.

(13) **fibul/o** refers to the *fibula (smaller, outer bone of lower leg)*. The fibula is not a weight-bearing bone but is important because muscles are attached and anchored to it.

(14) **calcane/o** refers to the *calcaneum (heel bone)*.

Competency Verification: Check your labeling of Figure 10–3 with Appendix B, Answer Key, page 532.

ALERT — You are not expected to know the combining forms and the names of the bones from memory. If needed, you can always refer to Figure 10–3, Appendix A: Glossary of Medical Word Elements, or a medical dictionary to obtain information about a bone or its combining form.

---

pain, head	**10-44** Words containing **cephal/o** refer to the *head*. Cephal/o/dynia is a _____ in the _____.
cephal/algia sĕf-ă-LĂL-gē-ă	**10-45** Cephal/o/dynia is the medical term for a headache. Construct another word meaning pain in the head: _____ / _____.

head **-meter**	**10-46** A meter is an instrument to measure. A cephal/o/meter is an instrument to measure the _____. In cephal/o/meter, the element meaning an instrument to measure is _____.
encephal/o	**10-47** The prefix en- means *in, within*. Combine en- + **cephal/o** to form a new combining form that refers to the brain: _____ / ____.
encephal/oma ĕn-sĕf-ă-LŌ-mă **encephal/itis** ĕn-sĕf-ă-LĪ-tĭs **encephal/o/malacia** ĕn-sĕf-ă-lō-mă-LĀ-sē-ă	**10-48** Use **encephal/o** to build words meaning tumor of the brain: _____ / _____. inflammation of the brain: _____ / _____. softening of the brain (tissue): _____ / ____ / _____.
encephal/itis ĕn-sĕf-ă-LĪ-tĭs	**10-49** Encephal/itis usually is caused by viruses (for example, *arborvirus, herpesvirus*). Less frequently, it may occur as a component of rabies and acquired immunodeficiency syndrome (AIDS) and as an aftereffect of systemic viral diseases, such as influenza, German measles, and chickenpox. The medical term for an inflammatory condition of the brain is _____ / _____.
disease **brain**	**10-50** Encephal/o/pathy is a _____ of the _____.
brain	**10-51** An encephal/o/cele is a protrusion of _____ substance through an opening of the skull.
inter- **cost** **-al**	**10-52** Inter/cost/al muscles, located between the ribs, move the ribs during the breathing process. Write the elements in this frame that mean in, within: _____. ribs: _____. pertaining to, relating to: _____.
under *or* **below** **ribs**	**10-53** Sub/cost/al refers to the area _____ the _____.
pain, rib	**10-54** Cost/algia is a _____ in a _____.

Fractures and Repairs

10–55 A fracture is a break or crack in the bone. Fractures are defined according to the type and extent of the break. A (1) **closed fracture** means the bone is broken with no open wound; surrounding tissue damage is minimal. An (2) **open fracture,** also called compound fracture, means the broken end of a bone pierces the skin creating an open wound. There may be extensive damage to surrounding blood vessels, nerves, and muscles. Label the closed and open fractures in Figure 10–4.

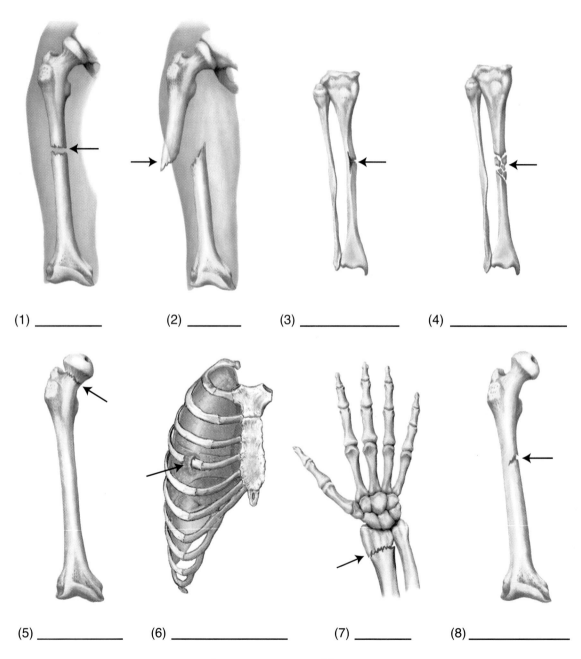

(1) _____   (2) _____   (3) _____   (4) _____

(5) _____   (6) _____   (7) _____   (8) _____

Figure 10-4   Types of fractures.

10-56 Discussion of examples of different types of fractures follows. A (3) **greenstick fracture** means there is an incomplete break of a soft bone; the bone is partially bent and partially broken. These fractures usually occur in children because their bones tend to splinter rather than break completely. A (4) **comminuted fracture** occurs when the bone is broken into pieces. In an (5) **impacted fracture,** the broken ends of a bone are forced into one another; many bone fragments may be created by such a fracture. A (6) **complicated fracture** involves extensive soft tissue injury, such as when a broken rib pierces a lung. A (7) **Colles fracture** is a break of the lower end of the radius, which occurs just above the wrist. It causes displacement of the hand and usually occurs as a result of flexing a hand to cushion a fall. An (8) **incomplete fracture** is when the line of fracture does not include the whole bone. Label and study the different types of fractures in Figure 10–4.

Competency Verification: Check your labeling of Figure 10–4 in Appendix B, Answer Key, page 538.

10-57 Refer to Figure 10–4 to complete this frame.

Identify the following fractures:

Bone pierces the skin and causes extensive damage to surrounding blood

| open, compound |
| closed |

vessels: _____ or _____.

Bone is broken with no external wound present: _____

Bone is partially bent and partially broken; found more commonly in

| greenstick |

children: _____.

Broken ends of bone segments are wedged into one another:

| impacted |
| ĭm-PĂK-tĕd |

_____.

Vertebral Column

10-58 The vertebr/al or spin/al column (see Figure 10–5) supports the body and provides a protective bony canal for the spinal cord.

Another name for the vertebr/al column is

| spin/al column |
| SPĪ-năl KŎL-ŭm |

_____ / _____ _____.

From the word spin/al, construct the combining form for the spine:

| spin/o |

_____ / ___.

10-59 **Spondyl/o** and **vertebr/o** are combining forms that refer to the

| vertebra |
| VĔR-tĕ-bră |

vertebrae (backbone). The singular form of vertebrae is _____.

| vertebra |
| VĔR-tĕ-bră |

10-60 Vertebr/ectomy is an excision of a _____.

| vertebra |
| VĔR-tĕ-bră |

Spondyl/o/dynia is a painful condition of a _____.

10-61 Change the following words from singular to plural form by retaining the *a* and adding an *e*.

Singular   Plural

vertebrae
VĔR-tĕ-brē

vertebra   _____

bursae
BĔR-sē

bursa   _____

pleurae
PLOO-rē

pleura   _____

10-62   **Spondyl/o** is used to form words about the condition of the structure. Build medical words meaning

spondyl/itis
spŏn-dĭl-Ī-tĭs

inflammation of the vertebrae: _____ / _____.

disease of the vertebrae:

spondyl/o/pathy
spŏn-dĭl-ŎP-ă-thē

_____ / _____ / _____.

softening of the vertebrae:

spondyl/o/malacia
spŏn-dĭl-ō-mă-LĀ-shē-ă

_____ / _____ / _____.

10-63   **Vertebr/o** is used to form words that describe the vertebral structure. For example, vertebr/o/cost/al means pertaining to a

vertebra

_____ and a rib; vertebr/o/stern/al means pertaining to a

vertebra
VĔR-tĕ-bră

_____ and the sternum or chest plate.

10-64   Vertebrae are separate and cushioned from each other by (1) **intervertebral disks** composed of cartilage. Label Figure 10–5 as you learn about the vertebr/al or spin/al column.

10-65   Determine the elements in inter/vertebr/al that mean

inter-

between: _____.

vertebr/o

vertebrae (backbone): _____ / _____.

-al

pertaining to, relating to: _____.

10-66   The vertebr/al column, also called the spin/al column or backbone, is composed of 26 bones known as vertebrae (singular, vertebra). There are five regions of these bones in the vertebr/al column, each of which derives its name from its location along the length of the spin/al column. Seven (2) **cervical vertebrae** form the skeletal framework of the neck. The first cervic/al vertebra is called the (3) **atlas** and supports the skull. The second, the (4) **axis**, makes possible rotation of the skull on the neck. Label these structures in Figure 10–5

10-67   **Cervic/o** is the combining form for the *neck* and the *cervix uteri*

neck

(*neck of the uterus*). Cervic/o/facial refers to the face and _____.

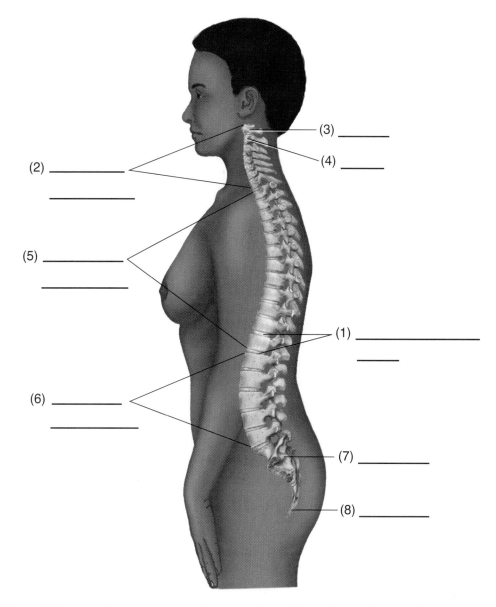

Figure 10-5   Vertebral column, lateral view. Regions of the spine as shown with normal curves.

atlas ĂT-lăs **cervic/al** SĔR-vi-kăl	**10-68** The first cervic/al vertebra is the _____. A term meaning pertaining to the neck is _____ / _____.
C5 *or* **C₅**	**10-69** In medical reports, the first cervical vertebra is designated as **C1**. The fifth cervical vertebra is designated as _____.

	10-70 When the radi/o/logist interprets an x-ray film and indicates a herniation or rupture at C3 to C4 disk in a report, he or she is referring to a herniation or rupture of the inter/vertebr/al disk between C3 and C4.
	When the radi/o/logist indicates a herniation at C4 to C5 disk in a report, he or she is referring to a herniation of the inter/vertebr/al disk between
C5 *or* **C₅**	C4 and _____.
C2 *or* **C₂**	**10-71** The second vertebra is identified as _____.
seven	**10-72** There are a total of _____ cervic/al vertebrae.
	10-73 Twelve (5) **thoracic vertebrae** support the chest and serve as a point of articulation for the ribs. The next five vertebrae are the (6) **lumbar vertebrae**. These are situated in the lower back and carry most of the weight of the torso. Label these structures in Figure 10–5.
articulation ăr-tĭk-ū-LĀ-shŭn **thorac/ic** thō-RĂS-ĭk	**10-74** Identify the terms in Frame 10–73 that mean a place where two bones meet: _____. pertaining to the chest: _____ / _____.
pertaining to *or* **relating to** **back**	**10-75** The combining form **lumb/o** refers to the *loins (lower back)*. Lumb/ar means _____ the loin or lower _____.
pain	**10-76** Lumb/o/dynia is a _____ in the lower back.
lumbar, five LŬM-băr	**10-77** Examine the position of the five lumbar vertebrae in Figure 10–5. These are designated as L1 to L5 in medical reports. An obese person with weak abdominal muscles tends to experience pain in the lower back area, or L1 to L5. L5 refers to _____ vertebra _____.
	10-78 Below the lumbar vertebrae are five **sacral vertebrae** that are fused into a single bone in the adult and are referred to as the (7) **sacrum** and the tail of the vertebral column, the (8) **coccyx.** Label the sacrum and coccyx in Figure 10–5.
pain **sacr/um** SĀ-krŭm **spine**	**10-79** **Sacr/o** is the combining form for the *sacr/um*. The suffix in the term sacr/um refers to a *structure, thing*. Sacr/o/dynia is a _____ in the sacrum. Sacr/o/spin/al refers to the _____ / _____ and _____.

S5 or S₅

10-80 To designate the exact position of abnormalities on the sacrum, the label S1 to S5 is used. The first vertebra of the sacrum is designated as S1. The fifth vertebra of the sacrum is designated as _____.

lumbar, sacrum
LŬM-băr, SĀ-krŭm

10-81 A ruptured disk can cause severe pain, muscle weakness, or numbness in either leg. The disk that most often ruptures is the L5 to S1 disk. L5 refers to _____ five; S1 refers to _____ one.

Competency Verification: Check your labeling of Figure 10–5 in Appendix B, Answer Key, page 532.

Listen and Learn, the audio CD-ROM that accompanies this book, will help you master the pronunciation of selected medical words. Use it to practice pronunciations of selected terms from frames 10–1 to 10–81 and for instructions to complete the *Listen and Learn* exercise on the CD-ROM for this section.

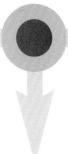

SECTION REVIEW 10 – 3

Using the following table, write the combining form or suffix that matches its definition in the space provided to the left of the definition. There may be more than one word element that matches a definition.

Combining Forms	Suffixes
arthr/o	-centesis
cephal/o	-ectomy
cervic/o	-osis
cost/o	-pathy
encephal/o	-um
lumb/o	
oste/o	
sacr/o	
spondyl/o	
thorac/o	
vertebr/o	

1. _____ abnormal condition; increase (used primarily with blood cells)
2. _____ bone
3. _____ brain
4. _____ chest
5. _____ disease
6. _____ excision, removal
7. _____ head
8. _____ joint
9. _____ loins (lower back)
10. _____ neck; cervix uteri (neck of uterus)
11. _____ structure, thing
12. _____ ribs
13. _____ sacrum
14. _____ surgical puncture
15. _____ vertebrae (backbone)

Competency Verification: Check your answers in Appendix B, Answer Key, page 532. If you are not satisfied with your level of comprehension, go back to Frame 10–35 and rework the frames.

Correct Answers _____ × 6.67 = _____% Score

Muscular System

The human body is composed of hundreds of skeletal muscles, overlapping each in intricate layers. Muscles usually are described in groups according to their anatomical location and cooperative function. Selected muscles of the body are illustrated in Figure 10–6.

All muscles, through contraction, provide the body with motion or body posture. The less apparent motions provided by muscles include the passage and elimination of food through the digestive system, propulsion of blood through the arteries, and contraction of the bladder to eliminate urine. In addition, muscles function in body movements in several different ways to allow a range of motion for the contraction and relaxation of muscle fibers.

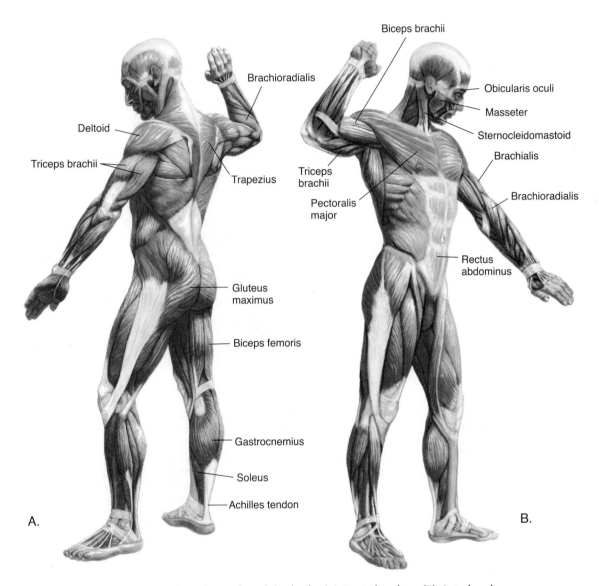

Figure 10-6   Selected muscles of the body. (A) Posterior view. (B) Anterior view.

Word Elements

This section introduces combining forms related to the muscular system. Included are key suffixes; prefixes are defined in the right-hand column as needed. Review the following table, and pronounce each word in the word analysis column aloud before you begin to work the frames.

Word Element	Meaning	Word Analysis
COMBINING FORMS		
lumb/o	loins (lower back)	lumb/o/cost/al (lŭm-bō-KŎS-tăl): pertaining to the lumbar region and the ribs *cost:* ribs *-al:* pertaining to, relating to
my/o	muscle	my/o/rrhexis (mī-or-ĔK-sĭs): tearing of a muscle; rupture of a muscle *-rrhexis:* rupture
ten/o	tendon	ten/o/tomy (tĕn-ŎT-ō-mē): total or partial severing of a tendon *-tomy:* incision *Tenotomy is performed to correct a muscle imbalance, such as in the correction of strabismus of the eye or in clubfoot.*
tend/o		tend/o/lysis (tĕn-DŎL-ĭ-sĭs): release of a tendon from adhesions; also called tenolysis *-lysis:* separation; destruction; loosening
tendin/o		tendin/itis (tĕn-dĭn-Ī-tĭs): inflammation of a tendon, usually resulting from strain; also called tendonitis *-itis:* inflammation
SUFFIXES		
-algia	pain	my/algia (mī-ĂL-jē-ă): tenderness or pain in the muscles; muscular rheumatism *my:* muscle
-pathy	disease	my/o/pathy (mī-ŎP-ă-thē): any abnormal condition or disease of the muscular tissues; commonly designates a disorder involving skeletal muscle *my/o:* muscle
-plegia	paralysis	hemi/plegia (hĕm-ē-PLĒ-jē-ă): paralysis of one side of the body *hemi-:* one half *Types of hemiplegia include cerebral hemiplegia and facial hemiplegia.*

Word Element	Meaning	Word Analysis
-rrhaphy	suture	my/o/rrhaphy (mī-OR-ă-fē): suturing of a wound in a muscle *my/o*: muscle
-rrhexis	rupture	my/o/rrhexis (mī-or-ĔK-sĭs): tearing of any muscle *my/o*: muscle
-sarcoma	malignant tumor of connective tissue	my/o/sarcoma (mī-ō-sar-KŌ-mă): malignant tumor of muscular tissue *my/o*: muscle
-tomy	incision	chondr/o/tomy (kŏn-DRŎT-ō-mē): incision for dividing a cartilage *chondr/o*: cartilage

 Listen and Learn, the audio CD-ROM that accompanies this book, will help you master the pronunciation of selected medical words. Use it to practice pronunciations of the above-listed medical terms and for instructions to complete the *Listen and Learn* exercise on the CD-ROM for this section.

For the following medical terms, first write the suffix and its meaning. Then translate the meaning of the remaining elements starting with the first part of the word. The first word is an example that is completed for you.

Term	Meaning
1. my/o/sarcoma	-sarcoma: malignant tumor of connective tissue; muscle
2. my/o/rrhaphy	_____
3. hemi/plegia	_____
4. ten/o/tomy	_____
5. cost/o/chondr/itis	_____
6. tend/o/lysis	_____
7. my/o/pathy	_____
8. lumb/o/cost/al	_____
9. tendin/itis	_____
10. my/algia	_____

Competency Verification: Check your answers in Appendix B, Answer Key, page 533. If you are not satisfied with your level of comprehension, review the vocabulary and retake the review.

Correct Answers _____ × 10 = _____% Score

muscle(s)	**10–82** The fibers within each muscle are characteristically arranged into specific patterns that provide specific functional capabilities. Most skeletal muscles lie between the skin and the skeleton. My/o/genesis is the embryonic formation of _____.
my/o/plasty MĪ-ō-plăs-tē **my/o/rrhaphy** mī-OR-ă-fē **my/o/tomy** mī-ŎT-ō-mē	**10–83** Practice building medical words meaning surgical repair of muscle: _____ / _____ / _____. suture of muscle: _____ / _____ / _____. incision of muscle: _____ / _____ / _____.

my/o/rrhexis
mī-or-ĔK-sĭs

10-84   Often, sports-related injuries are caused by the tremendous stress exerted on certain parts of musculoskeletal structures. In many instances, these types of athletic injuries may result in a torn muscle.

Form a word meaning rupture (tear) of a muscle.

_____ / _____ / _____ .

---

hepat/o/rrhexis
hĕp-ă-tō-RĔKS-ĭs
cyst/o/rrhexis
sĭs-tō-RĔKS-ĭs
enter/o/rrhexis
ĕn-tĕr-ō-RĔKS-ĭs

10-85   Use -rrhexis to practice building words with the following organs.

rupture of the liver: _____ / _____ / _____ .

rupture of the bladder: _____ / _____ / _____ .

rupture of the intestine: _____ / _____ / _____ .

---

my/algia
mī-ĂL-jē-ă

10-86   My/o/dynia is a muscle pain. Form another word that means muscle pain: _____ / _____ .

---

my/o/pathy
mī-ŎP-ă-thē

10-87   The medical term meaning any disease of muscle is

_____ / _____ / _____ .

---

muscle

10-88   The term my/o/genesis refers to forming, producing, or origin of _____ .

---

hardening

sclera

10-89   The combining form **scler/o** refers to _____ , _____ (white of eye).

---

scler/osis
sklĕ-RŌ-sĭs

my/o/scler/osis
mī-ō-sklĕr-Ō-sĭs

10-90   An abnormal condition of hardening is called

_____ / _____ ; an abnormal condition of muscle hardening is known as:

_____ / _____ / _____ / _____ .

---

anterior

posterior

10-91   To become familiar with the names of the major muscles of the body, study Figure 10–6A and B. Identify the words in the Figure 10–6 caption that mean

in front of: _____ .

back (of body), behind: _____ .

---

tendon

10-92   **Tend/o** is a combining form for *tendon*, which is the fibrous connective tissue that attaches muscles to bone.

Tend/o/plasty is a surgical repair of a _____ .

tend/o/tome TĔN-dō-tōm **tend/o/tomy** tĕn-DŎT-ō-mē **tend/o/plasty** TĔN-dō-plăs-tē	**10–93** Use **tend/o** to form words meaning: instrument to cut a tendon: _____ / ___ / _____ . incision of a tendon: _____ / ___ / _____ . surgical repair of a tendon: _____ / ___ / _____ .
inferior	**10–94** The *Achilles tendon* is attached to a muscle in the lower leg. Locate the Achilles tendon in Figure 10–6A. It is located (superior, inferior) _____ to the gastrocnemius muscle.
paralysis pă-RĂL-ĭ-sĭs	**10–95** The prefix quadri- refers to *four.* Quadri/plegia is a _____ of all four extremities.
paralysis pă-RĂL-ĭ-sĭs	**10–96** The prefix hemi- means *one half.* Hemi/plegia is a _____ of half the body.
	10–97 With the exception of rotations of the body, other types of body movements occur in pairs as summarized in Table 10–1 and illustrated in Figure 10–7.

Table 10–1. Types of Movements Produced by Muscles

This table examines movements and their actions, grouped in pairs of antagonistic (or opposite) functions.

Movement	Action
Flexion (FLĔK-shŭn) **Extension** (ĕks-TĔN-shŭn)	bending and extension of a limb
Abduction (ăb-DŬK-shŭn) **Adduction** (ă-DŬK-shŭn)	movement away from and toward the body
Rotation (rō-TĀ-shŭn)	circular movement around an axis
Pronation (prō-NĀ-shŭn) **supination** (sū-pĭn-Ā-shŭn)	turning the hand to a palm down or palm up position
Dorsiflexion (dor-sĭ-FLĔK-shŭn) **plantar flexion** (PLĂN-tăr FLĔK-shŭn)	bending the foot or toes upward or downward
Eversion (ē-VĔR-zhŭn) **Inversion** (ĭn-VĔR-zhŭn)	moving the sole of the foot outward or inward

Listen and Learn, the audio CD-ROM that accompanies this book, will help you master the pronunciation of selected terms. Use it to practice pronunciations of selected terms from frames 10–82 to 10–97 and for instructions to complete the *Listen and Learn* exercise on the CD-ROM for this.

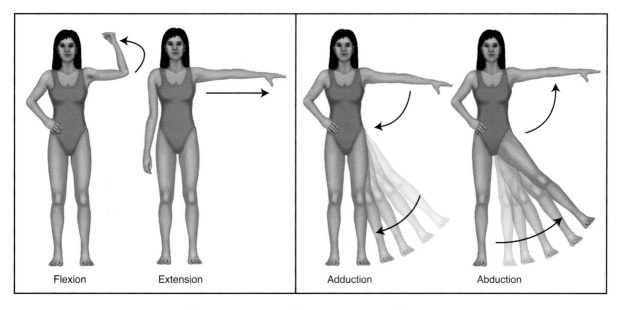

Flexion   Extension   Adduction   Abduction

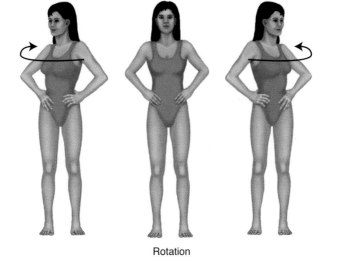

Rotation

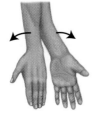

Pronation   Supination

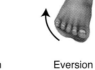

Eversion   Inversion

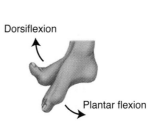

Dorsiflexion

Plantar flexion

Figure 10-7   Body movements generated by muscles.

Using the following table, write the combining form, suffix, or prefix that matches its definition in the space provided to the left of the definition. There may be more than one word element that matches a definition.

Combining Forms	Suffixes	Prefixes
chondr/o	-cyte	hemi-
cyst/o	-genesis	quadri-
enter/o	-lysis	
hepat/o	-osis	
my/o	-plasty	
scler/o	-plegia	
tendin/o	-rrhaphy	
tend/o	-rrhexis	
ten/o	-sarcoma	
	-tome	
	-tomy	

1. _____ abnormal condition; increase (used primarily with blood cells)

2. _____ bladder

3. _____ cell

4. _____ four

5. _____ one half

6. _____ hardening; sclera (white of eye)

7. _____ incision

8. _____ intestine (usually small intestine)

9. _____ liver

10. _____ muscle

11. _____ paralysis

12. _____ forming, producing, origin

13. _____ rupture

14. _____ surgical repair

15. _____ suture

16. _____ tendon

17. _____ instrument to cut

18. _____ cartilage

19. _____ malignant tumor of connective tissue

20. _____ separation; destruction; loosening

Competency Verification: Check your answers in Appendix B, Answer Key, page 533. If you are not satisfied with your level of comprehension, go back to Frame 10–82 rework the frames.

Correct Answers _____ × 5 = _____ % Score

Abbreviations

This section introduces musculoskeletal system–related abbreviations and their meanings. Included are abbreviations contained in the medical record activities that follow.

Abbreviation	Meaning	Abbreviation	Meaning
AE	above the elbow	HD	hip disarticulation; hemodialysis; hearing distance
AIDS	acquired immunodeficiency syndrome	HNP	herniated nucleus pulposus (herniated disk)
AK	above the knee	IM	intramuscular
AP	anteroposterior	L1, L2 to L5	first lumbar vertebra, second lumbar vertebra, and so on
BE	below the elbow	ORTH, Ortho	orthopedics
BK	below the knee	RA	rheumatoid arthritis
C1, C2 to C7	first cervical vertebra, second cervical vertebra, and so on	S1, S2 to S5	first sacral vertebra, second sacral vertebra, and so on
CT	computed tomography	T1, T2 to T12	first thoracic vertebra, second thoracic vertebra, and so on
CTS	carpal tunnel syndrome	TKR	total knee replacement
Fx	fracture		

Pathological, Diagnostic, and Therapeutic Terms

The following are additional terms related to the musculoskeletal system. Recognizing and learning these terms will help you understand the connection between a pathological condition, its diagnosis, and the rationale behind the method of treatment selected for a particular disorder.

Pathological

Bones and Joints

ankylosis (ăng-kĭ-LŌ-sĭs): immobility of a joint.

carpal tunnel syndrome (KĂR-păl TŬN-ĕl SĬN-drōm): pain or numbness resulting from compression of the median nerve within the carpal tunnel (wrist canal through which the flexor tendons and median nerve pass).

contracture (kŏn-TRAK-chŭr): fibrosis of connective tissue in skin, fascia, muscle, or joint capsule that prevents normal mobility of the related tissue or joint.

crepitation (krĕp-ĭ-TĀ-shŭn): grating sound made by movement of bone ends rubbing together, indicating a fracture or joint destruction.

Ewing sarcoma (Ū-ĭng săr-KŌ-mă): malignant tumor that develops from bone marrow, usually in long bones or the pelvis. It occurs most frequently in adolescent boys.

gout (gowt): hereditary metabolic disease that is a form of acute arthritis characterized by excessive uric acid in the blood and around the joints.

herniated disk (HĔR-nē-āt-ĕd): herniation or rupture of the nucleus pulposus (center gelatinous material within an intervetebral disk) between two vertebrae (see Figure 10–8).

Displacement of the disk irritates the spinal nerves, causing muscle spasms and pain.

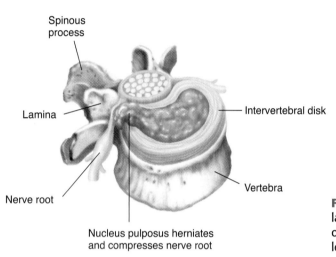

Figure 10-8   A herniated disk, also called a prolapsed disk, places pressure on a spinal root nerve or the spinal cord. It occurs most frequently in the lower spine.

osteoporosis (ŏs-tē-ō-pōr-Ō-sĭs): decrease in bone density with an increase in porosity, causing bones to become brittle and increasing the risk of fractures.

Paget disease (PĂJ-ĕt dĭ-ZĒZ): skeletal disease affecting elderly people that causes chronic inflammation of bones, resulting in thickening and softening of bones and bowing of long bones; also called *osteitis deformans.*

rheumatoid arthritis (ROO-mă-toyd ăr-THRĪ-tĭs): chronic, systemic disease characterized by inflammatory changes in joints and related structures that result in crippling deformities (see Figure 10–9).

sequestrum (sē-KWĔS-trŭm): fragment of a necrosed bone that has become separated from surrounding tissue.

Spinal Disorders

kyphosis (kī-FŌ-sĭs): increased curvature of the thoracic region of the vertebral column, leading to a humpback posture.

Kyphosis may be caused by poor posture, arthritis, or osteomalacia; commonly known as hunchback (see Figure 10–10).

lordosis (lōr-DŌ-sĭs): forward curvature of the lumbar region of the vertebral column, leading to a swayback posture.

Lordosis may be caused by increased weight in the abdomen such as during pregnancy (see Figure 10–10).

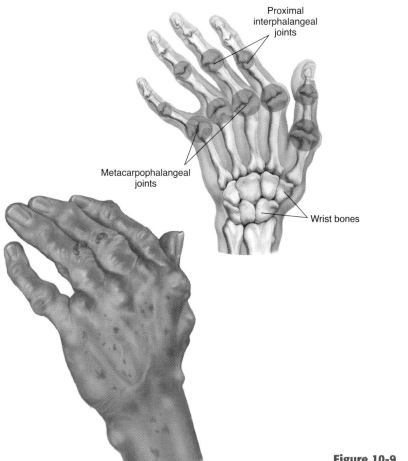

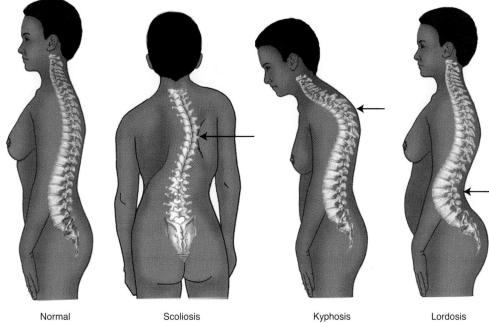

Figure 10-9   Rheumatoid arthritis.

Normal   Scoliosis   Kyphosis   Lordosis

Figure 10-10   Spinal curvatures.

scoliosis (skō-lē-Ō-sĭs): abnormal sideward curvature of the spine, either to the left or to the right (see Figure 10–10).

Scoliosis eventually causes back pain, disk disease, or arthritis. It is often a congenital disease, but may result from poor posture.

Muscular Disorders

muscular dystrophy (MŬS-kū-lăr DĬS-trō-fē): group of hereditary diseases characterized by gradual atrophy and weakness of muscle tissue.

There is no cure, and most individuals die before age 20. Duchenne dystrophy is the most common form.

myasthenia gravis (mī-ăs-THĒ-nē-ă GRĂV-ĭs): autoimmune neuromuscular disorder characterized by severe muscular weakness and progressive fatigue.

rotator cuff injuries: injuries to the capsule of the shoulder joint, which is reinforced by muscles and tendons; also called *musculotendinous rotator cuff injuries.*

Shoulder joint injuries occur in sports in which there is a complete abduction of the shoulder, followed by a rapid and forceful rotation and flexion of the shoulder (see Figure 10–7). This occurs most frequently in baseball injuries when the player throws a baseball. Although less frequent, it also occurs in tennis injuries when the player is serving or completing an overhead stroke.

sprain: trauma to a joint that causes injury to the surrounding ligament, accompanied by pain and disability.

strain: trauma to a muscle from overuse or excessive forcible stretch.

talipes (TĂL-ĭ-pēz): congenital deformity of the foot; also called *clubfoot* (see Figure 10–11,).

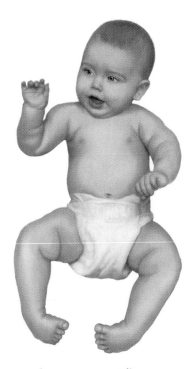

Figure 10-11 Talipes.

tendonitis (těn-dĭn-Ī-tĭs): inflammation of a tendon usually caused by injury or overuse; also called *tendinitis.*

torticollis (tōr-tĭ-KŎL-ĭs): spasmodic contraction of the neck muscles causing stiffness and twisting of the neck that may be congenital or acquired; also called *wryneck.*

Diagnostic

arthrocentesis (ăr-thrō-sĕn-TĒ-sĭs): puncture of a joint space with a needle to remove fluid.

Arthrocentesis is performed to obtain samples of synovial fluid for diagnostic purposes. It also may be used to instill medications and to remove accumulated fluid from joints simply to relieve pain.

rheumatoid factor (ROO-mă-toyd): blood test to detect the presence of rheumatoid factor, a substance presence in patients with rheumatoid arthritis.

Therapeutic

arthroplasty (ĂR-thrō-plăs-tē): surgical reconstruction or replacement of a painful, degenerated joint to restore mobility in rheumatoid or osteoarthritis or to correct a congenital deformity.

arthroscopy (ăr-THRŎS-kō-pē): visual examination of the interior of a joint performed by inserting an endoscope through a small incision.

Arthroscopy is performed to repair and remove joint tissue, especially of the knee, ankle, and shoulder.

sequestrectomy (sē-kwěs-TRĚK-tō-mē): excision of a necrosed piece of bone *(sequestrum).*

total hip arthroplasty (ĂR-thrō-plăs-tē): replacement of the femur and acetabulum with metal components. The acetabulum is plastic coated to avoid metal-to-metal articulating surfaces (see Figure 10–12).

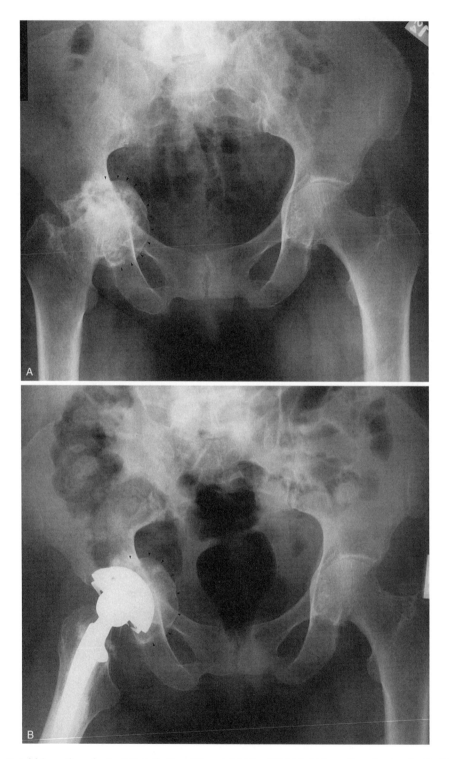

Figure 10-12   Total hip arthroplasty. (A) Arthritis of the right hip. (B) Total hip arthroplasty of arthritic hip. From McKinnis, LN: Fundamentals of Orthopedic Radiology, page 133. FA Davis, 1997, with permission.

Listen and Learn, the audio CD-ROM that accompanies this book, will help you master the pronunciation of selected medical words. Use it to practice pronunciations of the above-listed medical terms and for instructions to complete the *Listen and Learn* exercise on the CD-ROM for this section.

PATHOLOGICAL, DIAGNOSTIC, AND THERAPEUTIC TERMS REVIEW

Match the medical term(s) below with the definitions in the numbered list.

ankylosis   crepitation   lordosis   rheumatoid arthritis   sprain
arthroplasty   Ewing sarcoma   muscular dystrophy   rheumatoid factor   strain
arthroscopy   gout   myasthenia gravis   scoliosis   talipes
carpal tunnel syndrome herniated disk osteoporosis   sequestrectomy   tendonitis
contracture   kyphosis   Paget disease   sequestrum   torticollis

1. _____ means decrease in bone density and an increase in porosity, causing the risk of fractures.

2. _____ means inflammation of a tendon.

3. _____ refers to trauma to a joint, causing injury to the surrounding ligament.

4. _____ refers to trauma to a muscle that results from overuse or excessive, forcible stretch.

5. _____ means hunchback or humpback.

6. _____ is a malignant tumor that develops from bone marrow, usually in long bones or the pelvis; occurs most frequently in adolescent boys.

7. _____ means wryneck.

8. _____ is a disease characterized by excessive uric acid in the blood and around the joints.

9. _____ is a disease characterized by inflammatory changes in joints and related structures that result in crippling deformities.

10. _____ is a skeletal disease of the elderly with chronic inflammation of bones, resulting in thickening and softening of bones and bowing of long bones; osteitis deformans.

11. _____ is a fragment of necrosed bone that has become separated from surrounding tissue.

12. _____ means replacement of a joint.

13. _____ is a grating sound made by the ends of bone rubbing together.

14. _____ is a neuromuscular disorder characterized by muscular weakness and progressive fatigue.

15. _____ means forward curvature of the lumbar spine; swayback.

16. _____ refers to a group of hereditary diseases characterized by gradual atrophy and weakness of muscle; the most common form is called *Duchenne*.

449

17. _____ is connective tissue fibrosis that prevents normal mobility of the related tissue or joint.

18. _____ means immobility of a joint.

19. _____ refers to rupture of the nucleus pulposus between two vertebrae.

20. _____ is pain or numbness resulting from compression of the median nerve within the carpal tunnel.

21. _____ is excision of a necrosed piece of bone.

22. _____ is a blood test to detect a substance present in the blood of patients with rheumatoid arthritis.

23. _____ is a congenital foot deformity; clubfoot.

24. _____ means visual examination of a joint.

25. _____ is abnormal sideward curvature of the spine, either to the left or to the right

Competency Verification: Check your answers in Appendix B, Answer Key, page 533. If you are not satisfied with your level or comprehension, review the pathological, diagnostic, and therapeutic terms and retake the review.

Correct Answers: _____ × 4 _____% Score

Medical Record Activities

The following medical records reflect common real-life clinical scenarios using medical terminology to document patient care. The physician who specializes in the treatment of musculoskeletal disorders is an *orthopedic surgeon;* the medical specialty concerned in the diagnoses and treatment of musculoskeletal disorders is called *orthopedics.* Complete the medical record activities in the following sections.

✓ MEDICAL RECORD ACTIVITY 10–1. Degenerative, Intervertebral Disk Disease

Terminology

The terms listed in the chart come from the medical record *Degenerative, Intervertebral Disk Disease* that follows. Use a medical dictionary such as *Taber's Cyclopedic Medical Dictionary,* the appendices of this book, or other resources to define each term. Then practice reading the pronunciations aloud for each term.

Term	Definition
anteroposterior ăn-tĕr-ō-PŌ-stĭr-ē-or	
bilateral bī-LĂT-ĕr-ăl	
degenerative dĕ-JĔN-ĕr-ă-tĭv	
hypertrophic hī-pĕr-TRŌF-ĭk	
intervertebral ĭn-tĕr-VĔRT-ĕ-brĕl	
L5	
laminectomies lăm-ĭ-NĔK-tĕ-mēz	
lateral views LĂT-ĕr-ăl	
lumbar LŬM-băr	
lumbosacral lŭm-bō-SĀ-krĕl	
S1	
sacroiliac sā-krō-ĬL-ē-ăk	
sacrum SĀ-krŭm	

 Listen and Learn Online! will help you master the pronunciation of selected medical words from this medical record activity. Visit www.fadavis.com/gylys/simplified for instructions in completing the *Listen and Learn Online!* exercise for this section and then to practice pronunciations.

DEGENERATIVE, INTERVERTEBRAL DISK DISEASE

Reading

Practice pronunciation of medical terms by reading the following medical report aloud.

Anteroposterior and lateral views of the lumbar spine and an AP view of the sacrum show a placement of L5 on S1. The L5 to S1 intervertebral disk space contains a slight shadow of decreased density. There is now slight narrowing of the L3 to L4 and L4 to L5 spaces. Bilateral laminectomies appear to have been done at L5 to S1. Slight hypertrophic lipping of the upper lumbar vertebral bodies is now seen, as is slight lipping of the upper margin of the body of L4. The sacroiliac joint spaces are well preserved. Lateral views of the lumbosacral spine taken with the spine in flexion and extension show slight motion at all of the lumbar and lumbosacral levels.

IMPRESSION: 1. Degenerative, intervertebral disk disease at L5 to S1, now also accompanied by slight narrowing of the L3 to L4 and L4 to L5 disk spaces.
2. Slight motion at all of the lumbar and lumbosacral levels.

Evaluation

Review the medical record to answer the following questions.

1. Why does the x-ray show a decreased density at L5 to S1?

_____

_____

2. What is the most common cause of degenerative intervertebral disk disease?

_____

_____

3. What happens to the gelatinous material of the disk as aging occurs?

_____

_____

4. What is the probable cause of the narrowing of the L3 to L4 and L4 to L5 spaces?

_____

_____

✓ MEDICAL RECORD ACTIVITY 10–2. Rotator Cuff Tear, Right Shoulder

Terminology

The terms listed in the chart come from the medical record *Rotator Cuff Tear, Right Shoulder* that follows. Use a medical dictionary such as *Taber's Cyclopedic Medical Dictionary*, the appendices, or other resources to define each term. Then practice reading the pronunciations aloud for each term.

Term	Definition
AC joint	
acromial ăk-RŌ-mē-ăl	
acromioclavicular ă-krō-mē-ō-klă-VĬK-ū-lăr	
arthritis ăr-THRĪ-tĭs	
arthroscopy ăr-THRŎS-kō-pē	
biceps BĪ-sĕps	
bursectomy bŭr-SĔK-tō-mē	
calcification kăl-sĭ-fĭ-KĀ-shŭn	
degenerative dĕ-JĔN-ĕr-ă-tĭv	
glenohumeral glē-nō-HŪ-mĕr-ăl	
glenoid GLĒ-noyd	
gouty GOW-tē	
intra-articular ĭn-tră-ăr-TĬK-ū-lăr	
labra (singular, labrum) LĂ-bră	
osteoarthritis ŏs-tē-ō-ăr-THRĪ-tĭs	

(Continued)

Term	Definition *(Continued)*
osteophyte ŎS-tē-ō-fīt	
spur SPŬR	
subacromial sŭb-ă-KRŌ-mē-ăl	
tendonitis tĕn-dĭn-Ī-tĭs	
tuberosity tū-bĕr-ŎS-ĭ-tē	

Listen and Learn Online! will help you master the pronunciation of selected medical words from this medical record activity. Visit www.fadavis.com/gylys/simplified for instructions in completing the *Listen and Learn Online!* exercise for this section and then to practice pronunciations.

ROTATOR CUFF TEAR, RIGHT SHOULDER

Reading

Practice pronunciation of medical terms by reading the following medical report aloud.

PREOPERATIVE AND POSTOPERATIVE DIAGNOSIS: Rotator cuff tear, right shoulder. Degenerative arthritis, right acromioclavicular joint. Calcific tendinitis at the level of the superior glenoid tuberosity, right shoulder. Early degenerative osteoarthritis of the right shoulder. History of gouty arthritis.

OPERATION: Open repair of rotator cuff, open incision outer end of clavicle, anterior acromioplasty, glenohumeral and subacromial arthroscopy with arthroscopic bursectomy.

FINDINGS: A glenohumeral arthroscopy revealed the superior, anterior, inferior, and posterior glenoid labra were intact. There was some fraying of the anterior glenoid labrum. The long head of the biceps was intact. We were unable to visualize any intra-articular calcification. We observed the takeoff of the long head of the biceps from the posterior superior edge of the glenoid labrum and the glenoid tuberosity. There was an osteophyte inferiorly on the humeral head. There was a deep surface tear of the rotator cuff at the posterior superior corner of the greater tuberosity of the humerus at the infraspinatus insertion. There was an extremely dense subacromial bursal scar. There was prominence of the inferior edge of the AC joint, with inferior AC joint and anterior acromial spurs.

Evaluation

Review the medical record to answer the following questions.

1. What type of arthritis did the patient have?

_____

_____

2. Did the patient have calcium deposits in the right shoulder?

_____

_____

3. What type of instrument did the physician use to visualize the glenoid labra?

_____

_____

4. What are labra?

_____

_____

5. Did the patient have any outgrowths of bone? If so, where?

_____

_____

6. Did they find any deposits of calcium salts within the shoulder joint?

_____

_____

Chapter Review

Word Elements Summary

The following table summarizes combining forms, suffixes, and prefixes related to the musculoskeletal system.

Word Element	Meaning
COMBINING FORMS	
arthr/o	joint
calc/o	calcium
calcane/o	calcaneum (heel bone)
carp/o	carpus (wrist bones)
cephal/o	head
cervic/o	neck; cervix uteri (neck of uterus)
chondr/o	cartilage
cost/o	ribs
crani/o	cranium (skull)
encephal/o	brain
femor/o	femur (thigh bone)
fibul/o	fibula (smaller, outer bone of lower leg)
humer/o	humerus (upper arm bone)
lumb/o	loin (lower back)
metacarp/o	metacarpus (hand bones)
myel/o	bone marrow; spinal cord
my/o	muscle
oste/o	bone
patell/o	patella (kneecap)
sacr/o	sacrum
spin/o	spine
spondyl/o, vertebr/o	vertebrae (backbone)
stern/o	sternum (breastbone)
tend/o	tendon
tibi/o	tibia (larger inner bone of lower leg)

Word Element	Meaning
OTHER COMBINING FORMS	
cyt/o	cell
cyst/o	bladder
dist/o	far, farthest
enter/o	intestine (usually small intestine)
hepat/o	liver
proxim/o	near
radi/o	radiation, x-ray; radius (lower arm bone on thumb side)
roentgen/o	x-rays
scler/o	hardening; sclera (white of eye)
SUFFIXES	
SURGICAL	
-centesis	surgical puncture
-ectomy	excision, removal
-plasty	surgical repair
-rrhaphy	suture
-tomy	incision
DIAGNOSTIC, SYMPTOMATIC, AND RELATED	
-algia, -dynia	pain
-cele	hernia, swelling
-cyte	cell
-emia	blood condition
-genesis	forming, producing, origin
-gram	record, writing
-graphy	process of recording
-ist	specialist
-itis	inflammation
-logist	specialist in study of
-malacia	softening
-meter	instrument for measuring
-oma	tumor

(Continued)

Word Element	Meaning *(Continued)*
-osis	abnormal condition
-pathy	disease
-plegia	paralysis
-rrhexis	rupture
REFIXES	
en-	in, within
hemi-	one half
hypo-	under, below, deficient
inter-	between
peri-	around
quadri-	four

WORD ELEMENTS REVIEW

After you review the word elements summary, complete this activity by writing the meaning of each element in the space provided.

Word Element	Meaning
COMBINING FORMS	
1. arthr/o	
2. calc/o	
3. calcane/o	
4. carp/o	
5. cephal/o	
6. cervic/o	
7. chondr/o	
8. cost/o	
9. crani/o	
10. encephal/o	
11. femor/o	
12. fibul/o	
13. humer/o	
14. lumb/o	
15. metacarp/o	
16. myel/o	
17. my/o	
18. oste/o	
19. patell/o	
20. sacr/o	
21. spin/o	
22. spondyl/o	
23. vertebr/o	
24. stern/o	
25. tend/o	
26. tibi/o	

(Continued)

459

Word Element	Meaning *(Continued)*
OTHER COMBINING FORMS	
27. proxim/o	
28. radi/o	
SUFFIXES	
SURGICAL	
29. -centesis	
30. -ectomy	
31. -plasty	
DIAGNOSTIC, SYMPTOMATIC, AND RELATED	
32. -cyte	
33. -genesis	
34. -gram	
35. -graphy	
36. -ist	
37. -itis	
38. -logist	
39. -malacia	
40. -meter	
41. -oma	
42. -osis	
43. -pathy	
44. -plegia	
PREFIXES	
45. en-	
46. hemi-	
47. hypo-	
48. inter-	
49. peri-	
50. quadri-	

Competency Verification: Check your answers in Appendix A, Glossary of Medical Word Elements, page 497 If you are not satisfied with your level of comprehension, review the word elements and retake the review.

Correct Answers: _____ × 2 _____% Score

Chapter 10 Vocabulary Review

Match these medical word(s) below with the definitions in the numbered list.

AP	bone marrow	distal	proximal
arthrocentesis	cephalometer	intervertebral	quadriplegia
articulation	cervical vertebrae	myelogram	radiologist
atlas	closed fracture	myorrhexis	radiology
bilateral	diaphysis	open fracture	spondylomalacia

1. _____ is the study of x-rays and radioactive substances used for diagnosing and treating diseases.

2. _____ means shaft or main part of the bone.

3. _____ means passing from the front to the rear.

4. _____ is a fracture in which the bone is broken, but there is no external wound; surrounding tissue damage is minimal.

5. _____ means pertaining to or affecting two sides.

6. _____ means near the point of attachment to the trunk.

7. _____ is the place of union between two or more bones; a joint.

8. _____ is a fracture in which the broken end of a bone has moved so that it pierces the skin; possible extensive damage to surrounding blood vessels, nerves, and muscles.

9. _____ is the first cervical vertebra, which supports the skull.

10. _____ is a surgical puncture of a joint to remove fluid.

11. _____ is soft tissue that fills the medullary cavities of long bones.

12. _____ is an instrument used to measure the head.

13. _____ refers to a radiograph of the spinal canal after injection of a contrast medium.

14. _____ means rupture of a muscle.

15. _____ means softening of vertebrae.

16. _____ is a directional term that means farthest from the point of attachment to the trunk.

17. _____ is a physician who specializes in the use of x-rays for diagnosis and the treatment of disease.

18. _____ are bones that form the skeletal framework of the neck.

19. _____ is situated between two adjacent vertebrae.

20. _____ means paralysis of all four extremities.

Competency Verification: Check your answers in Appendix B, Answer Key, page 534. If you are not satisfied with your level of comprehension, review the chapter vocabulary and retake the review.

Correct Answers: _____ × 5 _____% Score

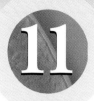

Special Senses:
The Eyes and Ears

OBJECTIVES

Upon completion of this chapter, you will be able to:

- Describe the sensory organs of seeing and hearing and explain their primary functions.
- Identify the major structures of the eyes and ears.
- Describe pathological, diagnostic, therapeutic, and other terms related to the sensory organs of seeing and hearing.
- Recognize, define, pronounce, and spell terms correctly by completing the audio CD-ROM exercises.
- Demonstrate your knowledge of this chapter by successfully completing the frames, reviews, and medical report evaluations.

The major senses of the body are sight, hearing, smell, taste, touch, and balance. These sensations are identified with specific body organs. The senses of smell and taste were discussed in previous chapters; the senses of sight, hearing, and balance are discussed in this chapter. Other senses of the body not attributed to any specific organ include hunger, thirst, pain, and temperature. This chapter provides information about the eyes and ears.

Eye

The eyes and their accessory structures are the receptor organs that provide vision. As one of the most important sense organs of the body, the eyes provide us not only with most of the information about what we see, but also of what we learn from printed material. Similar to other sensory organs, the eyes are constructed to detect stimuli in the environment and to transmit those observations to the brain for visual interpretation.

Word Elements

This section introduces combining forms related to the eye. Included are key suffixes; prefixes are defined in the right-hand column as needed. Review the following table, and pronounce each word in the word analysis column aloud before you begin to work the frames.

Word Element	Meaning	Word Analysis
COMBINING FORMS		
blephar/o	eyelid	blephar/o/spasm (BLĔF-ă-rō-spăzm): involuntary contraction of eyelid muscles *-spasm:* involuntary contraction, twitching *Blepharospasm may be due to eye strain or nervous irritability.*
choroid/o	choroid	choroid/o/pathy (kō-roy-DŎP-ă-thē): noninflammatory degeneration of the choroid *-pathy:* disease *The choroid is a thin, highly vascular layer of the eye between the retina and sclera.*
corne/o	cornea	corne/itis (kōr-nē-Ī-tĭs): inflammation of the cornea; also called keratitis *-itis:* inflammation
cor/o	pupil	aniso/cor/ia (ăn-ī-sō-KŌ-rē-ă): inequality of the size of the pupils *aniso-:* unequal, dissimilar *-ia:* condition *Anisocoria may be congenital or associated with a neurological injury or disease.*
core/o		core/o/meter (kō-rē-ŎM-ĕ-tĕr): instrument for measuring the pupil *-meter:* instrument for measuring
dacry/o	tear; lacrimal apparatus (duct, sac, or gland)	dacry/o/rrhea (dăk-rē-ō-RĒ-ă): excessive secretion of tears *-rrhea:* discharge, flow
lacrim/o		lacrim/ation (lăk-rĭ-MĀ-shūn): secretion and discharge of tears *-ation:* process (of)
dipl/o	double	dipl/opia (dĭp-LŌ-pē-ă): two images of an object seen at the same time *-opia:* vision
irid/o	iris	irid/o/plegia (ĭr-ĭd-ō-PLĒ-jē-ă): paralysis of the sphincter of the iris *-plegia:* paralysis
kerat/o	horny tissue; hard; cornea	kerat/o/plasty (KĔR-ă-tō-plăs-tē): replacement of a cloudy cornea with a transparent one, typically derived from an organ donor; corneal grafting *-plasty:* surgical repair

Word Element	Meaning	Word Analysis
ocul/o	eye	intra/ocul/ar (ĭn-tră-ŎK-ū-lăr): within the eyeball *intra-:* in, within *-ar:* pertaining to, relating to
ophthalm/o		ophthalm/o/scope (ŏf-THĂL-mō-skōp): instrument used for examining the interior of the eye especially the retina *-scope:* instrument for examining
opt/o	eye, vision	opt/ic (ŎP-tĭk): pertaining to the eye or to sight *-ic:* pertaining to, relating to
retin/o	retina	retin/o/pathy (rĕt-ĭn-ŎP-ă-thē): any disease of the retina *-pathy:* disease
scler/o	hardening; sclera (white of eye)	scler/itis (sklĕ-RĪ-tĭs): superficial and deep inflammation of the sclera *-itis:* inflammation
SUFFIXES		
-opia	vision	ambly/opia (ăm-blē-Ō-pē-ă): reduction or dimness of vision with no apparent pathological condition *ambly:* dull, dim
-opsia		heter/opsia (hĕt-ĕr-ŎP-sē-ă): inequality of vision in the two eyes *heter-:* different
-ptosis	prolapse, downward displacement	blephar/o/ptosis (blĕf-ă-rō-TŌ-sĭs): drooping of the upper eyelid *blephar/o:* eyelid

 Listen and Learn, the audio CD-ROM that accompanies this book, will help you master the pronunciation of selected medical words. Use it to practice pronunciations of the above-listed medical terms and for instructions to complete the *Listen and Learn* exercise on the CD-ROM for this section.

For the following medical terms, first write the suffix and its meaning. Then translate the meaning of the remaining elements starting with the first part of the word. The first word is an example that is completed for you.

Term	Meaning
1. aniso/cor/ia	-ia: condition; unequal, dissimilar; pupil
2. blephar/o/ptosis	_____
3. ambly/opia	_____
4. retin/o/pathy	_____
5. scler/itis	_____
6. ophthalm/o/scope	_____
7. intra/ocul/ar	_____
8. dacry/o/rrhea	_____
9. dipl/opia	_____
10. blephar/o/spasm	_____

Competency Verification: Check your answers in Appendix B, Answer Key, page 535. If you are not satisfied with your level of comprehension, review the vocabulary and retake the review.

Correct Answers _____ × 10 = _____ % Score

11-1   The eye is a globe-shaped, hollow structure set within a bony cavity. The bony cavity, or orbit, houses the eyeball and associated structures, such as the eye muscles, nerves, and blood vessels. Most of the eyeball is protected from trauma by the orbit's bony cavity. The wall of the eyeball is composed of three layers: the (1) **sclera**, the white outer layer of the eyeball, is composed of fibrous connective tissue. On the most anterior portion of the eye, the sclera forms a transparent, domed structure called the (2) **cornea.** The cornea also protects the front part of the eye from injury and is the first part of the eye that refracts light rays. In addition, the cornea is avascular (without blood vessels or capillaries), but is well supplied with nerve endings, most of which are pain fibers. For this reason, some people can never adjust to wearing contact lenses. Label the structures in Figure 11–1 as you observe the location and layers of the eyeball.

466

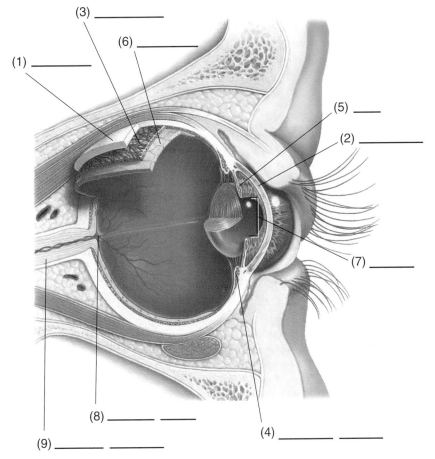

(3) _____

(6) _____

(1) _____

(5) ____

(2) _____

(7) _____

(8) _____ _____

(4) _____ _____

(9) _____ _____

Figure 11-1   Eye structures.

11-2   The (3) **choroid** layer lies below the sclera. It contains blood vessels and a dark pigmented tissue that prevents glare within the eyeball by absorbing light. The anterior portion of the choroid is modified and forms the (4) **ciliary body** (or muscle) and the (5) **iris**, the colored portion of the eye. The (6) **retina** lines the posterior two thirds portion of the eyeball and contains rods and cones, the sensory receptors for vision. Rods perceive only the presence of light, whereas cones perceive the different wavelengths of light as colors. The primary function of the retina is image formation. Continue to label the structures in Figure 11–1 as you observe the location and layers of the eyeball.

11-3   The combining form **scler/o** refers to *hardening; sclera (white of eye);* **choroid/o** refers to the *choroid;* and **retin/o** refers to the *retina.* Use these combining forms to build medical terms that mean inflammation of the

scler/itis
sklĕ-RĪ-tĭs

sclera: _____ / _____.

choroid/itis
kō-royd-Ī-tĭs

choroid: _____ / _____.

retin/itis
rĕt-ĭ-NĪ-tĭs

retina: _____ / _____.

choroid/o/pathy
kō-roy-DŎP-ă-thē
retin/o/pathy
rĕt-ĭn-ŎP-ă-thē

11-4 Practice building medical words that mean disease of the

choroid: _____ / ____ / _____.

retina: _____ / ____ / _____.

---

kerat/o/rrhexis
kĕr-ă-tō-RĔK-sĭs
irid/o/cele
ĭ-RĬD-ō-sēl

11-5 The combining form **kerat/o** refers to *horny tissue; hard; cornea.* The combining form **irid/o** refers to the *iris.* Use these combining forms to build medical terms that mean

rupture of the cornea:

_____ / ____ / _____.

herniation of the iris: _____ / ____ / _____.

---

kerat/o

11-6 Kerat/itis, a vision-threatening infection, can occur if contact lenses are not cleaned and disinfected properly.

From kerat/itis, construct the combining form for cornea.

_____ / ____.

---

scler/itis
sklĕ-RĪ-tĭs

scler/o/malacia
sklĕ-rō-mă-LĀ-shē-ă

11-7 Form medical words meaning

inflammation of the sclera: _____ / _____.

softening of the sclera:

_____ / ____ / _____.

---

cornea
KŌR-nē-ă

11-8 A kerat/o/tome is an instrument for incising the

_____.

---

kerat/o/tomy
kĕr-ă-TŎT-ō-mē

11-9 In some cases, laser kerat/o/tomy is being used to correct vision, eliminating the need for contact lenses or glasses. Shallow, bloodless, hairline, radial incisions are made using a laser in the outer portion of the cornea, where they will not interfere with vision. This allows the cornea to flatten and helps to correct nearsightedness.

About two thirds of patients are able to eliminate the use of glasses or contact lenses by undergoing the surgical procedure called laser

_____ / ____ / _____.

11-10 The opening in the center of the iris is called the (7) **pupil.** The amount of light entering the eye is controlled by contractions and dilations of the pupil. Constriction of the pupil permits a sharper near vision. It is also a reflex that protects the retina from intense light. Label the pupil in Figure 11–1.

11-11   The sensory receptors of vision, the rods and cones, contain light-sensitive molecules *(photopigments)* that convert light energy into electrical impulses. Impulses generated by the rods and cones are transmitted by retinal nerve fibers to areas of the brain that are responsible for processing visual information. The retinal nerve fibers unite at the (8) **optic disk** and cut across through the wall of the eyeball as the (9) **optic nerve.** Because the optic disk has no rods or cones, it is known as the *blind spot.* Label the structures in Figure 11–1 as you learn about the location and role these structures play in providing vision.

Competency Verification: Check your labeling of Figure 11–1 with Appendix B, Answer Key, page 535.

ŏf-THĂL-mō	**11-12** Words with **ophthalm/o** *(eye)* may be difficult to pronounce when you first encounter them. To avoid confusion, write the pronunciation ŏf-**THĂL-mō** and practice saying it aloud: _____.
instrument	**11-13** An ophthalm/o/scope is an _____ for examining the interior of the eye.
ophthalm/o/scopy ŏf-thăl-MŎS-kō-pē	**11-14** The word meaning visual examination of the eye is _____ / ____ / _____.
ophthalm/algia ŏf-thăl-MĂL-jē-ă	**11-15** High blood pressure may cause ophthalm/o/dynia or _____ / _____.
eye(s)	**11-16** An ophthalm/o/logist is a physician who specializes in disorders and treatment of the _____.
ophthalm/ectomy ŏf-thăl-MĔK-tō-mē ophthalm/o/malacia ŏf-thăl-mō-mă-LĀ-shē-ă ophthalm/o/plegia ŏf-thăl-mō-PLĒ-jē-ă	**11-17** Use **ophthalm/o** to build words meaning surgical excision of the eye: _____ / _____. softening of the eye: _____ / ____ / _____. paralysis of the eye: _____ / ____ / _____.
ophthalm/o/plegia ŏf-thăl-mō-PLĒ-jē-ă	**11-18** A stroke can prevent eye movement and cause paralysis of the eye muscles. A person with paralysis of the eye (muscles) has a condition called _____ / ____ / _____.
eyelid(s)	**11-19** A twitching eyelid may result from a neurological disorder. Another disorder, blephar/edema, is a swelling and baggy appearance of the _____.

blephar/o/plasty
BLĔF-ă-rō-plăs-tē

11-20 Blephar/o/plasty, also called an eye tuck, is a surgical procedure to remove wrinkles from the eyelids for medical or cosmetic reasons.

Surgical repair of the eyelid(s) is known as

_____ / ____ / _____ .

---

blephar/o/plasty
BLĔF-ă-rō-plăs-tē

11-21 When a person has an eye tuck, small portions of the eyelids are removed to tighten the skin, removing wrinkles.

The surgical procedure for an eye tuck is called

_____ / ____ / _____ .

---

blephar/ectomy
blĕf-ă-RĔK-tō-mē
blephar/o/tomy
blĕf-ă-RŎT-ō-mē

blephar/o/spasm
BLĔF-ă-rō-spăzm

blephar/o/plegia
blĕf-ă-rō-PLĒ-jē-ă

11-22 Form medical words meaning

excision of part or all of the eyelid:

_____ / _____ .

surgical incision of the eyelid: _____ / ____ / _____ .

twitching or spasm of the eyelid:

_____ / ____ / _____ .

paralysis of an eyelid:

_____ / ____ / _____ .

---

red

yellow

11-23 The suffix -opia is used in words to mean *vision*.

Erythr/opia is a condition in which objects that are not red appear to be

_____ .

Xanth/opia is a condition in which objects that are not yellow appear to be

_____ .

---

dipl/opia
dĭp-LŌ-pē-ă

11-24 The elements dipl- and **dipl/o** mean *double*. Dipl/opia occurs when both eyes are used but are not in focus.

A person with double vision has a condition called

_____ / _____ .

---

dipl/opia
dĭp-LŌ-pē-ă

11-25 Dipl/opia can occur with brain tumors, strokes, head trauma, and migraine headaches.

Write the word in this frame that means double vision:

_____ / _____ .

hyper- **-opia** **my/o**	**11-26** Two common vision defects are my/opia (nearsightedness) and hyper/opia (farsightedness). See Figure 11–2 to compare a normal eye (emmetropia) with my/opia and hyper/opia. Write the element in this frame that means excessive, above normal: _____. vision: _____. muscle: _____ / ____.
nearsightedness	**11-27** Hyper/opia is farsightedness; my/opia is _____.
hyper/opia hī-pĕr-Ō-pē-ă	**11-28** The opposite of my/opia is _____ / _____.
my/opia mī-Ō-pē-ă	**11-29** If the eyeball is too long, the image falls in front of the retina (see Figure 11–2). This condition is called nearsightedness, or _____ / _____.
hyper/opia hī-pĕr-Ō-pē-ă	**11-30** If the eyeball is too short, the image falls behind the retina (see Figure 11–2). This condition is called farsightedness, or _____ / _____.
blephar/o/plasty BLĔF-ă-rō-plăs-tē **blephar/o/spasm** BLĔF-ă-rō-spăzm **blephar/o/ptosis** blĕf-ă-rō-TŌ-sĭs	**11-31** Eyelids shade the eyes during sleep, protect them from excessive light and foreign objects, and spread lubricating secretions over the eyeballs. Use **blephar/o** (*eyelid*) to construct medical words meaning surgical repair of the eyelid: _____ / ____ / _____. twitching of an eyelid: _____ / ____ / _____. prolapse of an eyelid: _____ / ____ / _____.
blephar/o **-ptosis**	**11-32** Blephar/o/ptosis is often seen after a stroke because the muscles leading to the eyelids become paralyzed. Denote the elements in this frame that mean eyelid: _____ / ____. prolapse, downward displacement: _____.
	11-33 The (1) **lacrimal gland** is located above the outer corner of each eye. These glands produce tears, which keep the eyeballs moist. The (2) **nasolacrimal duct** collects and drains tears into the (3) **lacrimal sac**. Label the lacrimal structures in Figure 11–3.

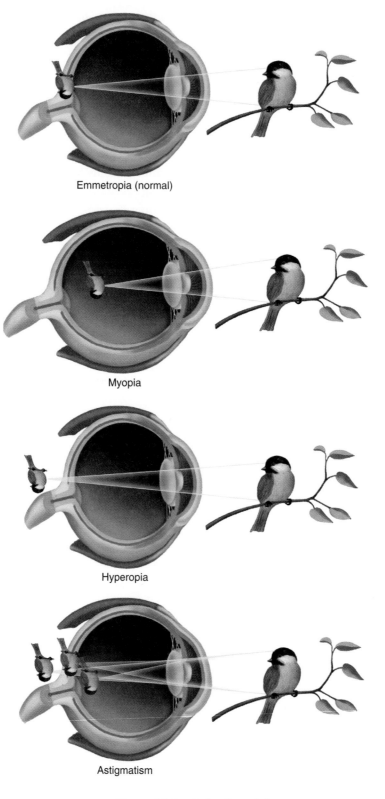

Emmetropia (normal)

Myopia

Hyperopia

Astigmatism

Figure 11-2 Refraction of the eye.

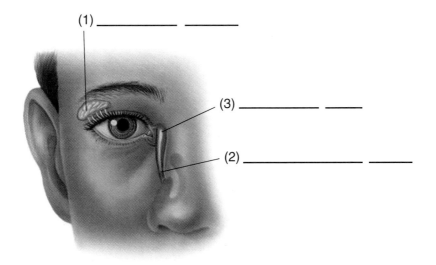

(1) _____ _____

(3) _____ _____

(2) _____ _____

Figure 11-3 Lacrimal apparatus.

tears	**11-34** The combining form **dacry/o** is used in words to mean *tear; lacrimal sac.* Dacry/o/rrhea is an excessive flow of _____.
pain	**11-35** Dacry/aden/algia is a _____ in a tear gland.
tear gland	**11-36** Dacry/aden/itis is an inflammation of a _____ _____.

Competency Verification: Check your labeling of Figure 11–3 with the answers in Appendix B, Answer Key, page 535.

Listen and Learn, the audio CD-ROM that accompanies this book, will help you master the pronunciation of selected medical words. Use it to practice pronunciations of *selected terms from frames 11–1 to 11–36* and from the word elements table. Listen for instructions to complete the *Listen and Learn* exercise on the CD-ROM for this section.

Ear

The ears and their accessory structures are the receptor organs that enable us to hear and to maintain our balance. Each ear consists of three divisions—the external ear, the middle ear, and the inner ear. The external and middle ear conduct sound waves through the ear; the inner ear contains auditory structures that receive the sound waves and transmits them to the brain for interpretation. The inner ear also contains specialized receptors that maintain balance and equilibrium regardless of changes in body position or motion.

Word Elements

This section introduces combining forms related to the ear. Included are key suffixes; prefixes are defined in the right-hand column as needed. Review the following table and pronounce each word in the word analysis column aloud before you begin to work the frames.

Word Element	Meaning	Word Analysis
COMBINING FORMS		
acous/o	hearing	acous/tic (ă-KOOS-tik): pertaining to sound or the sense of hearing *-tic:* pertaining to, relating to
audi/o		audi/o/meter (aw-dē-ŎM-ĕ-tĕr): an instrument for testing hearing *-meter:* instrument for measuring
myring/o	tympanic membrane (eardrum)	myring/o/tomy (mĭr-ĭn-GŎT-ō-mē): incision of the tympanic membrane *-tomy:* incision
tympan/o		tympan/o/plasty (tĭm-păn-ō-PLĂS-tē): surgical repair of the tympanic membrane *Any one of several surgical procedures designed either to cure a chronic inflammatory process in the middle ear or to restore function to the sound-transmitting mechanism of the middle ear.* *-plasty:* surgical repair
ot/o	ear	ot/o/rrhea (ō-tō-RĒ-ă): inflammation of the ear with purulent discharge *-rrhea:* discharge, flow

salping/o	tube (usually fallopian or eustachian [auditory] tubes)	salping/o/pharyng/eal (săl-pĭng-gō-fă-RĬN-jē-ăl): concerning the eustachian tube and the pharynx
		   pharyng: pharynx (throat)
		   -eal: pertaining to, relating to

SUFFIXES		
-acusis	hearing	an/acusis (ăn-ă-KŪ-sĭs): total deafness *an-:* without, not
-tropia	turning	hyper/tropia (hī-pĕr-TRŌ-pē-ă): an ocular deviation with one eye located higher than the other *hyper-:* excessive, above normal

Listen and Learn, the audio CD-ROM that accompanies this book, will help you master the pronunciation of selected medical words. Use it to practice pronunciations of the above-listed medical terms and for instructions to complete the *Listen and Learn* exercise on the CD-ROM for this section.

SECTION REVIEW 11-2

For the following medical terms, first write the suffix and its meaning. Then translate the meaning of the remaining elements starting with the first part of the word. The first word is an example that is completed for you.

Term	Meaning
1. tympan/o/centesis	-centesis: surgical puncture; tympanic membrane (eardrum)
2. acous/tic	_____
3. hyper/tropia	_____
4. ot/o/rrhea	_____
5. an/acusis	_____
6. myring/o/tomy	_____
7. tympan/o/plasty	_____
8. audi/o/meter	_____
9. ot/o/scope	_____
10. salping/o/pharyng/eal	_____

Competency Verification: Check your answers in Appendix B, Answer Key, page 536. If you are not satisfied with your level of comprehension, review the vocabulary and retake the review.

Correct Answers _____ × 10 = _____ % Score

Making a set of flash cards from key word elements in this chapter for each section review can help you remember the elements. Make a flash card by writing a word element on one side of a 3 × 5 or 4 × 6 index card. On the other side, write the meaning of the element. Do this for all word elements in the section reviews. Use your flash cards to review each section. You also might use the flash cards to prepare for the chapter review at the end of this chapter.

11-37 The ear can be divided into three anatomical sections—external, middle, and inner. The external ear includes the (1) **auricle,** which directs sound waves to the (2) **ear canal**. Eventually the sound waves hit the (3) **tympanic membrane** (eardrum) and make the eardrum vibrate. The transmission of sound waves ultimately generates impulses that are transmitted to and interpreted by the brain as sound. Label Figure 11–4 as you learn about the ear.

11-38 Swimmer's ear, resulting from infection transmitted in the water of a swimming pool, may cause severe ot/o/dynia or

_____ / _____ .

ot/algia
ō-TĂL-jē-ă

eardrum	**11-39** The combining forms **tympan/o** and **myring/o** refer to the *tympanic membrane (eardrum)*. Tympan/itis is an inflammation of the tympanic membrane (_____).
tympan/o, myring/o	**11-40** The tympan/ic membrane is stretched across the end of the ear canal and vibrates when sound waves strike it. The combining forms for the tympanic membrane (eardrum) are _____ / _____ and _____ / _____.
	11-41 The vibrations of the tympanic membrane are transmitted to the three auditory bones in the middle ear: the (4) **malleus**, the (5) **incus**, and the (6) **stapes**. The (7) **eustachian (auditory) tube** leads from the middle ear to the nasopharynx and permits air to enter or leave the middle ear cavity. Label and review the position of the middle ear structures in Figure 11-4.
salping/itis săl-pĭn-JĪ-tĭs	**11-42** The combining form **salping/o** means *tube (usually fallopian or eustachian [auditory] tubes)*. An inflammation of the eustachian tube would be diagnosed as _____ / _____.
salping/o/scope săl-PĬNG-gō-skōp **salping/o/scopy** săl-pĭng-GŎS-kō-pē **salping/o/stenosis** săl-pĭng-gō-stĕn-NŌ-sĭs	**11-43** The eustachian tube equalizes the air pressure in the middle ear with that of the outside atmosphere. Air pressure must be equalized for the eardrum to vibrate properly. Build medical words meaning instrument for examining the eustachian tube: _____ / _____ / _____. visual examination of the eustachian tube: _____ / _____ / _____. narrowing or stricture of the eustachian tube: _____ / _____ / _____.
	11-44 Components of the inner ear include the (8) **cochlea** for hearing, the (9) **semicircular canals** for equilibrium, and the (10) **vestibule**, which is a chamber that joins the cochlea and semicircular canals. Label the inner ear structures in Figure 11-4.
	11-45 The inner ear, also called the labyrinth, consists of complicated mazelike structures (see Figure 11-5), all of which contain the functional organs for hearing and equilibrium. Use your medical dictionary to define *labyrinth* and list two types of inner ear labyrinths. _____ _____

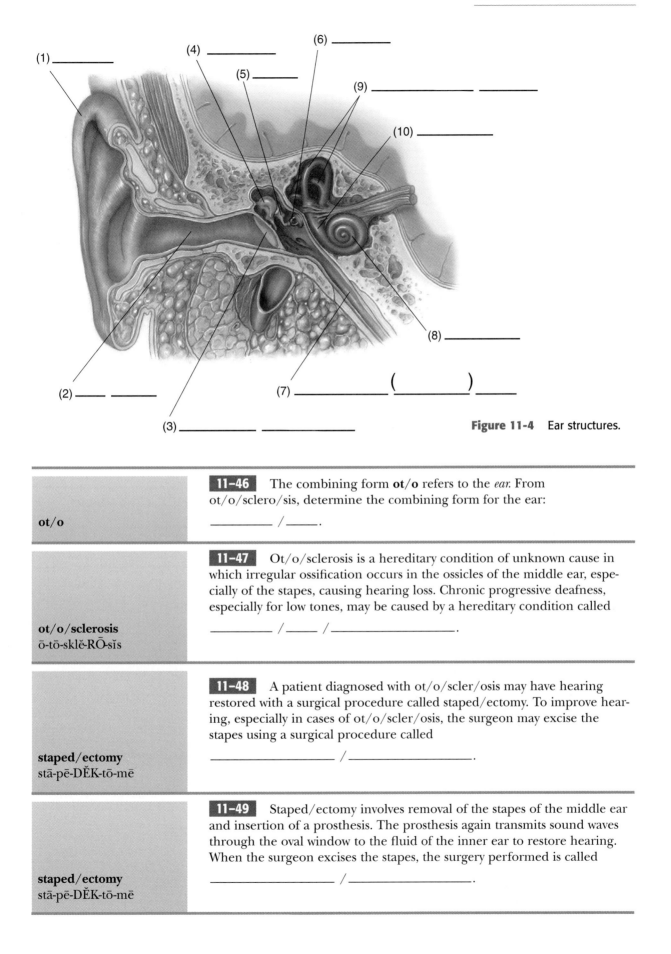

(1) _____

(4) _____

(5) _____

(6) _____

(9) _____ _____

(10) _____

(2) ____ ____

(8) _____

(7) _____ (_____) ____

(3) _____ _____

Figure 11-4 Ear structures.

---

ot/o

11-46 The combining form **ot/o** refers to the *ear*. From ot/o/sclero/sis, determine the combining form for the ear:

_____ / ____ .

---

ot/o/sclerosis
ō-tō-sklĕ-RŌ-sĭs

11-47 Ot/o/sclerosis is a hereditary condition of unknown cause in which irregular ossification occurs in the ossicles of the middle ear, especially of the stapes, causing hearing loss. Chronic progressive deafness, especially for low tones, may be caused by a hereditary condition called

_____ / ____ / _____ .

---

staped/ectomy
stā-pē-DĔK-tō-mē

11-48 A patient diagnosed with ot/o/scler/osis may have hearing restored with a surgical procedure called staped/ectomy. To improve hearing, especially in cases of ot/o/scler/osis, the surgeon may excise the stapes using a surgical procedure called

_____ / _____ .

---

staped/ectomy
stā-pē-DĔK-tō-mē

11-49 Staped/ectomy involves removal of the stapes of the middle ear and insertion of a prosthesis. The prosthesis again transmits sound waves through the oval window to the fluid of the inner ear to restore hearing. When the surgeon excises the stapes, the surgery performed is called

_____ / _____ .

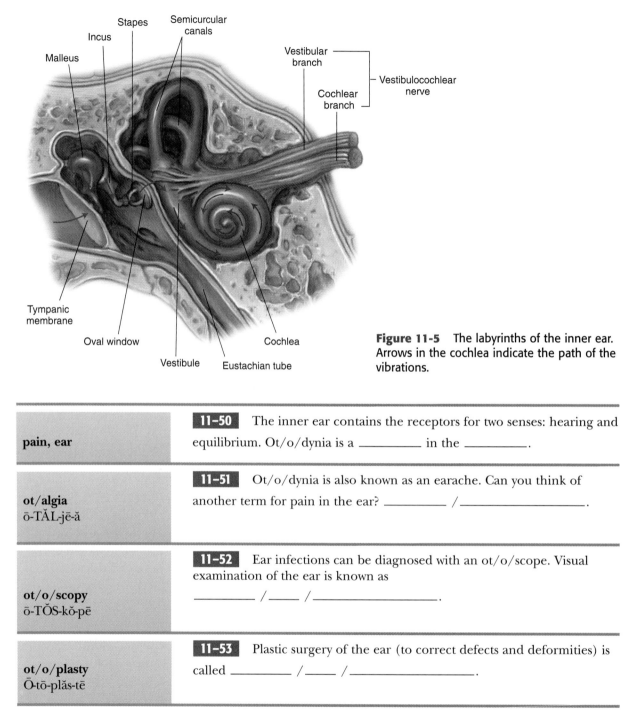

Malleus

Incus

Stapes

Semicircular canals

Vestibular branch

Cochlear branch

Vestibulocochlear nerve

Tympanic membrane

Oval window

Vestibule

Eustachian tube

Cochlea

Figure 11-5 The labyrinths of the inner ear. Arrows in the cochlea indicate the path of the vibrations.

pain, ear	**11-50** The inner ear contains the receptors for two senses: hearing and equilibrium. Ot/o/dynia is a _____ in the _____.
ot/algia ō-TĂL-jē-ă	**11-51** Ot/o/dynia is also known as an earache. Can you think of another term for pain in the ear? _____ / _____.
ot/o/scopy ō-TŎS-kŏ-pē	**11-52** Ear infections can be diagnosed with an ot/o/scope. Visual examination of the ear is known as _____ / ____ / _____.
ot/o/plasty Ō-tō-plăs-tē	**11-53** Plastic surgery of the ear (to correct defects and deformities) is called _____ / ____ / _____.

Competency Verification: Check your labeling of Figure 11–4 with the answers in Appendix B, Answer Key, page 536.

Listen and Learn, the audio CD-ROM that accompanies this book, will help you master the pronunciation of selected medical words. Use it to practice pronunciations *of selected term from frames 11–37 to 11–53* and from the word elements table. Listen for instructions to complete the *Listen and Learn* exercise on the CD-ROM for this section.

Using the following table, write the combining form, suffix, or prefix that matches its definition in the space provided to the left of the definition. There may be more than one word element that matches a definition.

Combining Forms		Suffixes		Prefixes
aden/o	myring/o	-acusis	-spasm	dipl-
audi/o	ophthalm/o	-edema	-stenosis	hyper-
blephar/o	ot/o	-logist		
choroid/o	retin/o	-malacia		
corne/o	salping/o	-opia		
dacry/o	scler/o	-opsia		
dipl/o	tympan/o	-ptosis		
irid/o	xanth/o	-rrhexis		
kerat/o		-salpinx		

1. _____ excessive, above normal

2. _____ choroid

3. _____ horny tissue; hard; cornea

4. _____ double

5. _____ ear

6. _____ tube (usually fallopian or eustachian [auditory] tubes)

7. _____ eye

8. _____ eyelid

9. _____ gland

10. _____ hardening; sclera (white of eye)

11. _____ involuntary contraction, twitching

12. _____ iris

13. _____ prolapse, downward displacement

14. _____ specialist in study of

15. _____ retina

16. _____ rupture

17. _____ softening

18. _____ hearing

19. _____ narrowing, stricture

20. _____ swelling

21. _____ tear; lacrimal apparatus (duct, sac, or gland)

22. _____ tympanic membrane (eardrum)

23. _____ cornea

24. _____ vision

25. _____ yellow

Competency Verification: Check your answers in Appendix B, Answer Key, page 536. If you are not satisfied with your level of comprehension, go back to Frame 11–1 and rework the frames.

Correct Answers _____ × 4 = _____ % Score

Abbreviations

This section introduces abbreviations related to the eyes and ears and their meanings. Included are abbreviations contained in the medical record activities that follow.

Abbreviation	Meaning	Abbreviation	Meaning
EYE			
ARMD	age-related macular degeneration	OD*	right eye
astigm	astigmatism	OS*	left eye
D	diopter (lens strength)	OU*	each eye; both eyes together
EOM	extraocular movement	REM	rapid eye movement
IOL	intraocular lens	ST	esotropia
IOP	intraocular pressure	VA	visual acuity
mix astig	mixed astigmatism	VF	visual field
Myop	myopia	XT	exotropia
EAR			
AD*	right ear	AU*	both ears
AS*	left ear	ENT	ear, nose, and throat
ABBREVIATIONS RELATED TO DIAGNOSTIC AND SURGICAL PROCEDURES			
ECG, EKG	electrocardiogram	MVR	massive vitreous retractor (blade)
mm	millimeter		

*Although these abbreviations currently are found in medical records and clinical notes, the Joint Commission on Accreditation of Healthcare Organizations (JCAHO) requires the discontinuance of the abbreviation. Instead, write out the meanings.

Pathological, Diagnostic, and Therapeutic Terms

The following are additional terms related to the eyes and ears. Recognizing and learning these terms will help you understand the connection between a pathological condition, its diagnosis, and the rationale behind the method of treatment selected for a particular disorder.

Pathological

Eye

achromatopsia (ă-krō-mă-TŎP-sē-ă): condition of color blindness that is more common in men.

astigmatism (ă-STĬG-mă-tĭzm): defective curvature of the cornea and lens, which causes light rays to focus unevenly over the retina rather than being focused on a single point, resulting in a distorted image (see Figure 11–2).

cataract (KĂT-ă-răkt): opacity (cloudiness) of the lens as a result of protein deposits on its surface that slowly build up until vision is lost.

Cataracts are a result of the aging process. Treatment usually consists of surgical removal of the lens.

conjunctivitis (kŏn-jŭnk-tĭ-VĪ-tĭs): inflammation of the conjunctiva that can be caused by bacteria, allergy, irritation, or a foreign body; also called *pinkeye*.

diabetic retinopathy (dī-ă-BĔT-ĭk rĕt-ĭn-ŎP-ă-thē): retinal damage marked by aneurismal dilation of blood vessels.

Diabetic retinopathy occurs in people with diabetes, manifested by small hemorrhages, edema, and formation of new vessels leading to scarring and eventual loss of vision.

esotropia (ĕs-ō-TRŌ-pē-ă): strabismus in which there is deviation of the visual axis of one eye toward that of the other eye resulting in diplopia; also called *cross-eye* and *convergent strabismus* (see Figure 11–6).

exotropia (ĕks-ō-TRŌ-pē-ă): strabismus in which there is deviation of the visual axis of one eye away from that of the other, resulting in diplopia; also called *wall-eye* and *divergent strabismus* (see Figure 11–6).

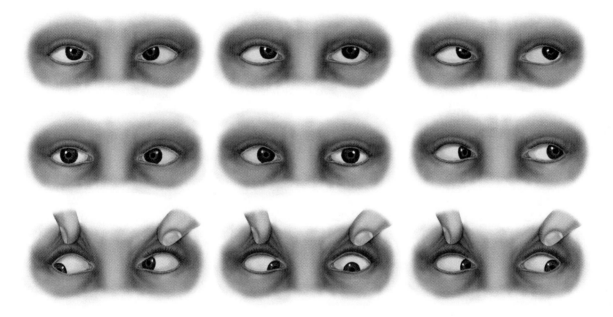

Figure 11-6   Types of Strabismus.

glaucoma (glaw-KŌ-mă): increased intraocular pressure caused by the failure of the aqueous humor to drain, which results in atrophy of the optic nerve and eventually may lead to blindness.

hordeolum (hor-DĒ-ō-lŭm): small purulent inflammatory infection of a sebaceous gland of the eyelid; also called *sty*.

macular degeneration (MĂK-ū-lăr): breakdown of the tissues in the macula resulting in loss of central vision.

Macular degeneration is the most common cause of visual impairment in persons over age 50 (see Figure 11–7).

photophobia (fō-tō-FŌ-bē-ă): unusual intolerance and sensitivity to light; occurs in diseases such as meningitis, inflammation of the eyes, measles, and rubella.

retinal detachment (RĔT-ĭ-năl): separation of the retina from the choroid, which disrupts vision and results in blindness if not repaired.

Retinal detachment may follow trauma, choroidal hemorrhages, or tumors and may be associated with diabetes mellitus.

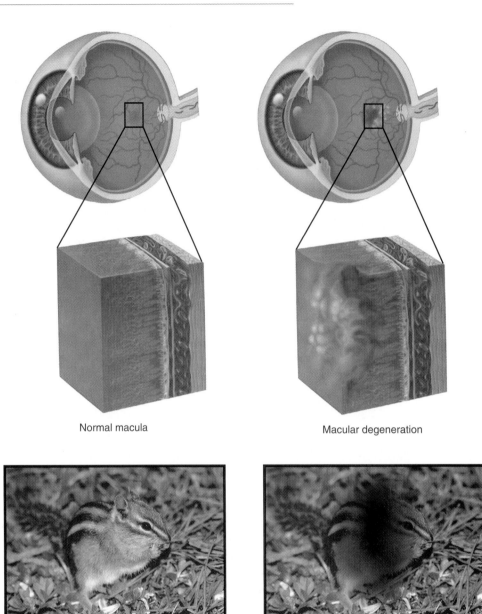

Normal macula

Macular degeneration

Normal vision

Central vision loss

Figure 11-7 Macular degeneration

strabismus (strǎ-BĬZ-mǔs): muscular eye disorder in which the eyes turn from the normal position so that they deviate in different directions.

In children, strabismus is associated with the lazy-eye syndrome. Various forms of strabismus are referred to as tropias, their direction being indicated by the appropriate prefix, as esotropia and exotropia (see Figure 11–6).

Ear

acoustic neuroma (a-KOOS-tĭk nū-RŌ-mǎ): benign tumor that develops from the eighth cranial (vestibulo-cochlear) nerve and grows within the auditory canal.

Depending on the location and size of the tumor, progressive hearing loss, headache, facial numbness, dizziness, and an unsteady gait may result.

anacusis (ăn-ă-KŪ-sĭs): total deafness; complete hearing loss.

conductive hearing loss: hearing loss due to an impairment in the transmission of sound because of an obstruction of the ear canal or damage to the eardrum or ossicles.

Méniére disease (měn-ē-ĀR): rare disorder of unknown etiology within the labyrinth of the inner ear that can lead to a progressive loss of hearing.

Symptoms of Méniére disease include vertigo, hearing loss, tinnitus, and the sensation of pressure in the ear.

otitis media (ō-TĪ-tĭs MĒ-dē-ă): middle ear infection, usually a result of bacterial infection.

Otitis media is most frequently seen in children.

otosclerosis (ō-tō-sklĕ-RŌ-sĭs): progressive deafness due to ossification in the bony labyrinth of the inner ear.

Stapedectomy or stapedotomy is usually successful in restoring hearing.

presbycusis (prĕz-bĭ-KŪ-sĭs): impairment of hearing resulting from the aging process.

tinnitus (tĭn-Ī-tĭs): ringing in the ears.

vertigo (VĔR-tĭ-gō): sensation of moving around in space; a feeling of spinning or dizziness.

Vertigo usually results from inner ear structure damage associated with balance and equilibrium.

Diagnostic

Eye

tonometry (tōn-ŎM-ĕ-trē): measuring of intraocular pressure by determining the resistance of the eyeball to indentation by an applied force; used to detect glaucoma (see Figure 11–8).

visual acuity test (ă-KŪ-ĭ-tē): standard test of visual acuity in which a person is asked to read letters and numbers on a chart 20 feet away with the use of the Snellen chart; also called an *E chart.*

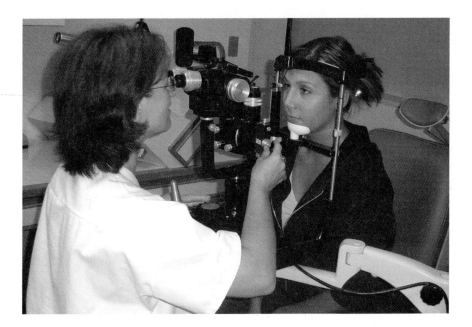

Figure 11-8 Tonometry. The slit-lamp examination is used to measure intraocular pressure (Courtesy of Richard H. Koop. MD).

Ear

audiometry (ăw-dē-ŎM-ĕ-trē): test that measures hearing acuity of various sound frequencies.

An instrument called an audiometer delivers acoustic stimuli at different frequencies, and the results are plotted on a graph called an audiogram.

otoscopy (ō-TŎS-kŏ-pē): visual examination of the ear, especially the eardrum, using an otoscope.

Rinne test (RĬN): hearing acuity test that is performed with a vibrating tuning fork placed on the mastoid process, then in front of the external auditory canal to test bone and air conduction.

The Rinne test is useful for differentiating between conductive and sensoneural hearing loss.

Therapeutic

Eye

cataract surgery (KĂT-ă-răkt): excision of cataracts by surgical removal of the lens. To correct the visual deficit when the eye is without a lens (aphakic), the insertion of an artificial lens (intraocular lens transplant) or the use of eyeglasses or contact lenses is needed. Several surgical techniques involving cataract removal are described below (see Figure 11–9).

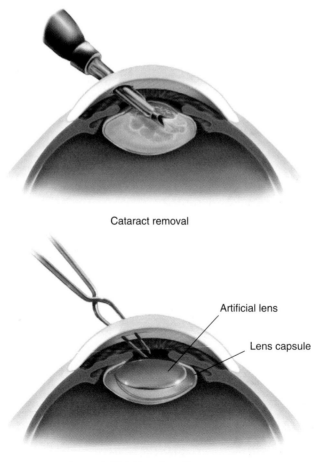

Cataract removal

Artificial lens

Lens capsule

Artificial lens insertion

Figure 11-9 Cataract surgery. Phacoemulsification.

corneal transplant (KŎR-nē-ĕl): surgical transplantation of a donor cornea (from a cadaver) into the eye of a recipient; also called keratoplasty.

extracapsular surgery (ĕks-tră-KĂP-sū-lăr): excision of most of the lens, followed by insertion of an intraocular lens transplant.

iridectomy (ĭr-ĭ-DĔK-tĕ-mē): excision of a portion of the iris.

> *Iridectomy is a surgical procedure that usually is performed to create an opening through which aqueous humor can drain; used to relieve intraocular pressure in patients with glaucoma.*

phacoemulsification (FĂK-ō-ē-mŭl-sĭ-fĭ-kā-shŭn): excision of the lens by ultrasonic vibrations that break the lens into tiny particles, which are suctioned out of the eye (see Figure 11–9).

Ear

cochlear implant (KŎK-lē-ĕr): electronic transmitter that is surgically implanted into the cochlea of a deaf individual; performed to restore hearing loss.

myringoplasty (mĭr-ĬN-gō-plăst-ē): surgical repair of a perforated eardrum with a tissue graft.

> *Myringoplasty is performed to correct hearing loss; also called tympanoplasty.*

myringotomy (mĭr-ĭn-GŎT-ō-mē): incision of the eardrum to relieve pressure and release pus or serous fluid from the middle ear or to insert tympanostomy tubes surgically in the eardrum.

> *Tympanostomy tubes provide ventilation and drainage of the middle ear when repeated ear infections do not respond to antibiotic treatment and are used when persistent severely negative middle ear pressure is present.*

 Listen and Learn, the audio CD-ROM that accompanies this book, will help you master the pronunciation of selected medical words. Use it to practice pronunciations of the above-listed medical terms and for instructions to complete the *Listen and Learn* exercise on the CD-ROM for this section.

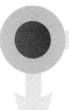

PATHOLOGICAL, DIAGNOSTIC, AND THERAPEUTIC TERMS REVIEW

Match the medical term(s) below with the definitions in the numbered list.

achromatopsia
acoustic neuroma
anacusis
astigmatism
cataract

conductive hearing loss
conjunctivitis
diabetic retinopathy
glaucoma
hordeolum

iridectomy
macular degeneration
Méniére disease
myringotomy
otitis media

otosclerosis
phacoemulsification
photophobia
presbycusis
retinal detachment

Rinne test
strabismus
tinnitus
tonometry
vertigo

1. _____ means ringing in the ears.

2. _____ is progressive deafness due to ossification in the bony labyrinth of the inner ear.

3. _____ means color blindness.

4. _____ is a rare disorder characterized by progressive deafness, vertigo, and tinnitus, possibly caused by swelling of membranous structures within the labyrinth.

5. _____ is a disorder in which both eyes cannot focus on the same point, resulting in looking in different directions at the same time; also called *lazy eye* or *cross-eye*.

6. _____ means total deafness.

7. _____ refers to middle ear infection that is most commonly seen in young children.

8. _____ refers to pink-eye.

9. _____ means intolerance or unusual sensitivity to light.

10. _____ is hearing loss due to old age.

11. _____ refers to increased intraocular pressure caused by the failure of the aqueous humor to drain, which results in atrophy of the optic nerve and eventually may lead to blindness.

12. _____ refers to a feeling of spinning or dizziness.

13. _____ refers to separation of the retina from the choroids.

14. _____ is another term for sty.

15. _____ is abnormal curvature of the cornea, which causes light rays to focus unevenly over the retina rather than focus on a single point, resulting in a distorted image.

16. _____ is a benign tumor of the eighth cranial nerve that may or may not produce symptomatic changes.

17. _____ measures intraocular pressure; used to diagnose glaucoma.

18. _____ refers to excision of a portion of the iris.

486

19. _____ is hearing loss caused by an impairment in sound transmission because of damage to the eardrum or ossicles or obstruction of the ear canal.

20. _____ refers to opacity (cloudiness) of the lens as a result of protein deposits on its surface.

21. _____ is a type of cataract surgery.

22. _____ is a hearing acuity test that is performed with a vibrating tuning fork.

23. _____ refers to retinal damage marked by aneurysmal dilation of blood vessels.

24. _____ refers to macular tissue breakdown causing loss of central vision; most common cause of visual impairment in persons older than age 50.

25. _____ is an incision of the eardrum to relieve pressure and release pus or serous fluid from the middle ear.

Competency Verification: Check your answers in Appendix B, Answer Key, page 536. If you are not satisfied with your level of comprehension, review the pathological, diagnostic, and therapeutic terms and retake the review.

Correct Answers: _____ × 4 _____% Score

Medical Record Activities

The following medical records reflect common real-life clinical scenarios using medical terminology to document patient care. The physician who specializes in the treatment of the eyes is an *ophthalmologist;* the medical specialty concerned in the diagnoses and treatment of eye disorders is called *ophthalmology.* The physician who specializes in the treatment of the ear, nose, and throat disorders is an *otolaryngologist,* or an *ENT* specialist; the medical specialty concerned in the diagnoses and treatment of the ear, nose, and throat disorders is called *otolaryngology.* Ophthalmologists, otolaryngologists, and ENT physicians specialize in medical and surgical treatment of diseases and disorders in their respective areas of specialization.

✓ MEDICAL RECORD ACTIVITY 11–1. Retinal Detachment

Terminology

The terms listed in the chart come from the medical record *Retinal Detachment* that follows. Use a medical dictionary such as *Taber's Cyclopedic Medical Dictionary,* the appendices of this book, or other resources to define each term. Then practice reading the pronunciations aloud for each term.

Term	Definition
akinesia ă-kĭ-NĒ-zē-ă	
anesthesia ăn-ĕs-THĒ-zē-ă	
anteriorly ăn-TĒR-ē-or-lē	
cannula KĂN-ū-lă	
conjunctival kŏn-jŭnk-TĬ-văl	
EKG	
hemorrhage HĔM-ĕ-rĭj	
IV	
limbus LĬM-bŭs	
mm	
MVR	
retinal detachment RĔT-ĭ-năl	
retinitis rĕt-ĭ-NĪ-tĭs	
retrobulbar rĕt-rō-BŬL-băr	

Term	Definition
sclerotomy sklĕ-RŎT-ō-mē	
vitrectomy vĭ-TRĔK-tō-mē	

 Listen and Learn Online! will help you master the pronunciation of selected medical words from this medical record activity. Visit www.fadavis.com/gylys/simplified for instructions in completing the *Listen and Learn Online!* exercise for this section and then to practice pronunciations.

RETINAL DETACHMENT

Reading

Practice pronunciation of medical terms by reading the following medical report aloud.

DIAGNOSIS: Total retinal detachment, left eye, secondary to complications of retinitis.

PROCEDURE: The patient was taken to the operating room, placed on the operating table, IV line begun, EKG lead monitor attached, and retrobulbar anesthetic given, achieving good anesthesia and akinesia. The patient was scrubbed, prepped, and draped in a standard sterile fashion for retinal surgery. A 360-degree conjunctival opening was made and 2–0 silk sutures were placed around each rectus muscle. Four millimeters from the limbus, a mark in the sclera was made and preplaced 5–0 Mersiline suture was passed; MVR stab incision made, and 4-mm infusion cannula was slipped into position and visualized inside the eye. Similar sclerotomy sites were made superior nasally and superior temporally. Trans pars plana vitrectomy was undertaken. Dense vitreous hemorrhage and debris were found, which were removed. There was incomplete posterior vitreous attachment. The retina was almost totally detached, and a small amount of nasal retina was still attached. A linear retinal break was seen just above the disk along a vessel. Gradually all the peripheral vitreous was removed.

The air-fluid exchange was performed with some difficulty because some sort of vitreous was found anteriorly, which loculated the bubble. It gave me a peculiar view, but slowly the retina became totally flat, and we treated the retinal break with the diode laser. A 240 band was wrapped around the eye and fixed with the Watke's sleeve superior temporally. The sclerotomies were all sewn closed. Before the last sclerotomy was closed, the air was exchanged for silicone. The eye was left soft because the patient had poor perfusion.

Evaluation

Review the medical record above to answer the following questions.

1. Where is the retina located?

_____

_____

2. Was the anesthetic administered behind or in front of the eyeball?

_____

_____

3. How much movement remained in the eye following anesthesia?

_____

_____

4. Where was the hemorrhage located?

_____

_____

5. What type of vitrectomy was undertaken?

_____

_____

6. Why was the eye left soft?

_____

_____

✓ MEDICAL RECORD ACTIVITY 11–2. Otitis Media

Terminology

The terms listed in the chart come from the medical record _Otitis Media_ that follows. Use a medical dictionary such as _Taber's Cyclopedic Medical Dictionary,_ the appendices of this book, or other resources to define each term. Then practice reading the pronunciations aloud for each term.

Term	Definition
cholesteatoma kō-lē-stē-ă-TŌ-mă	
ENT	
general anesthesia ăn-ĕs-THĒ-zē-ă	
mucoserous mū-kō-SĒR-ŭs	
otitis media ō-TĪ-tĭs MĒ-dē-ă	
postoperatively pōst-ŎP-ĕr-ă-tĭv-lē	
tympanoplasty tĭm-păn-ō-PLĂS-tē	

Listen and Learn Online! will help you master the pronunciation of selected medical words from this medical record activity. Visit www.fadavis.com/gylys/simplified for instructions in completing the _Listen and Learn Online!_ exercise for this section and then to practice pronunciations.

OTITIS MEDIA

Reading

Practice pronunciation of medical terms by reading the following medical report aloud.

A 25-year-old white woman with a diagnosis of mucoserous otitis media on the right ear was seen by the ENT specialist. The patient was admitted to the hospital and developed cholesteatoma. A tube was inserted for the chronic adhesive otitis media with secondary cholesteatoma. The patient progressed favorably postoperatively, but the cholesteatoma continued to enlarge in size. Currently she has been admitted to the hospital for a right tympanoplasty performed under general anesthesia.

Evaluation

Review the medical record to answer the following questions.

1. Where was the patient's infection located?

   _____

   _____

2. What complication developed while the patient was hospitalized?

   _____

   _____

3. What is the purpose of the tube placement?

   _____

   _____

4. What surgery is being performed to resolve the cholesteatoma?

   _____

   _____

5. Will the patient be asleep during the surgery?

   _____

   _____

Chapter Review

Word Elements Summary

The following table summarizes combining forms, suffixes, and prefixes related to the special senses.

Word Element	Meaning
COMBINING FORMS	
acous/o, audi/o	hearing
aden/o	gland
blephar/o	eyelid
choroid/o	choroid
corne/o	cornea
dacry/o, lacrim/o	tear; lacrimal apparatus (duct, sac, or gland)
dipl/o	double
irid/o	iris
kerat/o	horny tissue; hard; cornea
myring/o, tympan/o	tympanic membrane (eardrum)
ocul/o, ophthalm/o	eye
ot/o	ear
retin/o	retina
salping/o	tube (usually fallopian or eustachian [auditory] tubes)
scler/o	hardening; sclera (white of eye)
OTHER COMBINING FORMS	
erythr/o	red
my/o	muscle
xanth/o	yellow
SUFFIXES	
SURGICAL	
-ectomy	excision, removal
-tomy	incision
DIAGNOSTIC, SYMPTOMATIC, AND RELATED	
-acusis	hearing
-algia, -dynia	pain

Word Element	Meaning
-edema	swelling
-itis	inflammation
-logist	specialist in study of
-logy	study of
-malacia	softening
-opia	vision
-pathy	disease
-ptosis	prolapse, downward displacement
-rrhexis	rupture
-salpinx	tube (usually fallopian or eustachian [auditory] tubes)
-scope	instrument for examining
-spasm	involuntary contraction, twitching
-stenosis	narrowing, stricture
PREFIXES	
ana-	against; up; back
dipl-	double
exo-	outside, outward
hyper-	excessive, above normal

WORD ELEMENTS REVIEW

After you review the word elements summary, complete this activity by writing the meaning of each element in the space provided.

Word Element	Meaning
COMBINING FORMS	
1. acous/o, audi/o	
2. aden/o	
3. blephar/o	
4. choroid/o	
5. corne/o, kerat/o	
6. dacry/o, lacrim/o	
7. irid/o	
8. myring/o, tympan/o	
9. ocul/o, ophthalm/o	
10. ot/o	
11. retin/o	
12. salping/o	
13. scler/o	
SUFFIXES	
DIAGNOSTIC, SYMPTOMATIC, AND RELATED	
14. -acusis	
15. -edema	
16. -opia	
17. -pathy	
18. -ptosis	
19. -rrhexis	
20. -salpinx	
21. -stenosis	

Word Element	Meaning
PREFIXES	
22. ana-	
23. dipl-	
24. exo-	
25. hyper-	

Competency Verification: Check your answers in Appendix A, Glossary of Medical Word Elements, page 497. If you are not satisfied with your level of comprehension, review the word elements and retake the review.

Correct Answers: _____ × 4 _____% Score

Chapter 11 Vocabulary Review

Match the medical word(s) below with the definitions in the numbered list.

blepharoptosis	diplopia	labyrinth	otitis media
cholesteatoma	eustachian tube	mastoid surgery	postoperatively
chronic	general anesthetic	mucoserous	salpingostenosis
dacryorrhea	hyperopia	myopia	sclera
diagnosis	keratitis	ophthalmologist	tympanic membrane

1. _____ means double vision.

2. _____ refers to white of eye.

3. _____ is the eardrum; it vibrates when sound waves strike it.

4. _____ means excessive flow of tears.

5. _____ equalizes the air pressure in the middle ear with that of the outside atmosphere.

6. _____ refers to inflammation of the cornea due to a vision-threatening infection; sometimes occurs when contact lenses are not disinfected properly.

7. _____ is a process of determining the cause and nature of a pathological condition.

8. _____ means composed of mucus and serum.

9. _____ is inflammation of the middle ear.

10. _____ is a tumor-like sac filled with keratin debris most commonly found in the middle ear.

11. _____ is an operation on the mastoid process of the temporal bone.

12. _____ is anesthesia that affects the entire body with loss of consciousness.

13. _____ is a physician who specializes in the treatment of eye disorders.

14. _____ means of long duration; designating a disease showing little change or of slow progression

15. _____ means farsightedness.

16. _____ means occurring after surgery.

17. _____ is a system of intercommunicating canals, especially of the inner ear.

18. _____ is prolapse of an eyelid.

19. _____ is a narrowing or stricture of the eustachian tube.

20. _____ means nearsightedness.

Competency Verification: Check your answers in Appendix B, Answer Key, page 537. If you are not satisfied with your level of comprehension, review the chapter vocabulary and retake the review.

Correct Answers: _____ × 5 _____% Score

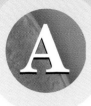

Glossary of Medical Word Elements

Medical Word Element	Meaning	Medical Word Element	Meaning
A		ana-	against; up; back
		andr/o	male
a-	without, not	aneurysm/o	a widening, a widened blood vessel
ab-	from, away from		
abdomin/o	abdomen	angi/o	vessel (usually blood or lymph)
abort/o	to miscarry		
-ac	pertaining to, relating to	aniso-	unequal, dissimilar
acous/o	hearing	ankyl/o	stiffness; bent, crooked
acr/o	extremity	ante-	before, in front of
acromi/o	acromion (projection of scapula)	anter/o	anterior, front
		anti-	against
-acusis	hearing	aort/o	aorta
-ad	toward	append/o	appendix
ad-	toward	appendic/o	appendix
aden/o	gland	aque/o	water
adenoid/o	adenoids	-ar	pertaining to, relating to
adip/o	fat		
adren/o	adrenal glands	-arche	beginning
adrenal/o	adrenal glands	arteri/o	artery
aer/o	air	arteriol/o	arteriole
agglutin/o	clumping, gluing	arthr/o	joint
-al	pertaining to, relating to	-ary	pertaining to, relating to
albin/o	white		
-algesia	pain	-asthenia	weakness, debility
-algia	pain	-ate	having the form of, possessing
alveol/o	alveolus (plural, alveoli)		
ambly/o	dull, dim	atel/o	incomplete; imperfect
amni/o	amnion (amniotic sac)	ather/o	fatty plaque
an-	without, not	-ation	process (of)
an/o	anus	atri/o	atrium
		audi/o	hearing

Medical Word Element	Meaning	Medical Word Element	Meaning
audit/o	hearing	circum-	around
aur/o	ear	cirrh/o	yellow
auricul/o	ear	-cision	a cutting
auto-	self, own	-clasia	to break; surgical fracture
axill/o	armpit		
azot/o	nitrogenous compounds	-clast	to break
		clavicul/o	clavicle (collar bone)
B		coccyg/o	coccyx (tailbone)
		cochle/o	cochlea
bacteri/o	bacteria	col/o	colon
balan/o	glans penis	colon/o	colon
bi-	two	colp/o	vagina
blephar/o	eyelid	conjunctiv/o	conjunctiva
-blast	embryonic cell	-continence	to hold back
blast/o	embryonic cell	core/o	pupil
brachi/o	arm	corne/o	cornea
brady-	slow	cor/o	pupil
bronch/o	bronchus (plural, bronchi)	cost/o	ribs
		crani/o	cranium (skull)
bronchi/o	bronchus (plural, bronchi)	cry/o	cold
		crypt/o	hidden
bronchiol/o	bronchiole	cutane/o	skin
		cyan/o	blue
C		cycl/o	ciliary body of eye; circular; cycle
		-cyesis	pregnancy
calc/o	calcium	cyst/o	bladder
calcane/o	calcaneum (heel bone)	cyt/o	cell
		-cyte	cell
carcin/o	cancer		
cardi/o	heart	**D**	
-cardia	heart condition		
carp/o	carpus (wrist bones)	dacry/o	tear; lacrimal apparatus (duct, sac, or gland)
caud/o	tail		
cauter/o	heat, burn		
-cele	hernia, swelling	dacryocyst/o	lacrimal sac
-centesis	surgical puncture	dactyl/o	fingers; toes
cephal/o	head	dent/o	teeth
-ception	conceiving	derm/o	skin
cerebell/o	cerebellum	-derma	skin
cerebr/o	cerebrum	dermat/o	skin
cervic/o	neck; cervix uteri (neck of uterus)	-desis	binding, fixation (of a bone or joint)
chol/e	bile, gall	di-	double
cholangi/o	bile vessel	dia-	through, across
cholecyst/o	gallbladder	dipl-	double
choledoch/o	bile duct	dipl/o	double
chondr/o	cartilage	dips/o	thirst
chori/o	chorion	-dipsia	thirst
choroid/o	choroid	dist/o	far, farthest
-cide	killing		

Medical Word Element	Meaning
dors/o	back (of body)
duct/o	to lead; carry
duoden/o	duodenum (first part of small intestine)
dur/o	dura mater; hard
-dynia	pain
dys-	bad; painful; difficult

E

Medical Word Element	Meaning
-eal	pertaining to, relating to
echo-	a repeated sound
-ectasis	dilation, expansion
ecto-	outside, outward
-ectomy	excision, removal
-edema	swelling
electr/o	electricity
-ema	state of; condition
embol/o	plug
-emesis	vomiting
-emia	blood condition
emphys/o	to inflate
en-	in, within
encephal/o	brain
end-	within
endo-	in, within
enter/o	intestine (usually small intestine)
epi-	above, upon
epididym/o	epididymis
epiglott/o	epiglottis
episi/o	vulva
erythem/o	red
erythemat/o	red
erythr/o	red
-esis	condition
esophag/o	esophagus
eu-	good, normal
ex-	out, out from
exo-	outside, outward
extra-	outside

F

Medical Word Element	Meaning
femor/o	femur (thigh bone)
fibr/o	fiber, fibrous tissue
fibul/o	fibula (smaller, outer bone of lower leg)

G

Medical Word Element	Meaning
galact/o	milk
gangli/o	ganglion (knot or knotlike mass)
gastr/o	stomach
-gen	forming, producing, origin
-genesis	forming, producing, origin
gen/o	forming, producing, origin
genit/o	organs of reproduction
gingiv/o	gum(s)
glauc/o	gray
gli/o	glue; neuroglial tissue
-glia	glue; neuroglial tissue
-globin	protein
glomerul/o	glomerulus
gloss/o	tongue
glott/o	glottis
gluc/o	sugar, sweetness
glyc/o	sugar, sweetness
-gnosis	knowing
gonad/o	gonads, sex glands
-graft	transplantation
-gram	record, writing
granul/o	granule
-graph	instrument for recording
-graphy	process of recording
-gravida	pregnant woman
gyn/o	woman, female
gynec/o	woman, female

H

Medical Word Element	Meaning
hem/o	blood
hemangi/o	blood vessel
hemat/o	blood
hemi-	one half
hepat/o	liver
hetero-	different
hidr/o	sweat
hist/o	tissue
histi/o	tissue
homeo-	same, alike
homo-	same
humer/o	humerus (upper arm bone)

Medical Word Element	Meaning	Medical Word Element	Meaning
hydr/o	water	iso-	same, equal
hyp-	under, below, deficient	-ist	specialist
hyper-	excessive, above normal	-isy	state of; condition
hypo-	under, below, deficient	-itic	pertaining to, relating to
hyster/o	uterus (womb)	-itis	inflammation
		-ive	pertaining to, relating to
I		-ization	process (of)
-ia	condition	**J**	
-iac	pertaining to, relating to		
-iasis	abnormal condition (produced by something specified)	jaund/o	yellow
		jejun/o	jejunum (second part of small intestine)
-iatry	medicine; treatment	**K**	
-ic	pertaining to, relating to		
-ical	pertaining to, relating to	kerat/o	horny tissue; hard; cornea
-ice	noun ending	kyph/o	hill, mountain
ichthy/o	dry, scaly	**L**	
-ician	specialist		
-icle	small, minute, little		
-ile	pertaining to, relating to	labi/o	lip
ile/o	ileum (third part of small intestine)	labyrinth/o	labyrinth (inner ear)
ili/o	ilium (lateral, flaring portion of hip bone)	lacrim/o	tear; lacrimal apparatus (duct, sac, or gland)
im-	not	lact/o	milk
immun/o	immune, immunity, safe	lamin/o	lamina (part of vertebral arch)
in-	in, not	-lampsia	to shine
-ine	pertaining to, relating to	lapar/o	abdomen
infer/o	lower, below	laryng/o	larynx (voice box)
infra-	under, below	later/o	side, to one side
inguin/o	groin	-lepsy	seizure
insulin/o	insulin	leuk/o	white
inter-	between	lingu/o	tongue
intestin/o	intestine	lip/o	fat
intra-	in, within	lipid/o	fat
-ion	the act of	-lith	stone, calculus
-ior	pertaining to, relating to	lith/o	stone, calculus
irid/o	iris	lob/o	lobe
-is	noun ending	log/o	study of
ischi/o	ischium (lower portion of hip bone)	-logist	specialist in study of
-ism	condition	-logy	study of
		lord/o	curve, swayback
		lumb/o	loins (lower back)
		lymph/o	lymph
		lymphaden/o	lymph gland (node)

Medical Word Element	Meaning	Medical Word Element	Meaning
lymphangi/o	lymph vessel	myos/o	muscle
-lysis	separation; destruction; loosening	myring/o	tympanic membrane (eardrum)

M

Medical Word Element	Meaning	Medical Word Element	Meaning
macro-	large		
mal-	bad		
-malacia	softening		
mamm/o	breast		
mast/o	breast		
mastoid/o	mastoid process		
maxill/o	maxilla (upper jaw bone)		
meat/o	opening, meatus		
medi-	middle		
medi/o	middle		
medull/o	medulla		
mega-	enlargement		
megal/o	enlargement		
-megaly	enlargement		
melan/o	black		
men/o	menses, menstruation		
mening/o	meninges (membranes covering brain and spinal cord)		
meningi/o	meninges (membranes covering brain and spinal cord)		
meso-	middle		
meta-	change, beyond		
metacarp/o	metacarpus (hand bones)		
metatars/o	metatarsus (foot bones)		
-meter	instrument for measuring		
metr/o	uterus (womb); measure		
metri/o	uterus (womb)		
-metry	act of measuring		
micr/o	small		
micro-	small		
mono-	one		
muc/o	mucus		
multi-	many, much		
muscul/o	muscle		
my/o	muscle		
myc/o	fungus		
myel/o	bone marrow; spinal cord		

N

Medical Word Element	Meaning
nas/o	nose
nat/o	birth
necr/o	death, necrosis
neo-	new
nephr/o	kidney
neur/o	nerve
nid/o	nest
noct/o	night
norm/o	normal; usual
nucle/o	nucleus
nulli-	none

O

Medical Word Element	Meaning
obstetr/o	midwife
ocul/o	eye
odont/o	teeth
-oid	resembling
-ole	small, minute
olig/o	scanty
-oma	tumor
onc/o	tumor
onych/o	nail
oophor/o	ovary
-opaque	obscure
ophthalm/o	eye
-opia	vision
-opsia	vision
-opsy	view of
opt/o	eye, vision
optic/o	eye, vision
or/o	mouth
orch/o	testis (plural, testes)
orchi/o	testis (plural, testes)
orchid/o	testis (plural, testes)
-orexia	appetite
orth/o	straight
-ory	pertaining to, relating to
-osis	abnormal condition; increase (used primarily with blood cells)
-osmia	smell
oste/o	bone

Medical Word Element	Meaning	Medical Word Element	Meaning
ot/o	ear	-plasty	surgical repair
-ous	pertaining to, relating to	-plegia	paralysis
		pleur/o	pleura
ovari/o	ovary	-plexy	stroke
-oxia	oxygen	-pnea	breathing
ox/o	oxygen	pneum/o	air; lung
		pneumon/o	air; lung
P		pod/o	foot
		-poiesis	formation, production
pancreat/o	pancreas	poli/o	gray; gray matter (of brain or spinal cord)
-para	to bear (offspring)		
para-	near, beside; beyond	poly-	many, much
parathyroid/o	parathyroid glands	polyp/o	small growth
-paresis	partial paralysis	-porosis	porous
patell/o	patella (kneecap)	post-	after, behind
path/o	disease	poster/o	back (of body), behind, posterior
-pathy	disease		
-pause	cessation	-potence	power
pector/o	chest	-prandial	meal
ped/i	foot; child	pre-	before, in front of
ped/o	foot; child	primi-	first
pelv/i	pelvis	pro-	before, in front of
pelv/o	pelvis	proct/o	anus, rectum
pen/o	penis	prostat/o	prostate gland
-penia	decrease, deficiency	proxim/o	near, nearest
-pepsia	digestion	pseudo-	false
per-	through	ptyal/o	saliva
peri-	around	-ptosis	prolapse, downward displacement
perine/o	perineum		
peritone/o	peritoneum	pub/o	pelvis bone (anterior part of pelvic bone)
-pexy	fixation (of an organ)		
phac/o	lens	pulmon/o	lung
phag/o	swallowing, eating	pupill/o	pupil
-phage	swallowing, eating	py/o	pus
-phagia	swallowing, eating	pyel/o	renal pelvis
phalang/o	phalanges (bones of fingers and toes)	pylor/o	pylorus
pharyng/o	pharynx (throat)	**Q**	
-phasia	speech		
phleb/o	vein	quadri-	four
-phobia	fear		
phon/o	voice, sound	**R**	
-phoresis	carrying, transmission		
phot/o	light	radi/o	radiation, x-ray; radius (lower arm bone on thumb side)
phren/o	diaphragm; mind		
-phylaxis	protection		
-physis	growth	rect/o	rectum
pil/o	hair	ren/o	kidney
pituitar/o	pituitary gland	retin/o	retina
-plasia	formation, growth	retro-	backward, behind
-plasm	formation, growth	rhabd/o	rod-shaped (striated)

Medical Word Element	Meaning	Medical Word Element	Meaning
rhabdomy/o	striated (skeletal) muscle	spondyl/o	vertebrae (backbone)
rhin/o	nose	squam/o	scale
roentgen/o	x-rays	staped/o	stapes
-rrhage	bursting forth (of)	-stasis	standing still
-rrhagia	bursting forth (of)	steat/o	fat
-rrhaphy	suture	sten/o	narrowing, stricture
-rrhea	discharge, flow	-stenosis	narrowing, stricture
-rrhexis	rupture	stern/o	sternum (breastbone)
		stomat/o	mouth
S		-stomy	forming an opening (mouth)
		sub-	under, below
sacr/o	sacrum	sudor/o	sweat
salping/o	tube (usually fallopian or eustachian [auditory] tubes)	super-	upper, above
		supra-	above; excessive; superior
-salpinx	tube (usually fallopian or eustachian [auditory] tubes)	synov/o	synovial membrane, synovial fluid
sarc/o	flesh (connective tissue)	**T**	
scapul/o	scapula (shoulder blade)	tachy-	rapid
-sarcoma	malignant tumor of connective tissue	ten/o	tendon
		tend/o	tendon
scler/o	hardening; sclera (white of eye)	tendin/o	tendon
		-tension	to stretch
scoli/o	crooked, bent	test/o	testis (plural, testes)
-scope	instrument for examining	thalam/o	thalamus
		-therapy	treatment
-scopy	visual examination	therm/o	heat
seb/o	sebum, sebaceous	thorac/o	chest
semi-	one half	-thorax	chest
sept/o	septum	thromb/o	blood clot
sequestr/o	a separation	thym/o	thymus gland
ser/o	serum	thyr/o	thyroid gland
sial/o	saliva, salivary gland	thyroid/o	thyroid gland
sigmoid/o	sigmoid colon	tibi/o	tibia (larger inner bone of lower leg)
sin/o	sinus, cavity	-tic	pertaining to, relating to
sinus/o	sinus, cavity	-tocia	childbirth, labor
son/o	sound	tom/o	to cut
-spadias	slit, fissure	-tome	instrument to cut
-spasm	involuntary contraction, twitching	-tomy	incision
		ton/o	tension
sperm/o	spermatozoa, sperm cells	tonsill/o	tonsils
		tox/o	poison
spermat/o	spermatozoa, sperm cells	-toxic	poison
		toxic/o	poison
spin/o	spine	trache/o	trachea (windpipe)
spir/o	breathe	trans-	through, across
splen/o	spleen	tri-	three

Medical Word Element	Meaning	Medical Word Element	Meaning
trich/o	hair	**V**	
-tripsy	crushing		
-trophy	development, nourishment	vagin/o	vagina
		valv/o	valve
-tropia	turning	varic/o	dilated vein
-tropin	stimulate	vas/o	vessel; vas deferens; duct
tubercul/o	a little swelling		
tympan/o	tympanic membrane (eardrum)	vascul/o	vessel
		ven/o	vein
		ventr/o	belly, belly side
U		ventricul/o	ventricle (of heart or brain)
-ula	small, minute	-verse	turning
-ule	small, minute	-version	turning
uln/o	ulna (lower arm bone on opposite side of thumb)	vertebr/o	vertebrae (backbone)
		vesic/o	bladder
		vesicul/o	seminal vesicle
ultra-	excess, beyond	vulv/o	vulva
-um	structure, thing		
umbilic/o	umbilicus, navel	**X**	
uni-	one		
ur/o	urine	xanth/o	yellow
ureter/o	ureter	xer/o	dry
urethr/o	urethra		
-uria	urine	**Y**	
urin/o	urine		
-us	condition; structure	-y	condition; process
uter/o	uterus (womb)		
uvul/o	uvula		

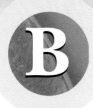

appendix

Answer Key

Chapter 1: Introduction to Programmed Learning and Medical Word Building

Frame 1–52

Medical Term	Combining Form (Root + o)	Word Root	Suffix
arthr/o/scop/ic	arthr/o	scop	-ic
ăr-thrōs-KŎP-ĭk			
erythr/o/cyt/osis	erythr/o	cyt	-osis
ĕ-rĭth-rō-sī-TŌ-sĭs			
append/ix		append	-ix
ă-PĔN-dĭks			
dermat/itis		dermat	-itis
dĕr-mă-TĪ-tĭs			
gastr/o/enter/itis	gastr/o	enter	-itis
găs-trō-ĕn-tĕr-Ī-tĭs			
orth/o/ped/ic	orth/o	ped	-ic
or-thō-PĒ-dĭk			
oste/o/arthr/itis	oste/o	arthr	-itis
ŏs-tē-ō-ăr-THRĪ-tĭs			
vagin/itis		vagin	-itis
văj-ĭn-Ī-tĭs			

Section Review 1–1

1. breve	3. long	5. pn	7. n	9. second
2. macron	4. short	6. hard	8. eye	10. separate

Section Review 1–2

Medical Word and Meaning	Prefix	Basic Elements of a Medical Word		
		Combining Form(s) (root + vowel)	Word Roots(s)	Suffix
1. **peri/dent/al** pĕr-ĭ-DĔN-tăl	peri-		dent	-al
2. **ab/norm/al** ăb-NŌR-măl	ab-		norm	-al
3. **hepat/itis** hĕp-ă-TĪ-tĭs			hepat	-itis
4. **supra/ren/al** soo-pră-RĒ-năl	supra-		ren	-al
5. **trans/vagin/al** trăns-VĂJ-ĭn-ăl	trans-		vagin	-al
6. **gastr/o/intestin/al** găs-trō-ĭn-TĔS-tĭ-năl		gastr/o	intestin	-al
7. **macro/cephal/ic** măk-rō-sĕf-ĂL-ĭk	macro-		cephal	-ic
8. **ren/o/pathy** rē-NŎP-ă-thē		ren/o		-pathy
9. **therm/o/meter** thĕr-MŎM-ĕ-tĕr		therm/o		-meter
10. **hepat/o/megaly** hĕp-ă-tō-MĔG-ă-lē		hepat/o		-megaly
11. **sub/stern/al** sŭb-STĔR-năl	sub-		stern	-al
12. **hypo/insulin/ism** hī-pō-ĬN-sū-lĭn-ĭzm	hypo-		insulin	-ism
13. **gastr/o/enter/o/pathy** găs-trō-ĕn-tĕr-Ŏ-pă-thē		gastr/o, enter/o		-pathy
14. **arteri/o/scler/osis** ăr-tē-rē-ō-sklĕ-RŌ-sĭs		arteri/o	scler	-osis
15. **hypo/derm/ic** hī-pō-DĔR-mĭk	hypo-		derm	-ic

Section Review 1–3

1. peridental
2. abnormal
3. hepatitis
4. suprarenal
5. transvaginal
6. gastrointestinal
7. macrocephalic
8. renopathy
9. thermometer
10. hepatomegaly
11. substernal
12. hypoinsulinism
13. gastroenteropathy
14. arteriosclerosis
15. hypodermic

Section Review 1–4

Singular	Plural	Rule
1. **sarcoma** săr-KŌ-mă	sarcomata	Retain the *ma* and add *ta*
2. **thrombus** THRŎM-bŭs	thrombi	Drop *us* and add *i*
3. **appendix** ă-PĔN-dĭks	appendices	Drop *ix* and add *ices*
4. **diverticulum** dī-vĕr-TĬK-ū-lŭm	diverticula	Drop *um* and add *a*
5. **ovary** Ō-vă-rē	ovaries	Drop *y* and add *ies*
6. **diagnosis** dī-ăg-NŌ-sĭs	diagnoses	Drop *is* and add *es*
7. **lumen** LŪ-mĕn	lumina	Drop *en* and add *ina*
8. **vertebra** VĔR-tĕ-bră	vertebrae	Retain the *a* and add *e*
9. **thorax** THŌ-răks	thoraces	Drop the *x* and add *ces*
10. **spermatozoon** spĕr-măt-ō-ZŌ-ŏn	spermatozoa	Drop *on* and add *a*

Chapter 2: Body Structure

Section Review 2–1

Term	Meaning
1. dist/al	*-al:* pertaining to, relating to; far, farthest
2. poster/ior	*-ior:* pertaining to, relating to; back (of body), behind, posterior
3. hist/o/logist	*-logist:* specialist in study of; tissue
4. dors/al	*-al:* pertaining to, relating to; back (of body)
5. anter/ior	*-ior:* pertaining to, relating to; anterior, front
6. later/al	*-al:* pertaining to, relating to; side, to one side
7. medi/ad	*-ad:* toward; middle
8. cyt/o/toxic	*-toxic:* poison; cell
9. proxim/al	*-al:* pertaining to, relating to; near, nearest
10. ventr/al	*-al:* pertaining to, relating to; belly, belly side

Section Review 2–2

1. hist/o
2. -al, -ior
3. medi/o
4. proxim/o
5. -logy
6. cyt/o
7. ventr/o
8. -toxic
9. -ad
10. caud/o
11. -logist
12. dist/o
13. infer/o
14. -lysis
15. later/o

Section Review 2–3

Term	Meaning
1. ili/ac	*-ac:* pertaining to, relating to; ilium (lateral, flaring portion of hip bone)
2. abdomin/al	*-al:* pertaining to, relating to; abdomen
3. inguin/al	*-al:* pertaining to, relating to; groin
4. spin/al	*-al:* pertaining to, relating to; spine
5. peri/umbilic/al	*-al:* pertaining to, relating to; around; umbilicus, navel
6. cephal/ad	*-ad:* toward; head
7. gastr/ic	*-ic:* pertaining to, relating to; stomach
8. thorac/ic	*-ic:* pertaining to, relating to; chest
9. cervic/al	*-al:* pertaining to, relating to; neck, cervix uteri (neck of uterus)
10. lumb/ar	*-ar:* pertaining to, relating to; loins (lower back)

Section Review 2–4

1. -ad
2. inguin/o
3. gastr/o
4. pelv/o
5. chondr/o
6. epi-
7. -ac, -al, ic, -ior
8. lumb/o
9. thorac/o
10. hypo-
11. crani/o
12. spin/o
13. ili/o
14. poster/o
15. abdomin/o

Chapter 2 Pathological, Diagnostic, and Therapeutic Terms Review

1. CT scan
2. fluoroscopy
3. US
4. MRI
5. PET
6. endoscope
7. anastomosis
8. SPECT
9. tomography
10. radiopharmaceutical
11. endoscopy
12. cauterize
13. adhesion
14. radiography
15. sepsis

Chapter 3: Integumentary System

Section Review 3–1

Term	Meaning
1. hypo/derm/ic	*-ic:* pertaining to, relating to; under, below, deficient; skin
2. melan/oma	*-oma:* tumor; black
3. kerat/osis	*-osis:* abnormal condition, increase (used primarily with blood cells); horny tissue, hard, cornea
4. cutane/ous	*-ous:* pertaining to, relating to; skin
5. lip/o/cyte	*-cyte:* cell; fat
6. onych/o/malacia	*-malacia:* softening; nail
7. scler/o/derma	*-derma:* skin; hardening, sclera (white of eye)
8. dia/phoresis	*-phoresis:* carrying, transmission; through, across
9. dermat/o/myc/osis	*-osis:* abnormal condition, increase (used primarily with blood cells); skin; fungus
10. cry/o/therapy	*-therapy:* treatment; cold

Competency Verification, Figure 3–2: Identifying Integumentary Structures (page 65)

1. epidermis
2. dermis
3. stratum corneum
4. basal layer
5. hair follicle
6. sebaceous (oil) gland
7. sudoriferous (sweat) gland
8. subcutaneous tissue

Competency Verification, Figure 3–3: Structure of a Fingernail (page 71)

1. nail root
2. matrix
3. cuticle
4. nail bed
5. nail body
6. lunula

Section Review 3–2

1. -pathy
2. xer/o
3. lip/o, adip/o, steat/o
4. -rrhea
5. trich/o, pil/o
6. scler/o
7. -cele
8. onych/o
9. derm/o, dermat/o, cutane/o, -derma
10. -malacia
11. -logist
12. epi-
13. -osis
14. hidr/o
15. hypo-

Section Review 3–3

1. melan/o	4. cyt/o, -cyte	7. -rrhea	10. -derma	13. xanth/o
2. cyan/o	5. -penia	8. erythr/o	11. -oma	14. necr/o
3. -emia	6. -pathy	9. auto-	12. leuk/o	15. -osis

Chapter 3 Pathological, Diagnostic, and Therapeutic Terms Review

1. wart	4. decubitus ulcer	7. biopsy	10. cryosurgery	13. alopecia
2. vitiligo	5. eczema	8. dermabrasion	11. debridement	14. comedo
3. tinea	6. urticaria	9. electrodesiccation	12. scabies	15. petechia

Medical Record Activity 3–1: Compound Nevus

Evaluation 3–1: Compound Nevus

1. What is a nevus?
   A mole; a type of skin tumor.

2. Locate the vermilion border on your lip. Where is it located?
   It is the edge of the red portion of the upper or lower lip.

3. Was the lesion limited to a certain area?
   Yes, the right side of the lower lip.

4. In the impression, the pathologist has ruled out melanoma. What does this mean?
   The nevus is not cancerous even though it appears to be.

5. Is a melanoma a dangerous condition? If so, explain why.
   Yes, it metastasizes rapidly.

Medical Record Activity 3–2: Psoriasis

Evaluation 3–2: Psoriasis

1. What causes psoriasis?
   The etiology is unknown, but heredity is a significant determining factor.

2. On what parts of the body does psoriasis typically occur?
   Scalp; elbows; knees; sacrum; around the nails, arms, and legs.

3. How is psoriasis treated?
   Mild to moderate psoriasis is treated with corticosteroids and phototherapy.

4. What is a histiocytoma?
   A tumor containing histiocytes, a macrophage present in all loose connective tissue.

Chapter 3 Vocabulary Review

1. subcutaneous
2. diaphoresis
3. trichopathy
4. autograft
5. Kaposi sarcoma
6. suction lipectomy
7. onychomycosis
8. decubitus ulcer
9. leukemia
10. ecchymosis
11. onychoma
12. hirsutism
13. pustule
14. papules
15. erythrocyte
16. xeroderma
17. melanoma
18. lipocele
19. xanthoma
20. onychomalacia

Chapter 4: Respiratory System

Section Review 4–1

Term	Meaning
1. laryng/o/scope	*-scope:* instrument for examining; larynx (voice box)
2. py/o/thorax	*-thorax:* chest; pus
3. hyp/oxia	*-oxia:* oxygen; under, below, deficient
4. trache/o/stomy	*-stomy:* forming an opening (mouth); trachea (windpipe)
5. a/pnea	*-pnea:* breathing; without, not
6. pulmon/o/logist	*-logist:* specialist in study of; lung
7. pneumon/ia	*-ia:* condition; air, lung
8. rhin/o/rrhea	*-rrhea:* discharge, flow; nose
9. an/osmia	*-osmia:* smell; without, not
10. pneum/ectomy	*-ectomy:* excision, removal; air, lung

Section Review 4–2

1. aer/o
2. para-
3. myc/o
4. -ectasis
5. -stomy
6. -tomy
7. -tome
8. laryng/o
9. -cele
10. neo-
11. nas/o, rhin/o
12. -plegia
13. pharyng/o
14. -stenosis
15. -phagia
16. trache/o
17. -therapy
18. a-, an-
19. -scopy
20. hydr/o

Competency Verification, Figure 4–2: Identifying the Upper and Lower Respiratory Tracts (page 107)

1. nasal cavity
2. pharynx (throat)
3. larynx (voice box)
4. epiglottis
5. trachea (windpipe)
6. right and left primary bronchi
7. bronchioles
8. left lung
9. alveoli
10. pulmonary capillaries
11. pleura
12. diaphragm

Section Review 4–3

1. -osis	6. bronch/o, bronchi/o	11. myc/o	16. macro-	21. orth/o
2. brady-	7. hem/o	12. eu-	17. tachy-	22. -stenosis
3. dys-	8. thorac/o	13. -cele	18. pneum/o, pneumon/o	23. -centesis
4. melan/o	9. -ectasis	14. -scope	19. pleur/o	24. a-
5. -pnea	10. -phobia	15. -spasm	20. micro-	25. chondr/o

Chapter 4 Pathological, Diagnostic, and Therapeutic Terms Review

1. stridor	6. cystic fibrosis	11. bronchodilators	16. pertussis
2. epistaxis	7. lung cancer	12. ARDS	17. CT scan
3. influenza	8. pleural effusion	13. MRI	18. SIDS
4. acidosis	9. pneumothorax	14. atelectasis	19. hypoxia
5. coryza	10. crackle	15. epiglottitis	20. rhonchi

Medical Record Activity 4–1: Papillary Carcinoma

Evaluation 4–1: Papillary Carcinoma

1. What types of patients are at risk for nasal polyps?
   Patients with chronic inflammation of the nasal and sinus mucosa that is usually due to allergies.

2. When is a polypectomy indicated?
   When the patient fails to respond to medical treatment or if there is severe nasal obstruction.

3. Were the patient's nasal polyps cancerous?
   No, polyps are benign.

4. What contributed to the patient's death?
   Papillary carcinoma that metastasized to the lymph node.

5. Why was a biopsy of the liver performed?
   To check for metastasis.

Medical Record Activity 4–2: Lobar Pneumonia

Evaluation 4–2: Lobar Pneumonia

1. What physical examination techniques are useful in this case?
   Inspection, palpation, percussion, and auscultation.

2. What explains the unilateral chest expansion?
   The affected lung doesn't expand with inspiration.

3. What explains the decrease in resonance and increase in tactile fremitus?
   The tissue underlying the chest wall in the affected region is dense.

4. What is the significance of bronchial breath sounds in this case?
   They are consistent with lung consolidation.

5. What laboratory data are useful to confirm the diagnosis?
   Chest x-ray, arterial blood gas analysis, sputum Gram stain with culture and sensitivity, and complete blood count.

Chapter 4 Vocabulary Review

1. pyothorax	7. apnea	12. anosmia	17. rhinoplasty
2. thoracentesis	8. aerophagia	13. pharyngoplegia	18. TB
3. asthma	9. aspirate	14. pleurisy	19. COLD
4. croup	10. chondroma	15. *Pneumocystis carinii*	20. pneumothorax
5. tracheostomy	11. atelectasis	16. catheter	
6. diagnosis			

Chapter 5: Cardiovascular and Lymphatic Systems

Section Review 5–1

Term	Meaning
1. endo/cardi/um	*-um:* structure, thing; in, within; heart
2. cardi/o/megaly	*-megaly:* enlargement; heart
3. aort/o/stenosis	*-stenosis:* narrowing, stricture; aorta
4. tachy/cardia	*-cardia:* heart condition; rapid
5. phleb/itis	*-itis:* inflammation; vein
6. thromb/o/lysis	*-lysis:* separation, destruction, loosening; blood clot
7. vas/o/spasm	*-spasm:* involuntary contraction, twitching; vessel, vas deferens, duct
8. ather/oma	*-oma:* tumor; fatty plaque
9. electr/o/cardi/o/graphy	*-graphy:* process of recording; electricity; heart
10. atri/o/ventricul/ar	*-ar:* pertaining to, relating to; atrium; ventricle (of heart or brain)

Competency Verification, Figure 5–2: Heart Structures (page 149)

1. endocardium	6. superior vena cava	11. right pulmonary veins
2. myocardium	7. inferior vena cava	12. left pulmonary veins
3. pericardium	8. pulmonary trunk	
4. aorta	9. right lung	
5. right atrium	10. left lung	

Competency Verification, Figure 5–3: Internal Structures of the Heart (page 151)

1. right atrium (RA)
2. left atrium (LA)
3. right ventricle (RV)
4. left ventricle (LV)
5. interventricular septum (IVS)
6. superior vena cava (SVC)
7. inferior vena cava (IVC)
8. tricuspid valve
9. pulmonary valve
10. right pulmonary artery; left pulmonary artery
11. right pulmonary veins; left pulmonary veins
12. mitral valve
13. aortic valve
14. aorta
15. branches of the aorta
16. descending aorta

Competency Verification, Figure 5–4: Heart Structures Depicting Valves and Cusps (page 159)

1. tricuspid valve
2. mitral valve
3. chordae tendineae
4. pulmonary valve
5. aortic valve
6. three cusps
7. two cusps

Section Review 5–2

1. -osis
2. epi-
3. aort/o
4. peri-
5. arteri/o
6. atri/o
7. hem/o, hemat/o
8. -pnea
9. -pathy
10. -ectasis
11. scler/o
12. cardi/o
13. -spasm
14. my/o
15. tachy-
16. -rrhexis
17. brady-
18. -ole, -ule
19. -rrhaphy
20. -stenosis
21. -phagia
22. tri-
23. bi-
24. phleb/o, ven/o
25. ventricul/o

Competency Verification, Figure 5–5: Conduction Pathway of the Heart (page 163)

1. sinoatrial (SA) node
2. right atrium (RA)
3. atrioventricular (AV) node
4. bundle of His
5. bundle branches
6. Purkinje fibers

Section Review 5–3

Term	Meaning
1. agglutin/ation	*-ation:* process (of); clumping, gluing
2. thym/oma	*-oma:* tumor; thymus gland
3. phag/o/cyte	*-cyte:* cell; swallowing, eating
4. lymphaden/itis	*-itis:* inflammation; lymph gland (node)
5. splen/o/megaly	*-megaly:* enlargement; spleen
6. aden/o/pathy	*-pathy:* disease; gland
7. ana/phylaxis	*-phylaxis:* protection; against, up, back
8. lymphangi/oma	*-oma:* tumor; lymph vessel
9. lymph/o/poiesis	*-poiesis:* formation, production; lymph
10. immun/o/gen	*-gen:* forming, producing, origin; immune, immunity, safe

Competency Verification, Figure 5–8: Lymphatic System (page 173)

1. lymph capillaries
2. lymph vessels
3. thoracic duct
4. right lymphatic duct
5. cervical nodes
6. axillary nodes
7. inguinal nodes

Section Review 5–4

1. aort/o
2. hem/o
3. thromb/o
4. -cyte
5. cerebr/o
6. necr/o
7. -pathy
8. electr/o
9. -megaly
10. cardi/o
11. lymph/o
12. my/o
13. -graphy
14. -gram
15. -al, -ic
16. -rrhexis
17. -lysis
18. -stenosis
19. -plasty
20. angi/o

Chapter 5 Pathological, Diagnostic, and Therapeutic Terms Review

1. varicose veins
2. mononucleosis
3. thrombolytic therapy
4. embolus
5. lymphadenitis
6. DVT
7. hypertension
8. arrhythmia
9. TIA
10. bruit
11. stroke
12. rheumatic heart disease
13. atherosclerosis
14. Holter monitor
15. Raynaud phenomenon
16. ischemia
17. Hodgkin disease
18. AIDS
19. heart failure (HF)
20. fibrillation
21. valvuloplasty
22. lymphangiography
23. tissue typing
24. troponin I
25. CABG

Medical Record Activity 5–1: Myocardial Infarction

Evaluation 5–1: Myocardial Infarction

1. What symptoms did the patient experience before admission to the hospital?
Generalized malaise, increased shortness of breath (SOB) while at rest, and dyspnea followed by periods of apnea and syncope.

2. What was found during clinical examination?
Irregular radial pulse, uncontrolled atrial fibrillation with evidence of a recent myocardial infarction (MI).

3. What is the danger of atrial fibrillation?
A decrease in cardiac output and promotion of thrombus formation in the upper chambers.

4. Did the patient have prior history of heart problems? If so, describe them.
Yes, sinus tachycardia attributed to preoperative anxiety and thyroiditis.

5. Was the patient's prior heart problem related to her current one?
No.

Medical Record Activity 5–2: Cardiac Catheterization

Evaluation 5–2: Cardiac Catheterization

1. What coronary arteries were under examination?
The left and right coronary arteries.

2. Which surgical procedure was used to clear the stenosis?
Balloon angioplasty.

3. What symptoms did the patient exhibit before balloon inflation?
The patient had significant ST elevations in the inferior leads and severe throat tightness and shortness of breath.

4. Why was the patient put on heparin?
To dissolve any blood clots that may be present and to prevent postsurgical clots from forming.

Chapter 5 Vocabulary Review

1. myocardium
2. tachypnea
3. arteriosclerosis
4. phagocyte
5. systole
6. diastole
7. EKG
8. malaise
9. desiccated
10. cardiomegaly
11. aneurysm
12. angina pectoris
13. MI
14. agglutination
15. tachyphagia
16. anaphylaxis
17. capillaries
18. hemangioma
19. arterioles
20. pacemaker

Chapter 6: Digestive System

Section Review 6–1

Term	Meaning
1. gingiv/itis	*-itis:* inflammation; gum(s)
2. dys/pepsia	*-pepsia:* digestion; bad, painful, difficult
3. pylor/o/tomy	*-tomy:* incision, pylorus
4. dent/ist	*-ist:* specialist; teeth
5. esophag/o/scope	*-scope:* instrument for examining; esophagus
6. gastr/o/scopy	*-scopy:* visual examination; stomach
7. dia/rrhea	*-rrhea:* discharge, flow; through, across
8. hyper/emesis	*-emesis:* vomiting; excessive, above normal
9. an/orexia	*-orexia:* appetite; without, not
10. sub/lingu/al	*-al:* pertaining to, relating to; under, below; tongue

Competency Verification, Figure 6–2: The Oral Cavity, Esophagus, Pharynx, and Stomach (page 203)

1. oral cavity
2. sublingual gland
3. submandibular gland
4. parotid gland
5. bolus
6. pharynx (throat)
7. esophagus
8. stomach

Section Review 6–2

1. -oma
2. -al, -ary, -ic
3. peri-
4. hypo-
5. -rrhea
6. myc/o
7. gingiv/o
8. pylor/o
9. dys-
10. hyper-
11. sial/o
12. gastr/o
13. -ist
14. orth/o
15. dent/o, odont/o
16. dia-
17. lingu/o, gloss/o
18. -scope
19. -tomy
20. -orexia
21. stomat/o, or/o
22. -algia, -dynia
23. -phagia
24. an-
25. -pepsia

Section Review 6–3

Term	Meaning
1. duoden/o/scopy	*-scopy:* visual examination; duodenum (first part of small intestine)
2. appendic/itis	*-itis:* inflammation; appendix
3. enter/o/pathy	*-pathy:* disease; intestine (usually small intestine)
4. col/o/stomy	*-stomy:* forming an opening (mouth); colon
5. rect/o/cele	*-cele:* hernia, swelling; rectum
6. sigmoid/o/tomy	*-tomy:* incision; sigmoid colon
7. proct/o/logist	*-logist:* specialist in study of; anus, rectum
8. jejun/o/rrhaphy	*-rrhaphy:* suture; jejunum (second part of small intestine)
9. append/ectomy	*-ectomy:* excision, removal; appendix
10. ile/o/stomy	*-stomy:* forming an opening (mouth); ileum (third part of small intestine)

Competency Verification, Figure 6–3: The Small Intestine and Colon (page 215)

1. duodenum
2. jejunum
3. ileum
4. ascending colon
5. transverse colon
6. descending colon
7. sigmoid colon
8. rectum
9. anus

Section Review 6–4

1. enter/o
2. -tome
3. rect/o
4. -spasm
5. ile/o
6. -scopy
7. jejun/o
8. col/o, colon/o
9. duoden/o
10. -stomy
11. proct/o
12. -stenosis
13. -rrhaphy
14. -tomy
15. sigmoid/o

Section Review 6–5

Term	Meaning
1. hepat/itis	*-itis:* inflammation; liver
2. hepat/o/megaly	*-megaly:* enlargement; liver
3. chol/e/lith*	*-lith:* stone, calculus; bile, gall
4. cholangi/ole	*-ole:* small, minute; bile vessel
5. cholecyst/ectomy	*-ectomy:* excision, removal; gallbladder
6. post/prandial	*-prandial:* meal; after, behind
7. chol/e/lith/iasis*	*-iasis:* abnormal condition (produced by something specified); bile, gall; stone, calculus
8. choledoch/o/tomy	*-tomy:* incision; bile duct
9. pancreat/o/lith	*-lith:* stone, calculus; pancreas
10. pancreat/o/lysis	*-lysis:* separation, destruction, loosening; pancreas

*The combining vowel *e* is used instead of *o.* This is an exception to the rule.

Competency Verification, Figure 6–6: The Liver, Gallbladder, Pancreas, and Duodenum with Associated Ducts and Blood Vessels (page 229)

1. liver
2. gallbladder
3. pancreas
4. duodenum
5. common bile duct
6. right hepatic duct
7. left hepatic duct
8. hepatic duct
9. cystic duct
10. pancreatic duct

Section Review 6–6

1. -osis
2. -iasis
3. choledoch/o
4. chol/e
5. cyst/o
6. -megaly
7. -ectomy
8. -stomy
9. cholecyst/o
10. therm/o
11. hepat/o
12. -algia, -dynia
13. pancreat/o
14. toxic/o, tox/o, -toxic
15. -graphy
16. -gram
17. -lith
18. -plasty
19. -rrhaphy
20. -emesis

Chapter 6 Pathological, Diagnostic, and Therapeutic Terms Review

1. hemoccult
2. nasogastric intubation
3. colonic polyposis
4. ascites
5. Crohn disease
6. lithotripsy
7. fistula
8. jaundice
9. barium enema
10. inflammatory bowel disease (IBD)
11. hematochezia
12. volvulus
13. cirrhosis
14. barium swallow
15. irritable bowel syndrome (IBS)

Medical Record Activity 6–1: Rectal Bleeding

Evaluation 6–1: Rectal Bleeding

1. What is the patient's symptom that made him seek medical help?
   Weight loss of 40 pounds since his last examination.

2. What surgical procedures were performed on the patient for his regional enteritis?
   Ileostomy and appendectomy.

3. What abnormality was found with the sigmoidoscopy?
   Dark blood and rectal bleeding.

4. What is causing the rectal bleeding?
   It could be due to a polyp, bleeding, diverticulum, or rectal carcinoma.

5. Write the plural form of diverticulum.
   Diverticula.

Medical Record Activity 6–2: Carcinosarcoma of the Esophagus

Evaluation 6–2: Carcinosarcoma of the Esophagus

1. What surgery was performed on this patient?
   Resection of the esophagus with anastomosis of the stomach; lymph node excision.

2. What diagnostic testing confirmed malignancy?
   Pathology tests on the biopsy specimen.

3. Where was the carcinosarcoma located?
   Middle third of the esophagus.

4. Why was the adjacent lymph node excised?
   Metastasis was suspected.

Chapter 6 Vocabulary Review

1. gastroscopy	11. cholecystectomy
2. dyspepsia	12. anastomosis
3. hematemesis	13. sigmoidotomy
4. ultrasound	14. rectoplasty
5. salivary glands	15. stomach
6. alimentary canal	16. ileostomy
7. stomatalgia	17. cholelithiasis
8. duodenotomy	18. friable
9. hepatomegaly	19. choledoch
10. dysphagia	20. sigmoid colon

Chapter 7: Urinary System

Section Review 7–1

Term	Meaning
1. glomerul/o/scler/osis	*-osis:* abnormal condition, increase (used primarily with blood cells); glomerulus; hardening, sclera (white of eye)
2. cyst/o/scopy	*-scopy:* visual examination; bladder
3. poly/uria	*-uria:* urine; many, much
4. lith/o/tripsy	*-tripsy:* crushing; stone, calculus
5. dia/lysis	*-lysis:* separation, destruction, loosening; through, across
6. ureter/o/stenosis	*-stenosis:* narrowing, stricture; ureter
7. meat/us	*-us:* condition, structure; opening, meatus
8. ur/emia	*-emia:* blood condition; urine
9. nephr/oma	*-oma:* tumor: kidney
10. ureter/o/cele	*-cele:* hernia, swelling; ureter

Section Review 7–2

1. -osis
2. -iasis
3. supra-
4. -pathy
5. -megaly
6. dia-
7. -pexy
8. scler/o
9. -tome
10. -tomy
11. nephr/o, ren/o
12. -ptosis
13. lith/o
14. -rrhaphy
15. poly-

Competency Verification, Figure 7–2: Urinary System (page 261)

1. right kidney
2. renal cortex
3. renal medulla
4. renal artery
5. renal vein
6. nephron
7. ureters
8. urinary bladder
9. urethra
10. urinary meatus

Section Review 7–3

1. -iasis
2. cyst/o, vesic/o
3. carcin/o
4. -pathy
5. -megaly
6. -ectomy
7. -ectasis
8. aden/o
9. -tomy
10. -itis
11. -scope
12. enter/o
13. pyel/o
14. rect/o
15. -lith
16. -plasty
17. -rrhaphy
18. -oma
19. ureter/o
20. urethr/o

Competency Verification, Figure 7–5: Nephron Structure (page 276)

1. renal cortex
2. renal medulla
3. glomerulus
4. collecting tubule
5. Bowman capsule

Section Review 7–4

1. cyst/o, vesic/o
2. hemat/o
3. cyt/o, -cyte
4. glomerul/o
5. scler/o
6. -ist
7. nephr/o, ren/o
8. py/o
9. erythr/o
10. pyel/o
11. olig/o
12. ureter/o
13. urethr/o
14. ur/o
15. leuk/o
16. -cele
17. poly-
18. -ptosis
19. intra-
20. a-, an-

Chapter 7 Pathological, Diagnostic, and Therapeutic Terms Review

1. urinalysis
2. Wilms tumor
3. azoturia
4. dysuria
5. diuresis
6. retrograde pyelography
7. hypospadias
8. interstitial nephritis
9. blood urea nitrogen
10. enuresis
11. catheterization
12. voiding cystourography
13. uremia
14. renal hypertension
15. CT scan

Medical Record Activity 7–1: Cystitis

Evaluation 7–1: Cystitis

1. What was found when the patient had a cystoscopy?
   Cystitis.

2. What are the symptoms of cystitis?
   Nocturia, urinary frequency, pelvic pain, and hematuria, in this case.

3. What is the patient's past surgical history?
   Cholecystectomy, choledocholithotomy, and incidental appendectomy.

4. What is the treatment for cystitis?
   Antibiotics and consumption of a lot of fluids.

5. What are the dangers of untreated cystitis?
   The spreading of infection to the kidneys or to the bloodstream (sepsis).

6. What instrument is used to perform a cystoscopy?
   A cystoscope.

Medical Record Activity 7–2: Benign Prostatic Hypertrophy

Evaluation 7–2: Benign Prostatic Hypertrophy

1. What prompted the consultation with the urologist, Dr. Moriarty?
   Preoperative catheterization was not possible and consultation with Dr. Moriarty was obtained.

2. What abnormality did the urologist discover?
   Mild to moderate benign prostatic hypertrophy.

3. Did the patient have any previous surgery on the prostate?
   No.

4. Where was the patient's hernia?
   In the groin and scrotum (hydrocele).

5. What in the patient's past medical history contributed to his present urological problem?
   Nothing in his past history contributed to his benign prostatic hypertrophy; he had a previous colon resection for carcinoma of the colon.

Chapter 7 Vocabulary Review

1. malignant	6. diuretics	11. nephroptosis	16. hematuria
2. nephrons	7. edema	12. ureteropyeloplasty	17. polyuria
3. cholelithiasis	8. benign	13. bilateral	18. oliguria
4. renal pelvis	9. nephrolithotomy	14. nocturia	19. anuria
5. IVP	10. acute renal failure	15. urinary incontinence	20. cystocele

Chapter 8: Reproductive Systems

Section Review 8–1

Term	Definition
1. primi/gravida	*-gravida:* pregnant woman; first
2. colp/o/scopy	*-scopy:* visual examination; vagina
3. gynec/o/logist	*-logist:* specialist in study of; woman, female
4. perine/o/rrhaphy	*-rrhaphy:* suture; perineum
5. hyster/ectomy	*-ectomy:* excision, removal; uterus (womb)
6. oophor/oma	*-oma:* tumor; ovary
7. dys/tocia	*-tocia:* childbirth, labor; bad, painful, difficult
8. endo/metr/itis	*-itis:* inflammation; in, within; uterus (womb), measure
9. mamm/o/gram	*-gram:* record, writing; breast
10. amni/o/centesis	*-centesis:* surgical puncture; amnion (amniotic sac)

Section Review 8–2

1. cyst/o	6. -tomy	11. muc/o	16. -oid
2. hemat/o, hem/o	7. -tome	12. oophor/o, ovari/o	17. -logist
3. -rrhage, -rrhagia	8. -scope	13. -arche	18. -logy
4. hyster/o, uter/o	9. salping/o, -salpinx	14. metr/o	19. -plasty
5. -cele	10. -pexy	15. -ptosis	20. colp/o, vagin/o

Competency Verification, Figures 8–2 and 8–3: Female Reproductive System, Lateral View; and Female Reproductive System, Anterior View (pages 308, 309)

1. ovary (singular)	6. labia minora
2. fallopian tube (singular)	7. clitoris
3. uterus	8. Bartholin gland
4. vagina	9. cervix
5. labia majora	

Competency Verification, Figure 8–5, Structure of Mammary Glands (page 321)

1. adipose tissue	4. lactiferous duct
2. glandular tissue	5. nipple
3. lobe	6. areola

Section Review 8–3

1. post-	11. -scopy
2. gynec/o	12. men/o
3. pre-	13. cervic/o
4. mamm/o, mast/o	14. -algia, -dynia
5. -pathy	15. -ary, -ous
6. -ectomy	16. -logist
7. -rrhea	17. salping/o
8. -itis	18. colp/o, vagin/o
9. -tome	19. vulv/o, episi/o
10. -scope	20. dys-

Section Review 8–4

Term	Meaning
1. vas/ectomy	*-ectomy:* excision, removal; vessel, vas deferens, duct
2. balan/itis	*-itis:* inflammation; glans penis
3. spermat/o/cide	*-cide:* killing; spermatozoa, sperm cells
4. gonad/o/tropin	*-tropin:* stimulate; gonads, sex glands
5. orchi/o/pexy	*-pexy:* fixation (of an organ); testis (plural, testes)
6. a/sperm/ia	*-ia:* condition; without, not; spermatozoa, sperm cells
7. vesicul/itis	*-itis:* inflammation; seminal vesicle
8. orchid/ectomy	*-ectomy:* excision, removal; testis (plural, testes)
9. andr/o/gen	*-gen:* forming, producing, origin; male
10. crypt/orch/ism	*-ism:* condition; hidden; testis (plural, testes)

Competency Verification, Figure 8–7: The Male Reproductive System (page 330)

1. testis (singular) or testicle (singular)
2. scrotum
3. epididymis
4. vas deferens
5. seminal vesicle
6. prostate gland
7. bulbourethral gland
8. penis
9. glans penis
10. foreskin

Section Review 8–5

1. -rrhaphy
2. dys-
3. cyst/o
4. carcin/o
5. -cyte
6. -pathy
7. -megaly
8. -cele
9. -itis
10. -tome
11. vas/o
12. muc/o
13. neo-
14. -genesis
15. prostat/o
16. test/o, orchi/o, orchid/o
17. olig/o
18. spermat/o, sperm/o
19. -pexy
20. hyper-

Chapter 8 Pathological, Diagnostic, and Therapeutic Terms Review

1. cryptorchidism
2. pyosalpinx
3. sterility
4. anorchism
5. candidiasis
6. chlamydia
7. circumcision
8. benign prostatic hypertrophy (BPH)
9. leukorrhea
10. endometriosis
11. mammography
12. gonorrhea
13. syphilis
14. toxic shock syndrome
15. trichomoniasis
16. dilation and curettage (D&C)
17. phimosis
18. impotence
19. oligomenorrhea
20. gonadotropins

Medical Record Activity 8–1: Postmenopausal Bleeding

Evaluation 8–1: Postmenopausal Bleeding

1. How many times has the patient been pregnant? How many children has the patient given birth to?
   Four; four.

2. Why is the patient being admitted to the hospital?
   To have a gynecological laparoscopy and diagnostic D&C, to rule out the neoplastic process.

3. What is a D&C?
   Dilation and curettage; a surgical procedure that expands the cervical canal of the uterus so that the surface lining of the uterine wall can be scraped.

4. What is the patient's past surgical history?
   Simple mastectomy last year.

5. At what sites did the patient have malignant growth?
   Left breast with metastases to the axilla, liver, and bone.

Medical Record Activity 8–2: Bilateral Vasectomy

Evaluation 8–2: Bilateral Vasectomy

1. What is the end result of a bilateral vasectomy?
   Sterilization.

2. Was the patient awake during the surgery? What type of anesthesia was used?
   Yes, 1% Xylocaine.

3. What was used to prevent bleeding?
   Hemostat.

4. What type of suture material was used to close the incision?
   3–0 chromic.

5. What was the patient given for pain relief at home?
   Darvocet-N 100.

6. Why is it important for the patient to go for a follow-up visit?
   To analyze his semen and confirm sterilization.

Chapter 8 Vocabulary Review

1. prostatomegaly
2. testopathy
3. testosterone
4. amenorrhea
5. estrogen, progesterone
6. oophoritis
7. aspermatism
8. gravida 4
9. uterus
10. prostatic cancer
11. epididymis
12. hydrocele
13. vas deferens
14. para 4
15. cervix uteri
16. dysmenorrhea
17. postmenopausal
18. aplasia
19. vasectomy
20. pelvic inflammatory disease (PID)

Chapter 9: Endocrine and Nervous Systems

Section Review 9–1

Term	Definition
1. toxic/o/logist	*-logist:* specialist in study of; poison
2. pancreat/itis	*-itis:* inflammation; pancreas
3. thyr/o/megaly	*-megaly:* enlargement; thyroid gland
4. hyper/trophy	*-trophy:* development, nourishment; excessive, above normal
5. gluc/o/genesis	*-genesis:* forming, producing, origin; sugar, sweetness
6. hypo/calc/emia	*-emia:* blood condition; under, below, deficient; calcium
7. adrenal/ectomy	*-ectomy:* excision, removal; adrenal glands
8. poly/dipsia	*-dipsia:* thirst; many, much
9. aden/oma	*-oma:* tumor; gland
10. thyroid/ectomy	*-ectomy:* excision, removal; thyroid gland

Section Review 9–2

1. -osis	6. calc/o	11. aden/o	16. radi/o
2. hyper-	7. -pathy	12. -tomy	17. -logist
3. poster/o	8. -megaly	13. -tome	18. poly-
4. dys-	9. acr/o	14. neur/o	19. thyroid/o, thyr/o
5. -emia	10. anter/o	15. toxic/o	20. hypo-

Competency Verification, Figure 9–3: Locations of Major Endocrine Glands (page 367)

1. pituitary gland	4. adrenal glands	7. thymus gland
2. thyroid gland	5. pancreas	8. ovaries
3. parathyroid glands	6. pineal gland	9. testes

Section Review 9–3

1. -iasis	6. -rrhea	11. -lysis	16. -dipsia
2. supra-	7. poly-	12. -lith	17. thym/o
3. adrenal/o, adren/o	8. para-	13. gluc/o, glyc/o	18. hypo-
4. -pathy	9. pancreat/o	14. -phagia	19. -uria
5. -pexy	10. -gen, -genesis	15. orch/o, orchi/o orchid/o	20. toxic/o

Section Review 9–4

Term	Meaning
1. meningi/oma	*-oma:* tumor; meninges
2. neur/o/lysis	*-lysis:* separation, destruction, loosening; nerve
3. hemi/paresis	*-paresis:* partial paralysis; one half
4. myel/algia	*-algia:* pain; bone marrow, spinal cord
5. cerebr/o/spin/al	*-al:* pertaining to, relating to; cerebrum; spine
6. a/phasia	*-phasia:* speech; without, not
7. mening/o/cele	*-cele:* hernia, swelling; meninges
8. encephal/itis	*-itis:* inflammation; brain
9. gli/oma	*-oma:* tumor; glue, neuroglial tissue
10. quadri/plegia	*-plegia:* paralysis; four

Section Review 9–5

1. -osis
2. dys-
3. thromb/o
4. vascul/o
5. encephal/o

6. -rrhage, -rrhagia
7. gli/o, -glia
8. scler/o
9. mening/o, meningi/o
10. neur/o

11. cerebr/o
12. -malacia
13. -phasia
14. myel/o
15. a-

Chapter 9 Pathological, Diagnostic, and Therapeutic Terms Review

1. Bell palsy
2. CVA
3. epilepsy
4. exophthalmos
5. Graves disease
6. insulinoma
7. myxedema
8. pheochromocytoma
9. Parkinson disease
10. poliomyelitis
11. sciatica
12. spina bifida
13. hydrocephalus

14. neuroblastoma
15. Alzheimer disease
16. MRI
17. type 1 diabetes
18. shingles
19. pituitarism
20. panhypopituitarism
21. Huntington chorea
22. Cushing syndrome
23. CT scan
24. thalamotomy
25. PET

Medical Record Activity 9–1: Diabetes Mellitus

Evaluation 9–1: Diabetes Mellitus

1. What symptoms of DM did the patient experience before his office visit?
   Glycosuria, elevated blood sugar of 400, polydipsia, and increased appetite.

2. What confirmed the patient's new diagnosis of DM?
   Elevated blood sugar and glycosuria.

3. What conditions had to be met before the patient could be discharged from the hospital?
   He had to be able to draw up and give his own insulin and perform fingersticks.

4. How many times a day does the patient have to take insulin?
   Two times, once in the morning and once in the afternoon.

5. Why does the patient have to perform fingersticks four times a day?
   To monitor his blood sugar levels closely and ensure they are within the normal range.

6. What is an ADA 3000-calorie diet? Why is it important?
   A 3000-calorie diet designed by the American Diabetic Association. Maintaining the same number of calories each day helps to control blood sugar levels.

Medical Record Activity 9–2: Cerebrovascular Accident

Evaluation 9–2: Cerebrovascular Accident

1. Did the patient have a history of cardiovascular problems before her CVA?
   No.

2. What symptoms did the patient experience just before her CVA?
   Paralysis of the right arm and left leg, aphasia, and diplopia.

3. What is the primary site of this patient's cancer?
   Head of the pancreas.

4. What is cerebrovascular disease?
   A disorder resulting from a change within the blood vessel(s) of the brain.

5. What is the probable cause of the patient's CVA?
   Metastatic lesion of the brain or cerebrovascular disease.

Chapter 9 Vocabulary Review

1. acromegaly
2. pancreatolysis
3. adenohypophysis
4. cerebral palsy
5. hypercalcemia
6. insulin
7. neurohypophysis
8. pancreatopathy
9. polyphagia
10. diabetes mellitus
11. hyperglycemia
12. pancreatolith
13. polydipsia
14. thyrotoxicosis
15. adrenalectomy
16. adrenaline
17. glycogenesis
18. meningocele
19. neuromalacia
20. pruritus
21. deglutition
22. vertigo
23. jaundice
24. metastasis
25. hormone

Chapter 10: Musculoskeletal System

Section Review 10–1

Term	Meaning
1. dia/physis	*-physis:* growth; through, across
2. sub/cost/al	*-al:* pertaining to, relating to; under, below; ribs
3. oste/o/malacia	*-malacia:* softening; bone
4. lamin/ectomy	*-ectomy:* removal; lamina (part of vertebral arch)
5. pelv/i/metry	*-metry:* act of measuring; pelvis
6. myel/o/cele	*-cele:* hernia, swelling; bone marrow, spinal cord
7. oste/o/porosis	*-porosis:* porous; bone
8. ankyl/osis	*-osis:* abnormal condition, increase (used primarily with blood cells); stiffness; bent, crooked
9. carp/o/ptosis	*-ptosis:* prolapse, downward displacement; carpus (wrist bones)
10. crani/o/tomy	*-tomy:* incision; cranium (skull)

Competency Verification, Figure 10–2: Longitudinal Section of a Long Bone (Femur) and Interior Bone Structure (page 417)

1. diaphysis
2. periosteum
3. compact bone
4. medullary cavity
5. distal epiphysis
6. proximal epiphysis
7. spongy bone

Section Review 10–2

1. hyper-
2. peri-
3. -emia
4. oste/o
5. chondr/o
6. calc/o
7. -cyte
8. dist/o
9. scler/o
10. -cele
11. -tomy
12. -itis
13. proxim/o
14. my/o
15. -algia, -dynia
16. -graphy
17. -genesis
18. -gram
19. -malacia
20. -logist
21. myel/o
22. -rrhaphy
23. -oma
24. hypo-
25. radi/o

Competency Verification, Figure 10–3: Anterior View of the Skeleton (page 425)

1. crani/o	6. carp/o	11. patell/o
2. stern/o	7. metacarp/o	12. tibi/o
3. cost/o	8. phalang/o	13. fibul/o
4. vertebr/o	9. pelv/i, pelv/o	14. calcane/o
5. humer/o	10. femor/o	

Competency Verification, Figure 10–4: Types of Fractures (page 428)

1. closed	5. impacted
2. open	6. complicated
3. greenstick	7. Colles
4. comminuted	8. incomplete

Competency Verification, Figure 10–5: Vertebral Column, Lateral View (page 431)

1. intervertebral disks	5. thoracic vertebrae
2. cervical vertebrae	6. lumbar vertebrae
3. atlas	7. sacrum
4. axis	8. coccyx

Section Review 10–3

1. -osis	9. lumb/o
2. oste/o	10. cervic/o
3. encephal/o	11. -um
4. thorac/o	12. cost/o
5. -pathy	13. sacr/o
6. -ectomy	14. -centesis
7. cephal/o	15. spondyl/o, vertebr/o
8. arthr/o	

Section Review 10–4

Term	Meaning
1. my/o/sarcoma	*-sarcoma:* malignant tumor of connective tissue; muscle
2. my/o/rrhaphy	*-rrhaphy:* suture; muscle
3. hemi/plegia	*-plegia:* paralysis; one half
4. ten/o/tomy	*-tomy:* incision; tendon
5. cost/o/chondr/itis	*-itis:* inflammation; ribs; cartilage
6. tend/o/lysis	*-lysis:* separation, destruction, loosening; tendon
7. my/o/pathy	*-pathy:* disease; muscle
8. lumb/o/cost/al	*-al:* pertaining to, relating to; loins (lower back); ribs
9. tendin/itis	*-itis:* inflammation; tendon
10. my/algia	*-algia:* pain; muscle

Section Review 10–5

1. -osis
2. cyst/o
3. -cyte
4. quadri-
5. hemi-
6. scler/o
7. -tomy
8. enter/o
9. hepat/o
10. my/o
11. -plegia
12. -genesis
13. -rrhexis
14. -plasty
15. -rrhaphy
16. ten/o, tendin/o, tend/o
17. -tome
18. chondr/o
19. -sarcoma
20. -lysis

Chapter 10 Pathological, Diagnostic, and Therapeutic Terms Review

1. osteoporosis
2. tendonitis
3. sprain
4. strain
5. kyphosis
6. Ewing sarcoma
7. torticollis
8. gout
9. rheumatoid arthritis
10. Paget disease
11. sequestrum
12. arthroplasty
13. crepitation
14. myasthenia gravis
15. lordosis
16. muscular dystrophy
17. contracture
18. ankylosis
19. herniated disk
20. carpal tunnel syndrome
21. sequestrectomy
22. rheumatoid factor
23. talipes
24. arthroscopy
25. scoliosis

Medical Record Activity 10–1: Degenerative, Intervertebral Disk Disease

Evaluation 10–1: Degenerative, Intervertebral Disk Disease

1. Why does the x-ray show a decreased density at L5 to S1?
   Appears that a bilateral laminectomy had been done.

2. What is the most common cause of degenerative intervertebral disk disease?
   Aging; this is a common finding in individuals 50 years old and older.

3. What happens to the gelatinous material of the disk as aging occurs?
   The gelatinous material is replaced by harder fibrocartilage.

4. What is the probable cause of the narrowing of the L3 to L4 and L4 to L5 spaces?
   Narrowing often occurs as a result of degenerative intervertebral disk disease.

Medical Record Activity 10–2: Rotator Cuff Tear, Right Shoulder

Evaluation 10–2: Rotator Cuff Tear, Right Shoulder

1. What type of arthritis did the patient have?
   Degenerative.

2. Did the patient have calcium deposits in the right shoulder?
   No.

3. What type of instrument did the physician use to visualize the glenoid labrums?
   Arthroscope.

4. What are labra?
   Liplike structures; in this case, edges or rims of bones.

5. Did the patient have any outgrowths of bone? If so, where?
   Yes, spurs were found at the inferior and anterior acromioclavicular calcifications.

6. Did they find any deposits of calcium salts within the shoulder joint?
   They were unable to visualize an intra-articular calcification.

Chapter 10 Vocabulary Review

1. radiology
2. diaphysis
3. AP
4. closed fracture
5. bilateral
6. proximal
7. articulation
8. open fracture
9. atlas
10. arthrocentesis
11. bone marrow
12. cephalometer
13. myelogram
14. myorrhexis
15. spondylomalacia
16. distal
17. radiologist
18. cervical vertebrae
19. intervertebral
20. quadriplegia

Chapter 11: Special Senses: The Eyes and Ears

Section Review 11–1

Term	Meaning
1. aniso/cor/ia	*-ia:* condition; unequal, dissimilar; pupil
2. blephar/o/ptosis	*-ptosis:* prolapse, downward displacement; eyelid
3. ambly/opia	*-opia:* vision; dull, dim
4. retin/o/pathy	*-pathy:* disease; retina
5. scler/itis	*-itis:* inflammation; hardening, sclera (white of eye)
6. ophthalm/o/scope	*-scope:* instrument for examining; eye
7. intra/ocul/ar	*-ar:* pertaining to, relating to; within, in; eye
8. dacry/o/rrhea	*-rrhea:* discharge, flow; tear, lacrimal apparatus (duct, sac, or gland)
9. dipl/opia	*-opia:* vision; double
10. blephar/o/spasm	*-spasm:* involuntary contraction, twitching; eyelid

Competency Verification, Figure 11–1: Eye Structures (page 467)

1. sclera
2. cornea
3. choroid
4. ciliary body
5. iris
6. retina
7. pupil
8. optic disk
9. optic nerve

Competency Verification, Figure 11–3: Lacrimal Apparatus (page 473)

1. lacrimal gland
2. nasolacrimal duct
3. lacrimal sac

Section Review 11–2

Term	Meaning
1. tympan/o/centesis	*-centesis:* surgical puncture; tympanic membrane (eardrum)
2. acous/tic	*-tic:* pertaining to, relating to; hearing
3. hyper/tropia	*-tropia:* turning; excessive, above normal
4. ot/o/rrhea	*-rrhea:* discharge, flow; ear
5. an/acusis	*-acusis:* hearing; without, not
6. myring/o/tomy	*-tomy:* incision; tympanic membrane (eardrum)
7. tympan/o/plasty	*-plasty:* surgical repair; tympanic membrane (eardrum)
8. audi/o/meter	*-meter:* instrument for measuring; hearing
9. ot/o/scope	*-scope:* instrument for examining; ear
10. salping/o/pharyng/eal	*-eal:* pertaining to, relating to; tube (usually fallopian or eustachian [auditory] tubes); pharynx (throat)

Competency Verification, Figure 11–4: Ear Structures (page 477)

1. auricle
2. ear canal
3. tympanic membrane
4. malleus
5. incus
6. stapes
7. eustachian (auditory) tube
8. cochlea
9. semicircular canals
10. vestibule

Section Review 11–3

1. hyper-
2. choroid/o
3. kerat/o
4. dipl/o, dipl-
5. ot/o
6. salping/o, -salpinx
7. ophthalm/o
8. blephar/o
9. aden/o
10. scler/o
11. -spasm
12. irid/o
13. -ptosis
14. -logist
15. retin/o
16. -rrhexis
17. -malacia
18. audi/o, -acusis
19. -stenosis
20. -edema
21. dacry/o
22. tympan/o, myring/o
23. corne/o
24. -opia, -opsia
25. xanth/o

Chapter 11 Pathological, Diagnostic, and Therapeutic Terms Review

1. tinnitus
2. otosclerosis
3. achromatopsia
4. Ménière disease
5. strabismus
6. anacusis
7. otitis media
8. conjunctivitis
9. photophobia
10. presbycusis
11. glaucoma
12. vertigo
13. retinal detachment
14. hordeolum
15. astigmatism
16. acoustic neuroma
17. tonometry
18. iridectomy
19. conductive hearing loss
20. cataract
21. phacoemulsification
22. Rinne test
23. diabetic retinopathy
24. macular degeneration
25. myringotomy

Medical Record Activity 11–1: Retinal Detachment

Evaluation 11–1: Retinal Detachment

1. Where is the retina located?
   The retina is the innermost layer of the eye.

2. Was the anesthetic administered behind or in front of the eyeball?
   Behind the eyeball (retrobulbar).

3. How much movement remained in the eye after anesthesia?
   None; akinesia.

4. Where was the hemorrhage located?
   In the orbit of the eye behind the lens, where the vitreous humor is located.

5. What type of vitrectomy was undertaken?
   Trans pars plana vitrectomy.

6. Why was the eye left soft?
   Because it had poor perfusion.

Medical Record Activity 11–2: Otitis Media

Evaluation 11–2: Otitis Media

1. Where was the patient's infection located?
   Right ear.

2. What complication developed while the patient was hospitalized?
   Cholesteatoma.

3. What is the purpose of the tube placement?
   It reduces the accumulation of fluid within the middle ear.

4. What surgery is being performed to resolve the cholesteatoma?
   Tympanoplasty, right ear.

5. Will the patient be asleep during the surgery?

   Yes, under general anesthesia.

Chapter 11 Vocabulary Review

1. diplopia	6. keratitis	11. mastoid surgery	16. postoperatively
2. sclera	7. diagnosis	12. general anesthetic	17. labyrinth
3. tympanic membrane	8. mucoserous	13. ophthalmologist	18. blepharoptosis
4. dacryorrhea	9. otitis media	14. chronic	19. salpingostenosis
5. eustachian tube	10. cholesteatoma	15. hyperopia	20. myopia

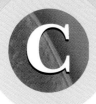
Diagnostic and Therapeutic Procedures

Diagnostic Procedures

This section provides a quick reference of the diagnostic and therapeutic procedures covered in the textbook. Pronunciations and brief descriptions of each procedure are included. Diagnostic procedures help the physician determine a patient's health status, evaluate the factors influencing that status, and determine a method of treatment. Therapeutic procedures are performed to treat a specific disorder that is diagnosed by the physician.

arterial blood gases (ăr-TĒ-rē-ăl): group of tests that measure the oxygen and carbon dioxide concentration in an arterial blood sample.

arthrocentesis (ăr-thrō-sĕn-TĒ-sĭs): puncture of a joint space with a needle to remove fluid.
Arthrocentesis is performed to obtain samples of synovial fluid for diagnostic purposes. It may also be used to instill medications and to remove accumulated fluid from joints simply to relieve pain.

arthroplasty (ĂR-thrō-plăs-tē): surgical reconstruction or replacement of a painful, degenerated joint to restore mobility in rheumatoid arthritis or osteoarthritis or to correct a congenital deformity.

arthroscopy (ăr-THRŎS-kō-pē): visual examination of the interior of a joint performed by inserting an endoscope through a small incision.
Arthroscopy is performed to repair and remove joint tissue, especially of knee, ankle, and shoulder.

barium enema (BĂ-rē-ŭm ĔN-ĕ-mă): radiographic examination of the rectum and colon after administration of barium sulfate (radiopaque contrast medium) into the rectum.
A barium enema is used for diagnosis of obstructions, tumors, or other abnormalities, such as ulcerative colitis.

barium swallow (BĂ-rē-ŭm): radiographic examination of the esophagus, stomach, and small intestine after oral administration of barium sulfate (radiopaque contrast medium).
Structural abnormalities of the esophagus and vessels, such as esophageal varices, may be diagnosed by use of this technique; also called upper GI series.

biopsy (BĪ-ŏp-sē): removal of a small piece of living tissue from an organ or other part of the body for microscopic examination to confirm or establish a diagnosis, estimate prognosis, or follow the course of a disease.
Types of biopsy include aspiration biopsy, needle biopsy, punch biopsy, and shave biopsy.

blood urea nitrogen (ū-RĒ-ă NĪ-trō-jĕn): laboratory test that measures the amount of urea (nitrogenous waste product) normally excreted by the kidneys into the blood. An increase in the blood urea nitrogen (BUN) level may indicate impaired kidney function.

539

bone marrow aspiration biopsy (ăs-pĭ-RĀ-shŭn BĪ-ŏp-sē): removal of living tissue, usually taken from the sternum or iliac crest, for microscopic examination of bone marrow tissue.
Bone marrow aspiration biopsy evaluates hematopoiesis by revealing the number, shape, and size of the red blood cells (RBCs) and white blood cells (WBCs) and platelet precursors.

cardiac catheterization (KĂR-dē-ăk kăth-ĕ-tĕr-ĭ-ZĀ-shŭn): insertion of a small tube (catheter) through an incision into a large vein, usually of an arm (brachial approach) or leg (femoral approach), that is threaded through a blood vessel until it reaches the heart.
A contrast medium also may be injected and x-rays taken (angiography). This procedure can accurately identify and assess many conditions, including congenital heart disease, valvular incompetence, blood supply, and myocardial infarction.

cardiac enzyme studies (KĂR-dē-ăk ĔN-zīm): battery of blood tests performed to determine the presence of cardiac damage.

cerebrospinal fluid analysis (sĕr-ĕ-brō-SPĪ-năl FLOO-ĭd ĕ-NĂL-ĭ-sĭs): cerebrospinal fluid obtained from a lumbar puncture is evaluated for the presence of blood, bacteria, malignant cells, and amount of protein and glucose present.

chest x-ray: radiograph of the chest taken from anteroposterior (AP), posteroanterior (PA), or lateral projections.
Chest x-rays are used to diagnose atelectasis, tumors, pneumonia, emphysema, and many other lung diseases.

colposcopy (kŏl-PŎS-kō-pē): examination of the vagina and cervix with an optical magnifying instrument (colposcope) to obtain biopsy specimens of the cervix; performed if the Papanicolaou (Pap) test results are abnormal.

computed tomography (CT) scan (kŏm-PŪ-tĕd tō-MŎG-ră-fē): radiographic technique that uses a narrow beam of x-rays, which rotates in a full arc around the patient to image the body in cross-sectional slices. A scanner and detector send the images to a computer, which consolidates all of the data it receives from the multiple x-ray views. It may be administered with or without a contrast medium.
CT scanning is used to detect tumor masses, cysts, bone displacement, accumulations of fluid, inflammation, abscesses, perforation, bleeding, and obstructions. It is also used to detect lesions in the lungs and thorax, blood clots, and pulmonary embolism.

digital rectal examination (dĭj-ĭ-TĂL RĔK-tăl): examination of the prostate gland by finger palpation through the rectum.
Digital rectal examination (DRE) is performed usually during physical examination to detect prostate enlargement.

echocardiography (ĕk-ō-kăr-dē-ŎG-ră-fē): ultrasound, also called ultrasonography, to visualize internal cardiac structures and motion of the heart.

electrocardiography (ē-lĕk-trō-KĂR-dē-ŏ-grăfē): creation and study of graphic records (electrocardiograms) produced by electric activity generated by the heart muscle; also called *cardiography*.
Electrocardiography (ECG, EKG) is analyzed by a cardiologist and is valuable in diagnosing cases of abnormal rhythm and myocardial damage.

endoscopy (ĕn-DŎS-kō-pē): visual examination of the interior of organs and cavities with a specialized lighted instrument called an *endoscope*.
Endoscopy also can be used to obtain tissue samples for cytologic and histologic examination (biopsy), for surgery, and to follow the course of a disease, as in the assessment of the healing of gastric and duodenal ulcers. The cavity or organ examined dictates the name of the endoscopic procedure. A camera or video recorder is frequently used during this procedure to provide a permanent record.

fluoroscopy (floo-or-ŎS-kō-pē): radiographic procedure that uses a fluorescent screen instead of a photographic plate to produce a visual image from x-rays that pass through the patient. The technique offers continuous imaging of the motion of internal structures and immediate serial images.

Fluoroscopy is invaluable in diagnostic and clinical procedures. It permits the radiographer to observe organs, such as the digestive tract and heart, in motion. It is also used during biopsy surgery, nasogastric tube placement, and catheter insertion during angiography.

Holter monitor (HŌL-tĕr): monitoring device worn on the patient for making prolonged electrocardiograph recordings (usually 24 hours) on a portable tape recorder while conducting normal daily activities.

Holter monitoring is particularly useful in obtaining a record of cardiac arrhythmia that would not be discovered by means of an ECG of only a few minutes' duration. Also, the patient may keep an activity diary for the purpose of comparing daily events with electrocardiograph tracings.

hysterosalpingography (hĭs-tĕr-ō-săl-pĭn-GŎG-ră-fē): radiography of the uterus and oviducts after injection of a contrast medium.

intravenous pyelogram (ĭn-tră-VĒ-nŭs PĪ-ĕ-lō-grăm): radiographic procedure in which a contrast medium is injected intravenously and serial x-ray films are taken to provide visualization and important information of the entire urinary tract: kidneys, ureters, bladder, and urethra; also called *intravenous urography (IVU)* or *excretory urogram* or *IVP*.

KUB: term used in a radiographic examination to determine the location, size, shape, and malformation of the kidneys, ureters, and bladder. Stones and calcified areas may be detected.

laparoscopy (lăp-ăr-ŎS-kō-pē): visual examination of the abdominal cavity with a laparoscope through one or more small incisions in the abdominal wall, usually at the umbilicus.

Laparoscopy is used for inspection of the ovaries and fallopian tubes, diagnosis of endometriosis, destruction of uterine leiomyomas, myomectomy, and gynecologic sterilization.

lymphangiography (lĭm-făn-jē-ŎG-ră-fē): radiographic examination of lymph glands and lymphatic vessels after an injection of a contrast medium.

Lymphangiography is used to show the path of lymph flow as it moves into the chest region.

magnetic resonance imaging (măg-NĔT-ĭc RĔZ-ĕn-ăns): radiographic technique that uses electromagnetic energy to produce multiplanar cross-sectional images of the body.

Magnetic resonance imaging (MRI) does not require a contrast medium, but it may be used to enhance internal structure visualization. MRI is regarded as superior to computed tomography for most central nervous system abnormalities, particularly of the brainstem and spinal cord, and abnormalities of the musculoskeletal and pelvic area. MRI is particularly useful in detecting abdominal masses and viewing images of abdominal structures and is used to produce scans of the chest and lungs.

mammography (măm-ŎG-ră-fē): radiography of the breast that is used to diagnose benign and malignant tumors.

nuclear scan (NŪ-klē-ăr): diagnostic technique that produces an image by recording the concentration of a *radiopharmaceutical* (a radioactive substance known as a *radionuclide* combined with another chemical) that is introduced into the body (ingested, inhaled, or injected) and specifically drawn to the area under study. A scanning device detects the shape, size, location, and function of the organ or structure under study to provide information about the structure and the function of an organ or system.

There are a variety of scans in nuclear medicine, such as bone scans, liver scans, and brain scans.

Papanicolaou (Pap) test (păp-ăh-NĬK-ĕ-lŏw): microscopic analysis of cells taken from the cervix and vagina to detect the presence of carcinoma. Cells are obtained after the insertion of a vaginal speculum and the use of a swab to scrape a small tissue sample from the cervix and vagina.

positron emission tomography (PŎZ-ĭ-trŏn ē-MĬSH-ŭn tō-MŎG-ră-fē): radiographic technique that combines computed tomography with the use of radiopharmaceuticals. Positron emission tomography (PET) produces a cross-sectional (transverse) image of the dispersement of radioactivity (through emission of positrons) in a section of the body to reveal the areas where the radiopharmaceutical is being metabolized and where there is a deficiency in metabolism.

PET is a type of nuclear scan used to diagnose disorders that involve metabolic processes. It can aid in the diagnosis of neurolgic disorders, such as brain tumors, epilepsy, stroke, Alzheimer disease, and abdominal and pulmonary disorders.

prostate-specific antigen (PSA) test (ĂN-tĭ-jĕn): blood test to screen for prostate cancer. Elevated levels of PSA are associated with prostate cancer and enlargement.

pulmonary function tests (PŬL-mō-nĕ-rē): include any of several tests to evaluate the condition of the respiratory system. Measures of expiratory flow and lung volume capacity are obtained.

radioactive iodine uptake (RAIU) test: imaging procedure that measures levels of radioactivity in the thyroid after administration of radioactive iodine either orally (po) or intravenously (IV).

RAIU is used to determine thyroid function by monitoring the thyroid's ability to take up (uptake) iodine from the blood.

radiography (rā-dē-ŎG-ră-fē): production of captured shadow images on photographic film through the action of ionizing radiation passing through the body from an external source.

Soft body tissue, such as the stomach or liver, appears black or gray on the radiograph; dense body tissue, such as bone, appears white on the radiograph, making it useful in diagnosing fractures.

radiopharmaceutical (rā-dē-ō-fărm-ă-SŪ-tĭ-kăl): drug that contains a radioactive substance that travels to an area or a specific organ that will be scanned.

Diagnostic, research, and therapeutic radiopharmaceuticals are available.

renal scan (RĒ-năl): imaging procedure that determines renal function and shape. A radioactive substance or radiopharmaceutical that concentrates in the kidney is injected intravenously. The radioactivity is measured as it accumulates in the kidneys and is recorded as an image. This is a nuclear medicine procedure.

retrograde pyelogram (RĔT-rō-grād PĪ-ĕ-lō-grăm): radiographic procedure in which a contrast medium is introduced through a cystoscope directly into the bladder and ureters, using small-caliber catheters.

Retrograde pyelogram provides detailed visualization of the urinary collecting system and is useful in locating obstruction in the urinary tract. It may also be used as a substitute for an IVP when a patient is allergic to the contrast medium.

rheumatoid factor (ROO-mă-toyd): blood test to detect the presence of rheumatoid factor, a substance present in patients with rheumatoid arthritis.

scan: technique for carefully studying an area, organ, or system of the body by recording and displaying an image of the area.

A concentration of a radioactive substance that has an affinity for a specific tissue may be administered intravenously to enhance the image. The liver, brain, and thyroid can be examined; tumors can be located; and function can be evaluated by various scanning techniques.

sequestrectomy (sē-kwĕs-TRĔK-tō-mē): excision of a necrosed piece of bone (*sequestrum*).

single-photon emission computed tomography (SĬNG-gŭl FŌ-tŏn ē-MĬSH-ŭn cŏm-PŪ-tĕd tō-MŎG-ră-fē): type of nuclear imaging study to scan organs after injection of a radioactive tracer. Single-photon emission computed tomography (SPECT) is similar to PET scans but employs a specialized gamma camera that detects emitted radiation to produce a three-dimensional image from a composite of numerous views.

Organs commonly studied by SPECT include the brain, heart, lungs, liver, spleen, bones, and in some cases joints.

skin test: method for determining induced sensitivity (allergy) by applying or inoculating a suspected allergen or sensitizer into the skin. Sensitivity (allergy) to the specific antigen is indicated by an inflammatory skin reaction to it.
The most commonly used skin tests are the intradermal, patch, and scratch tests.

spirometry (spī-RŎM-ĕ-trē): measures the breathing capacity of the lungs.

stool guaiac (GWĪ-ăk): test performed on feces using the reagent gum guaiac to detect the presence of blood in the feces that is not apparent on visual inspection; also called *hemoccult test.*

stress test: method of evaluating cardiovascular fitness. While exercising, usually on a treadmill, the individual is subjected to steadily increasing levels of work. At the same time, the amount of oxygen consumed is measured while an ECG is administered.

tissue typing: technique for determining the histocompatibility of tissues to be used in grafts and transplants with the recipient's tissues and cells; also called *histocompatibility testing.*

tomography (tō-MŎG-ră-fē): radiographic technique that produces a film representing a detailed cross-section of tissue structure at a predetermined depth.
Tomography is a valuable diagnostic tool for discovering and identifying space-occupying lesions, such as those found in the liver, brain, pancreas, and gallbladder. Various types of tomography include computed tomography (CT), positron emission tomography (PET), and single-photon emission computed tomography (SPECT).

tonometry (tōn-ŎM-ĕ-trē): measuring of intraocular pressure by determining the resistance of the eyeball to indentation by an applied force; used to detect glaucoma.

troponin I (TRŌ-pō-nĭn): blood test that measures protein that is released into the blood by damaged heart muscle (but not skeletal muscle) and is a highly sensitive and specific indicator of recent myocardial infarction.

total hip arthroplasty (ĂR-thrō-plăs-tē): replacement of the femur and acetabulum with metal components.

ultrasonography (ŭl-tră-sŏn-ŎG-ră-fē): imaging technique that uses high-frequency sound waves (ultrasound) that bounce off body tissues and are recorded to produce an image of an internal organ or tissue. Ultrasonic echoes are recorded and interpreted by a computer, which produces a detailed image of the organ or tissue being evaluated; also called *sonogram* or *echogram.*
In contrast to other imaging techniques, ultrasound (US) does not use ionizing radiation (x-ray). It is used to diagnose fetal development and internal structures of the abdomen, brain, and heart and musculoskeletal disorders. US visualization includes, but is not limited to, the liver, gallbladder, bile ducts, and pancreas. It is used to diagnose and locate cysts, tumors, and other digestive disorders and to guide the insertion of instruments during surgical procedures. Doppler US measures blood flow in blood vessels and allows the examiner to hear characteristic alterations in blood flow caused by vessel obstruction in various parts of an extremity. Pelvic US is used to evaluate the female reproductive organs; transvaginal US places the sound probe in the vagina instead of across the pelvis or abdomen, producing a sharper examination of normal and pathological structures within the pelvis.

urinalysis (ū-rĭ-NĂL-ĭ-sĭs): physical, chemical, or microscopic analysis of urine.

visual acuity test (ă-KŪ-ĭ-tē): standard test of visual acuity in which a person is asked to read letters and numbers on a chart 20 feet away with the use of the Snellen chart; also called an *E chart.*

voiding cystourethrography (sĭs-tō-ū-rē-THRŎG-ră-fē): radiography of the urinary bladder and urethra after the introduction of a contrast medium and during the process of voiding urine. The urinary bladder is filled with an opaque contrast medium before the procedure.

Therapeutic Procedures

The following terms are some of the therapeutic procedures used as methods of treatment for a particular disorder.

anastomosis (ă-năs-tō-MŌ-sĭs): connection between two vessels; surgical joining of two ducts, blood vessels, or bowel segments to allow flow from one to the other.

angioplasty (ĂN-jē-ō-plăs-tē): any endovascular procedure that reopens narrowed blood vessels and restores forward blood flow. The blocked vessel is usually opened by balloon dilation.

audiometry (ăw-dē-ŎM-ĕ-trē): test that measures hearing acuity of various sound frequencies.
An instrument called an audiometer delivers acoustic stimuli at different frequencies, and the results are plotted on a graph called an audiogram.

bronchodilators (brŏng-kō-DĪ-lā-tŏrz): drugs used to dilate the walls of the bronchi of the lungs to increase airflow.
Bronchodilators are used to treat asthma, emphysema, chronic obstructive lung disease (COLD), and exercise-induced bronchospasm.

bronchoscopy (brŏng-KŎS-kō-pē): direct visual examination of the interior bronchi using a bronchoscope (curved, flexible tube with a light).
A bronchoscopy may be performed to remove obstructions, obtain a biopsy, or to observe directly for pathological changes.

cataract surgery (KĂT-ă-răkt): excision of cataracts by surgical removal of the lens. To correct the visual deficit when the eye is without a lens (aphakic), the insertion of an artificial lens (intraocular lens transplant) or the use of eyeglasses or contact lenses is needed.
Several surgical techniques involving cataract removal are corneal transplant, extracapsular surgery, iridectomy, and phacoemulsification.

catheterization (kăth-ĕ-tĕr-ĭ-ZĀ-shŭn): insertion of a catheter (hollow flexible tube) into a body cavity or organ to instill a substance or remove fluid. The most common type is to insert a catheter through the urethra into the bladder to withdraw urine.

cauterize (KAW-tĕr-īz): process of burning tissue by thermal heat, including steam, electricity, or another agent, such a laser or dry ice, usually with the objective of destroying damaged or diseased tissues, preventing infections, or coagulating blood vessels.

cerclage (sār-KLŎZH): obstetric procedure in which a nonabsorbable suture is used for holding the cervix closed to prevent spontaneous abortion in a woman who has an incompetent cervix.

chemical peel: chemical removal of the outer layers of skin to treat acne scarring and general keratoses; also used for cosmetic purposes to remove fine wrinkles on the face; also called *chemabrasion.*

circumcision (sĕr-kŭm-SĬ-zhŭn): surgical removal of the foreskin or prepuce of the penis; usually performed on infants.

cochlear implant (KŎK-lē-ĕr): electronic transmitter that is surgically implanted into the cochlea of a deaf individual; performed to restore hearing loss.

corneal transplant (KŎR-nē-ĕl): surgical transplantation of a donor cornea (from a cadaver) into the eye of a recipient; also called *keratoplasty.*

coronary artery bypass graft (KŎR-ă-năr-ē ĂHR-tă-rē): surgery that involves bypassing one or more blocked coronary arteries to increase blood flow.
Cardiac catheterization is used to identify blocked coronary arteries. After the blockages are identified, coronary artery bypass graft (CABG) surgery is often performed. The operation involves the use of one or more of the patient's arteries or veins. Generally, the saphenous vein from the leg or the right or left internal mammary artery from the chest wall is used to bypass the blocked section.

corticosteroids (kor-tĭ-kō-STĒR-oydz): hormonal agents that reduce tissue edema and inflammation associated with chronic lung disease.

craniotomy (krā-nē-ŎT-ō-mē): surgical procedure to create an opening in the skull to gain access to the brain during neurosurgical procedures.
A craniotomy also is performed to relieve intracranial pressure, to control bleeding, or to remove a tumor.

cryosurgery (krī-ō-SĔR-jĕr-ē): use of subfreezing temperature (commonly with liquid nitrogen) to destroy abnormal tissue cells, such as unwanted, cancerous, or infected tissue.

debridement (dā-brēd-MŎNT): removal of foreign material and dead or damaged tissue, especially in a wound; used to promote healing and prevent infection.

dermabrasion (DĔRM-ă-brā-zhŭn): removal of acne scars, nevi, tattoos, or fine wrinkles on the skin through the use of sandpaper, wire brushes, or other abrasive materials on the epidermal layer.

dilation and curettage (DĬ-lā-shŭn and kū-rĕ-TĂZH): surgical procedure that expands the cervical canal of the uterus (dilation) so that the surface lining of the uterine wall can be scraped (curettage).
Dilation and curettage (D&C) is performed to stop prolonged or heavy uterine bleeding, diagnose uterine abnormalities, empty uterine contents of conception tissue, and obtain tissue for microscopic examination.

electrodessication (ē-lĕk-trō-dĕs-ĭ-KĀ-shŭn): process in which high-frequency electric sparks are used to dehydrate and destroy diseased tissue.

extracapsular surgery (ĕks-tră-KĂP-sū-lăr): excision of most of the lens, followed by insertion of an intraocular lens transplant.

extracorporeal shock-wave lithotripsy (ĕks-tră-kor-POR-ē-ăl LĬTH-ō-trĭp-sē): use of shock waves as a noninvasive method to destroy stones in the gallbladder and biliary ducts.
Ultrasound is used to locate the stones and to monitor their destruction. After extracorporeal shock-wave lithotripsy (ESWL), a course of oral dissolution drugs is used to ensure complete removal of all stones and stone fragments.

gonadotropins (gŏn-ă-dō-TRŌ-pĭnz): hormonal preparations used to increase the sperm count in infertility cases.

hormone replacement therapy: oral administration or injection of synthetic hormones to replace a hormone deficiency, such as of estrogen, testosterone, or thyroid hormone.

hysterosalpingo-oophorectomy (hĭs-tĕr-ō-săl-pĭng-gō-ō-ŏ-for-ĔK-tō-mē): surgical removal of a fallopian tube and an ovary.

incision and drainage (I&D): incision of a lesion, such as an abscess, followed by the drainage of its contents.

iridectomy (ĭr-ĭ-DĔK-tĕ-mē): excision of a portion of the iris.
Iridectomy is a surgical procedure that is usually performed to create an opening through which aqueous humor can drain; used to relieve intraocular pressure in patients with glaucoma.

lithotripsy (LĬTH-ō-trĭp-sē): procedure for eliminating a calculus in the gallbladder, renal pelvis, ureter, or bladder.
Stones may be crushed surgically or by using a noninvasive method, such as hydraulic, or high-energy, shock-wave or a pulsed-dye laser. The fragments may be expelled or washed out.

mastectomy (măs-TĔK-tŏ-mē): complete or partial surgical removal of one or both breasts, most commonly performed to remove a malignant tumor.
A mastectomy may be a simple, radical, or modified procedure depending on the extent of the malignancy and the amount of breast tissue excised.

myringoplasty (mĭr-ĬN-gō-plăst-ē): surgical repair of a perforated eardrum with a tissue graft.
Myringoplasty is performed to correct hearing loss; also called tympanoplasty.

myringotomy (mĭr-ĭn-GŎT-ō-mē): incision of the eardrum to relieve pressure and release pus or serous fluid from the middle ear or to insert tympanostomy tubes surgically in the eardrum.
Tympanostomy tubes provide ventilation and drainage of the middle ear when repeated ear infections do not respond to antibiotic treatment and are used when persistent severely negative middle ear pressure is present.

nasogastric intubation (nā-zō-GĂS-trĭk ĭn-tū-BĀ-shŭn): insertion of a nasogastric tube through the nose into the stomach.
Nasogastric intubation is used to relieve gastric distention by removing gas, gastric secretions, or food; to instill medication, food, or fluids; or to obtain a specimen for laboratory analysis.

nebulized mist treatment (NMT): use of a device for producing a fine spray (nebulizer) to deliver medication directly into the lungs.

otoscopy (ŏ-TŎS-kĕ-pē): visual examination of the ear, especially the eardrum, using an otoscope.

phacoemulsification (făk-ō-ē-MŬL-sĭ-fĭ-kā-shŭn): excision of the lens by ultrasonic vibrations that break the lens into tiny particles, which are then suctioned out of the eye.

postural drainage (PŎS-chur-ăl DRĀN-ăj): use of body positioning to assist in the removal of secretions from specific lobes of the lung, bronchi, or lung cavities.

renal transplantation (RĒ-năl trăns-plăn-TĀ-shŭn): surgical transfer of a complete kidney from a donor to a recipient.

Rinne test (RĬN): hearing acuity test that is performed with a vibrating tuning fork placed on the mastoid process, then in front of the external auditory canal to test bone and air conduction.
The Rinne test is useful for differentiating between conductive and sensorineural hearing loss.

thalamotomy (thăl-ă-MŎT-ō-mē): partial destruction of the thalamus to treat psychosis or intractable pain.

thrombolytic therapy (thrŏm-bō-LĬT-ĭk THĔR-ă-pē): administration of drugs to dissolve a blood clot(s).

tubal ligation (TŪ-băl lĭ-GĀ-shŭn): sterilization procedure that involves blocking both fallopian tubes by cutting or burning them and tying them off.

valvuloplasty (VĂL-vū-lō-plăs-tē): plastic or restorative surgery on a valve, especially a cardiac valve.
A special type of valvuloplasty is balloon valvuloplasty in which insertion of a balloon catheter to open a stenotic heart valve is performed. Inflating the balloon decreases the constriction.

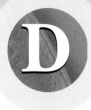

D

Drug Classifications

The following classifications of medication include prescription and over-the-counter drugs that are used for various medical purposes.

alkylate: drug used to treat certain types of malignancies.

analgesic, painkiller: drugs that relieve pain.

antacid: agent that neutralizes excess acid in the stomach and helps relieve gastritis and ulcer pain. Antacids also are used to relieve indigestion and reflux esophagitis (heartburn).

antianginal: agent used to relieve angina pectoris by vasodilation.

antibiotic: any of a variety of natural or synthetic substances that inhibit growth of or destroy microorganisms; used extensively in treatment of infectious diseases.

anticoagulant: agent that inhibits or delays the clotting process; used to prevent clots from forming in blood vessels.

anticonvulsant: substance that prevents or reduces the severity of epileptic or other convulsive seizures.

antidepressant: agent used to regulate mood and reduce symptoms of depression by affecting the amount of neurotransmitters in the brain.

antidiarrheal: agent used to relieve diarrhea either by absorbing the excess fluids that cause diarrhea or by lessening intestinal motility (slowing the movement of fecal material through the intestine), which allows more time for absorption of water.

antiemetic, antinauseant: agents that suppress nausea and vomiting, mainly by acting on the brain control centers to stop nerve impulses. There are many uses for these drugs, including the treatment of motion sickness and of dizziness associated with inner ear infections. Some antihistamines and tranquilizers have antiemetic properties.

antihistamine: drug that counteracts the effects of a histamine. Antihistamines are used to relieve the symptoms of allergic reactions, especially hay fever and other allergic disorders of the nasal passages.

antihyperlipidemic: agent that lowers cholesterol levels in the bloodstream, helping to prevent atherosclerosis (fatty buildup in the blood vessels).

antihypertensive: agent that lowers blood pressure.

anti-infective, antibacterial, antifungal: substances that eliminate or inhibit bacterial or fungal infections. They can be administered either topically or systemically.

anti-inflammatory, antipyretic: nonnarcotic analgesics used for relief of pain and fever. Many of these drugs have anti-inflammatory effects and are used to treat arthritis and gout. These drugs also are called *nonsteroidal anti-inflammatory drugs (NSAIDs)*.

anti-inflammatory, topical corticosteroid: topically applied drugs that relieve three common symptoms of skin disorders: pruritus or itching, vasodilation, and inflammation.

antimetabolite: agent that interferes with the use of enzymes required for cell division.

antipruritic: agent that prevents or relieves itching.

antiseptic: topically applied agent that destroys bacteria, preventing or treating the development of infections in cuts, scratches, and surgical incisions.

antispasmodic: agent that acts on the autonomic nervous system to slow peristalsis, relieving intestinal cramping.

antitussive: agent that prevents or relieves coughing.

astringent: agent used to shrink the blood vessels locally, dry up secretions from seepy lesions, and lessen skin sensitivity.

beta-adrenergic blocking agent: drug used to treat cardiac arrhythmias, angina pectoris, post–myocardial infarction hypertension, and migraine headaches.

beta-adrenergic: drug used in the treatment of glaucoma that lowers intraocular pressure by reducing the production of aqueous humor.

bronchodilator: agent that dilates the bronchi of the lungs to increase airflow.

calcium channel blocker: drug that selectively blocks the flow of calcium ions in the heart and is used to treat angina pectoris, certain arrhythmias, and hypertension.

contraceptive: any process, device, or method that prevents conception.

corticosteroid: replacement hormone for adrenal insufficiency (Addison disease). Corticosteroids are widely used for suppressing inflammation, controlling allergic reactions, reducing the rejection process in tissue and organ transplantation, and treating some cancers.

cycloplegic: agent that paralyzes the ciliary muscles and results in pupil dilation; used to facilitate certain eye examinations and surgical procedures.

cytotoxic: chemical agent that destroys cells or prevents their multiplication; used in cancer chemotherapy.

decongestant: agent that reduces congestion or swelling, especially in the nasal passages.

diuretic: agent that promotes the excretion of sodium and water; used to treat edema and hypertension.

emetic: substance used to induce vomiting, especially in cases of poisoning.

estrogen hormone: agent used in estrogen replacement therapy (ERT) during menopause to correct estrogen deficiency and as chemotherapy for some types of cancer, including tumors of the prostate.

expectorant: agent that promotes the expulsion of mucus from the respiratory tract.

fibrinolytic: agent that triggers the body to produce plasmin, an enzyme that dissolves clots; used to treat acute pulmonary embolism and, occasionally, deep vein thromboses.

gold therapy, chrysotherapy: therapy that uses gold compounds as a medicine; employed in treating rheumatoid arthritis.

gonadotropin: agent used to raise sperm count in infertility cases.

hemostatic: any drug, medicine, or blood component that serves to stop bleeding.

hypnotic: substance that induces sleep or hypnosis.

inotropic, cardiotonic: drugs that affect the force of contraction of the heart; used to treat cardiac arrhythmias and cardiac failure.

insulin: synthetic form of the insulin hormone for diabetes administered by injection to lower the glucose (sugar) level in the blood.

keratolytic: agent used to destroy and soften the outer layer of skin so that it is sloughed off or shed. Strong keratolytics are effective for removing warts and corns. Milder preparations are used to promote the shedding of scales and crusts in eczema, psoriasis, and seborrheic dermatitis. Weak keratolytics irritate inflamed skin, acting as tonics that speed up the healing process.

laxative (cathartic, purgative): agent that promotes bowel movements or defecation or both. When used in smaller doses, it relieves constipation. When used in larger doses, it evacuates the entire gasrointestinal tract, for example, before surgery or intestinal radiologic examinations.

miotic: any substance that constricts the pupil of the eye. These agents are used in the treatment of glaucoma.

mucolytic: group of agents that liquefy sputum or reduce its viscosity so that it can be coughed up more easily.

mydriatic: topical drug used to dilate the pupil and paralyze the muscles of accommodation of the iris; used to prepare the eye for internal examination and to treat inflammatory conditions of the iris.

nitrate: class of drugs used to treat angina.

opiate: narcotic drug that contains opium or its derivatives. Opiates are sometimes used for relieving severe pain.

oral contraceptive: pharmaceutically prepared chemical that is quite similar to natural hormones and act by preventing ovulation. When taken according to instructions, oral contraceptives are almost 100% effective; also called "the pill."

oxytocin: pharmaceutically prepared chemical that is similar to the pituitary hormone oxytocin. This hormone stimulates the uterus to contract, inducing labor, or to rid the uterus of an unexpelled placenta or a fetus that has died.

parasiticide: agent that, in its oral form, kills systemic parasites, such as pinworm or tapeworm.

protective: agent that functions by covering, cooling, drying, or soothing inflamed skin. Protectives do not penetrate or soften the skin but form a long-lasting film that protects the skin from air, water, and clothing during the natural healing process.

psychotropic: drug that affects and can alter psychic function, behavior, or experience. Psychotropics are often employed in the management of psychotic disorders.

relaxant: drug that reduces tension, such as a muscle relaxant or bowel relaxant.

sedative: agent that exerts a calming or tranquilizing effect.

spermicidal: substance that destroys sperm and is used within the woman's vagina for contraceptive purposes. Spermicidals consist of jellies, creams, and foams and do not require a prescription.

topical anesthetic: agent that is prescribed for pain on skin surfaces or mucous membranes that is caused by wounds, hemorrhoids, or sunburns. Topical anesthetics relieve pain and itching by numbing the skin layers and mucous membranes. They are applied directly by means of sprays, creams, gargles, suppositories, and other preparations; also used to numb the skin to make the injection of medication more comfortable.

tranquilizer: drug used to calm anxious or agitated people, ideally without decreasing their consciousness.

uricosuric: drug that increases the urinary excretion of uric acid, reducing the concentration of uric acid in the blood; used in the treatment of gout.

vasoconstrictor: drug that causes a narrowing of blood vessels; used to decrease blood flow.

vasodilator: drug that expands blood vessels; used in the treatment of angina pectoris and hypertension.

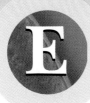

Abbreviations

Abbreviation	Meaning	Abbreviation	Meaning
A		**ALS**	amyotrophic lateral sclerosis; also called *Lou Gehrig disease*
AAA	abdominal aortic aneurysm	**ALT**	alanine aminotransferase (elevated in liver and heart disease); formerly *SGPT*
AB, ab	abnormal, abortion, antibody		
ABC	aspiration biopsy cytology		
ABO	blood groups A, AB, B, and O		
abd	abdomen	**AMD, ARMD**	age-related macular degeneration
ABGs	arterial blood gases	**AML**	acute myelogenous leukemia
ac	before meals	**ANS**	autonomic nervous system
AC	air conduction	**ant**	anterior
Acc	accommodation	**AP**	anteroposterior
AC joint	acromioclavicular joint	**APTT**	activated partial thromboplastin time
ACL	anterior cruciate ligament		
ACTH	adrenocorticotropic hormone	**ARDS**	acute respiratory distress syndrome; adult respiratory distress syndrome
AD	Alzheimer disease		
AD*	right ear		
ADA	American Diabetes Association	**ARF**	acute renal failure
ADH	antidiuretic hormone	**AS**	aortic stenosis
AE	above the elbow	**AS***	left ear
AF	atrial fibrillation	**ASD**	atrial septal defect
AFB	acid-fast bacillus (TB organism)	**ASHD**	arteriosclerotic heart disease
		AST	angiotensin sensitivity test; aspartate aminotransferase (cardiac enzyme, formerly called *SGOT*)
AGN	acute glomerulonephritis		
AI	artificial insemination		
AIDS	acquired immunodeficiency syndrome	**Ast**	astigmatism
AK	above the knee	**ATN**	acute tubular necrosis
alk phos	alkaline phosphatase	**AU***	both ears
ALL	acute lymphocytic leukemia	**AV**	atrioventricular, arteriovenous

*Although these abbreviations are currently found in medical records and clinical notes, the Joint Commission on Accreditation of Healthcare Organizations (JCAHO) requires their discontinuance. Instead, write out the meanings.

Abbreviation	Meaning	Abbreviation	Meaning
B		**CK**	creatine kinase (cardiac enzyme)
Ba	barium	**CLL**	chronic lymphocytic leukemia
BaE, BE	barium enema	**cm**	centimeter
baso	basophil (type of white blood cell)	**CML**	chronic myelogenous leukemia
BBB	bundle-branch block	**CNS**	central nervous system
BC	bone conduction	**CO₂**	carbon dioxide
BCC	basal cell carcinoma	**COLD**	chronic obstructive lung disease
BE	below the elbow	**COPD**	chronic obstructive pulmonary disease
BEAM	brain electrical activity mapping	**CP**	cerebral palsy
bid	twice a day	**CPD**	cephalopelvic disproportion
BK	below the knee	**CPR**	cardiopulmonary resuscitation
BM	bowel movement	**CS, C-section**	cesarean section
BMR	basal metabolic rate	**CSF**	cerebrospinal fluid
BNO	bladder neck obstruction	**CT**	computed tomography
BP	blood pressure	**CT scan, CAT scan**	computed tomography scan
BPH	benign prostatic hyperplasia; benign prostatic hypertrophy	**CTS**	carpal tunnel syndrome
BS	blood sugar	**CV**	cardiovascular
BSE	breast self-examination	**CVA**	cerebrovascular accident
BUN	blood urea nitrogen	**CVD**	cerebrovascular disease
Bx, bx	biopsy	**CVS**	chorionic villus sampling
		CWP	childbirth without pain
C		**CXR**	chest x-ray; chest radiograph
		cysto	cystoscopic examination
C&S	culture and sensitivity		
C1, C2 to C7	first cervical vertebra, second cervical vertebra, and so on	**D**	
CA	cancer; cardiac arrest; chronological age	**D**	diopter (lens strength)
Ca	calcium; cancer	**D&C**	dilation and curettage
CABG	coronary artery bypass graft	**decub**	decubitus
CAD	coronary artery disease	**derm**	dermatology
cath	catheterization; catheter	**DI**	diabetes insipidus; diagnostic imaging
CBC	complete blood count	**diff**	differential count (white blood cells)
cc	cubic centimeter	**DJD**	degenerative joint disease
CC	chief complaint	**DKA**	diabetic ketoacidosis
CCU	coronary care unit	**DM**	diabetes mellitus
CDH	congenital dislocation of the hip	**DOE**	dyspnea on exertion
CF	cystic fibrosis	**DPT**	diphteria, pertussis, tetanus
CHD	coronary heart disease	**DRE**	digital rectal examination
CHF	congestive heart failure (the term congestive heart failure is being replaced by the term *heart failure [HF]*)	**DSA**	digital subtraction angiography
		DUB	dysfunctional uterine bleeding
		DVT	deep vein thrombosis
Chol	cholesterol	**Dx, dx**	diagnoses (singular, diagnosis)

Abbreviation	Meaning
E	
EBV	Epstein-Barr virus
ECG, EKG	electrocardiogram
ECHO	echocardiogram; echoencephalogram
ED	emergency department; erectile dysfunction
EEG	electroencephalogram
EGD	esophagogastroduodenoscopy
Em	emmetropia
EMG	electromyogram
ENT	ears, nose, and throat
EOM	extraocular movement
eos	eosinophil (type of white blood cell)
ERCP	endoscopic retrograde cholangiopancreatography
ESR, sed rate	erythrocyte sedimentation rate; sedimentation rate
ESRD	end-stage renal disease
ESWL	extracorporeal shock-wave lithotripsy
EU	excretory urography; also called *intravenous pyelography (IVP)* or *intravenous urography (IVU)*
F	
FBS	fasting blood sugar
FECG; FEKG	fetal electrocardiogram
FHR	fetal heart rate
FHT	fetal heart tone
FH	family history
FS	frozen section
FSH	follicle-stimulating hormone
FTND	full-term normal delivery
FVC	forced vital capacity
Fx	fracture
G	
G	gravida (pregnant)
GB	gallbladder
GBS	gallbladder series
GC	gonorrhea
GC screen	gonococcal screen
GER	gastroesophageal reflux

Abbreviation	Meaning
GERD	gastroesophageal reflux disease
GH	growth hormone
GI	gastrointestinal
GTT	glucose tolerance test
GU	genitourinary
GYN	gynecology
H	
HAV	hepatitis A virus
Hb, Hg, Hgb	hemoglobin
HBV	hepatitis B virus
HCl	hydrochloric acid
HCT, Hct	hematocrit
HCV	hepatitis C virus
HD	hearing distance; hemodialysis; hip disarticulation
HDL	high-density lipoprotein
HDN	hemolytic disease of the newborn
HDV	hepatitis D virus
HEV	hepatitis E virus
HF	heart failure
HIV	human immunodeficiency virus
HMD	hyaline membrane disease
HNP	herniated nucleus pulposus (herniated disk)
HP	hemipelvectomy
HPV	human papillomavirus
HRT	hormone replacement therapy
HSG	hysterosalpingography
HSV	herpes simplex virus
Hx	history
I	
I&D	incision and drainage
IAS	interatrial septum
IBD	inflammatory bowel disease
IBS	irritable bowel syndrome
ICP	intracranial pressure
ICSH	interstitial cell–stimulating hormone
ID	intradermal

Abbreviation	Meaning	Abbreviation	Meaning
IDDM	insulin-dependent diabetes mellitus		dehydrogenase (cardiac enzyme)
Igs	immunoglobulins	LDL	low-density lipoprotein
IM	intramuscular; infectious mononucleosis	LH	luteinizing hormone
		LLQ	left lower quadrant
		LMP	last menstrual period
IMP	impression (synonymous with *diagnosis*)	LOC	loss of consciousness
		LP	lumbar puncture
IOL	intraocular lens	LSO	left salpingo-oophorectomy
IOP	intraocular pressure	Lt, lt	left
IPPB	intermittent positive-pressure breathing	LUQ	left upper quadrant
		LV	left ventricle
IRDS	infant respiratory distress syndrome	lymphos	lymphocytes
IS	intracostal space	**M**	
ITP	idiopathic thrombocytopenia purpura	MCH	mean cell hemoglobin (average amount of hemoglobin per cell); mean corpuscular hemoglobin
IUD	intrauterine device		
IUGR	intrauterine growth rate; intrauterine growth retardation		
IV, I.V.	intravenous	MCHC	mean cell hemoglobin concentration (average concentration of hemoglobin in a single red cell)
IVC	inferior vena cava; intravenous cholangiography		
IVF-ET	in vitro fertilization and embryo transfer	MCV	mean cell volume (average volume or size of a single red blood cell; high MCV = macrocytic cells; low MCV = microcytic cells)
IVP	intravenous pyelography; also called *excretory urography (EU)* or *intravenous urography (IVU)*		
IVS	interventricular septum	MEG	magnetoencephalography
IVU	intravenous urography; also called *excretory urography (EU)* or *intravenous pyelography (IVP)*	mg	milligram
		MG	myasthenia gravis
		MI	myocardial infarction
		mix astig	mixed astigmatism
K		mL, ml	milliliters
K	potassium	mm	millimeter
KD	knee disarticulation	mmHg	millimeters of mercury
KS	Kaposi sarcoma	MRA	magnetic resonance angiogram; magnetic resonance angiography
KUB	kidney, ureter, bladder		
L		MRI	magnetic resonance imaging
		MRI scan	magnetic resonance imaging scan
L1, L2 to L5	first lumbar vertebra, second lumbar vertebra, and so on	MS	mental status; mitral stenosis; multiple sclerosis; musculoskeletal
LA	left atrium		
LAT, lat	lateral		
LBW	low birth weight	MSH	melanocyte-stimulating hormone
LD	lactate dehydrogenase; lactic acid		

Abbreviation	Meaning	Abbreviation	Meaning
MVP	mitral valve prolapse	PCP	*Pneumocystis carinii* pneumonia
MVR	massive vitreous retractor (blade)	PCV	packed cell volume
		PE	physical examination
Myop	myopia	PE tube	pressure equalization tube (placed in eardrum)
N		PET	positron emission tomography
		PERLLA	pupils equal, round, and reactive to light and accommodation
Na⁺	sodium (an electrolyte)		
NB	newborn		
NCV	nerve conduction velocity	PFT	pulmonary function test
NG	nasogastric	PGH	pituitary growth hormone
NIDDM	non–insulin-dependent diabetes mellitus	pH	symbol for degree of acidity or alkalinity
NIHL	noise-induced hearing loss	PI	present illness
NMT	nebulized mist treatment	PID	pelvic inflammatory disease
NPH	neutral protamine Hagedorn (insulin)	PMH	polymorphonuclear leukocyte
		PMP	previous menstrual period
npo	nothing by mouth	PMS	premenstrual syndrome
NSAIDs	nonsteroidal anti-inflammatory drugs	PND	paroxysmal nocturnal dyspnea
O		po	by mouth (per os)
		PO₂	partial pressure oxygen
		poly,	polymorphonuclear leukocyte
O₂	oxygen	PMN,	
OB	obstetrics	PMNL	
OB-GYN	obstetrics and gynecology	post	posterior
OCPs	oral contraceptive pills	PRL	prolactin
OD*	right eye	prn	as required
oint	ointment	PSA	prostate-specific antigen
OR	operating room	PT	physical therapy; prothrombin time
ORTH,	orthopedics		
ortho		PTCA	percutaneous transluminal coronary angioplasty
OS*	left eye		
OU*	both eyes	PTH	parathyroid hormone
		PTT	partial thromboplastin time
P		PUD	peptic ulcer disease
		PVC	premature ventricular contraction
PA	posteroanterior		
PAC	premature atrial contraction	**Q**	
Pap	Papanicolaou test		
para 1, 2, 3	unipara, bipara, tripara (number of viable births)	q2h	every 2 hours
		q4h	every 4 hours
PAT	paroxysmal atrial tachycardia	qam, qm	every morning
pc, pp	after meals (postprandial)	qh	every hour
PCL	posterior cruciate ligament	qid	four times a day
PCNL	percutaneous nephrolithotomy	qod	every other day
PCO₂	partial pressure of carbon dioxide	qpm, qn	every night

*Although these abbreviations are currently found in medical records and clinical notes, the Joint Commission on Accreditation of Healthcare Organizations (JCAHO) requires their discontinuance. Instead, write out the meanings.

Abbreviation	Meaning	Abbreviation	Meaning
R		**ST**	esotropia
		stat	immediately
R/O	rule out	STD	sexually transmitted disease
RA	rheumatoid arthritis; right atrium	Sub-Q, subQ	subcutaneous (injection)
RAI	radioactive iodine	SVC	superior vena cava
RAIU	radioactive iodine uptake	Sx	symptom
RBC, rbc	red blood cell(s); red blood count	**T**	
RD	respiratory disease	T&A	tonsillectomy and adenoidectomy
RDS	respiratory distress syndrome	T_3	triiodothyronine (thyroid hormone)
REM	rapid eye movement		
RF	rheumatoid factor	T_4	thyroxine (thyroid hormone)
RK	radial keratotomy	T1, T2 to T12	first thoracic vertebra, second thoracic vertebra, and so on
RLQ	right lower quadrant		
ROM	range of motion	TAH	total abdominal hysterectomy
RP	retrograde pyelography	TB	tuberculosis
RSO	right salpingo-oophorectomy	TFT	thyroid function test
Rt	right	THA	total hip arthroplasty
RUQ	right upper quadrant	THR	total hip replacement
RV	right ventricle	TIA	transient ischemic attack
S		tid	three times a day
		TKA	total knee arthroplasty
S1, S2 to S5	first sacral vertebra, second sacral vertebra, and so on	TKR	total knee replacement
		TPR	temperature, pulse, and respiration
SA	sinoatrial (node)		
SaO_2	arterial oxygen saturation	TSE	testicular self-examination
SD	shoulder disarticulation	TSH	thyroid-stimulating hormone
segs	segmented neutrophils	TSS	toxic shock syndrome
SGOT	serum glutamic oxaloacetate transaminase; obsolete, now called AST	TUR, TURP	transurethral resection of the prostate
		TVH	total vaginal hysterectomy
SGPT	serum glutamic-pyruvic transaminase; obsolete, now called ALT	Tx	treatment
		U	
SICS	small incision cataract surgery	U&L, U/L	upper and lower
SIDS	sudden infant death syndrome	UA	urinalysis
SLE	systemic lupus erythematosus	UC	uterine contractions
SNS	sympathetic nervous system	UGI	upper gastrointestinal
SOB	shortness of breath	UGIS	upper gastrointestinal series
sono	sonogram	ung	ointment
sp. gr.	specific gravity	URI	upper respiratory infection
SPECT	single-photon emission computed tomography	US	ultrasound, ultrasonography
		UTI	urinary tract infection

Abbreviation	Meaning	Abbreviation	Meaning
V		**W**	
VA	visual acuity	**WBC**	white blood cell(s); white blood count
VC	vital capacity	**WNL**	within normal limits
VCUG	voiding cystourethrogram, voiding cystourethrography	**X**	
VD	venereal disease	**XDP, XP**	xeroderma pigmentosum
VF	visual field	**XT**	exotropia
VSD	ventricular septal defect	**XY**	male sex chromosomes
VT	ventricular tachycardia		

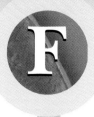

Medical Specialties

Medical Specialist	Medical Specialty	Description of Specialties
Allergist, Immunologist	Allergy or immunology	Diagnosis and treatment of body reactions resulting from hypersensitivity to foods, pollens, dusts, medicines, or other substances that do not normally cause a reaction
Anesthesiologist	Anesthesiology	Administration of a drug or gas to induce partial or complete loss of sensation with or without loss of consciousness
Cardiologist	Cardiology	Diagnosis and treatment of diseases of the heart, arteries, veins, and capillaries
Dermatologist	Dermatology	Diagnosis and treatment of diseases of the skin
Endocrinologist	Endocrinology	Diagnosis and treatment of the endocrine glands and their internal secretions
General practitioner	General practice or family practice	Diagnosis and treatment of disease by medical and surgical methods, without limitation to organ systems or body regions, to all members of a family regardless of age or sex
Geriatrician, Gerontologist	Geriatrics or gerontology	Diagnosis and treatment of diseases of the aged
Gynecologist	Gynecology	Diagnosis and treatment of diseases of the female reproductive organs
Hematologist	Hematology	Diagnosis and treatment of diseases of the blood and blood-forming tissues
Internist	Internal medicine	Diagnosis and treatment of internal organs by other than surgical means to adults

Medical Specialist	Medical Specialty	Description of Specialties
Neonatologist	Neonatology	Study and care of newborn infants
Neurologist	Neurology	Diagnosis and treatment of the nervous system and its diseases and abnormalities
Neurosurgeon	Neurological surgery	Surgery of the nervous system
Obstetrician	Obstetrics	Care of women during pregnancy, childbirth, and a short period after childbirth
Oncologist	Oncology	Diagnosis and treatment of tumors; the physician is a cancer specialist
Ophthalmologist	Ophthalmology	Diagnosis and treatment of eye diseases, including prescribing glasses
Orthopedist	Orthopedics	Prevention and correction of disorders involving locomotor structures of the body, especially the skeleton, joints, muscles, fascia, and other supporting structures such as ligaments and cartilage
Otolaryngologist	Otolaryngology	Diagnosis and treatment of diseases of the ear, nose, and throat
Pathologist	Pathology	Study and cause of disease; a pathologist usually specializes in autopsy or in clinical or surgical pathology
Pediatrician	Pediatrics	Diagnosis and treatment of children's diseases
Plastic surgeon	Plastic surgery	Surgery for the restoration, repair, or reconstruction of body structures
Physiatrist	Physiatrics	Treatment of disease by natural methods, especially physical therapy
Pulmonologist	Pulmonology	Diagnosis and treatment of diseases of the lungs
Psychiatrist	Psychiatry	Diagnosis, treatment, and prevention of mental illness
Radiologist	Radiology	Prevention, diagnosis, and treatment of diseases with radioactive substances, including x-rays
Rheumatologist	Rheumatology	Diagnosis and treatment of rheumatic diseases
Surgeon	Surgery	Treatment of deformities, injury, and disease with manual and operative procedures

Medical Specialist	Medical Specialty	Description of Specialties
Thoracic surgeon	Thoracic surgery	Surgery involving the rib cage and structures contained within the thoracic cage
Urologist	Urology	Diagnosis and treatment of the urinary tract in both sexes and of the male genital tract

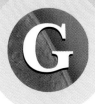

Spanish Translations

Introduction

The purpose of this appendix is to provide guidelines to help health-care practitioners identify and pronounce Spanish terms commonly used in the various medical specialties. Although the spelling of some Spanish terms resembles English terms, the terms are still pronounced with a Spanish accent. Because of these similarities, it is easier to learn the meaning and pronunciations of Spanish words. The first step in communicating with Spanish-speaking patients is to learn the Spanish sound system. The Spanish Sounds section that follows provides Spanish pronunciations of vowels and consonants. Practice the pronunciations in the Spanish Sounds table, and use the table as a reference when you review Spanish pronunciations in the Chapter Tables section.

Spanish Sounds

The following table lists vowels and their Spanish pronunciations. Practice the pronunciations before continuing with the other information in this appendix.

Vowel	Spanish Pronunciation Sounds Like
a	*ah* as in father
e	*eh* as in net
i	*ee* as in keep
o	*oh* as in no
u	*oo* as in spoon
y	*e* as in bee

(Continued)

Consonant *(Continued)*	
c (after an e or i)	*ss* as in lesson
g (after an e or i)	*h* as in hurry
h	silent; it is never pronounced
j	*h* as in hot
ll	*y* as in yellow
ñ	*ni* as in onion
qu	*k* as in kite
rr	"rolled" *r* sound
v	*b* as in boy
z	*s* as in sun

Chapter Tables

Many Spanish terms ending in the letter "a" denote the feminine gender of the noun being modified, as in *izquierda*; many Spanish terms ending in the letter "o" denote masculine gender of the noun being modified, as in *izquierdo*. These types of Spanish terms in this section are clearly identified. In summary, to change the feminine gender of the noun the adjective modifies, change the ending letter "a" (female) to "o" (male), as in the terms *izquierda* (female), *izquierdo* (male).

In the following tables, capitalization is used to indicate primary accent of Spanish words. The capital letters indicate that emphasis is placed on the respective syllable when pronouncing the Spanish word. For example, the pronunciation of **an-te-re-OR** indicates emphasis on the last syllable.

Chapter 2: Body Structure

This section introduces English and translated Spanish terms and their respective pronunciations commonly used throughout all of the medical specialties, including radiology and physical therapy.

English	Spanish	Spanish Pronunciation
abdomen	abdomen	**ab-DOH-men**
anterior	anterior	**an-te-re-OR**
arm	brazo	**BRAH-so**
belly	vientre	**BEE-en-tre**
cell	célula	**CEL-loo-lah**
chest	pecho	**PE-cho**

English	Spanish	Spanish Pronunciation
diaphragm	diafragma	**de-ah-FRAHG-ma**
far	lejos	**LE-hos**
groin	ingle	**IN-gle**
head	cabeza	**cah-BEY-sah**
hip	cadera	**ca-DE-rah**
inferior	inferior	**in-fe-re-OR**
lateral	lateral	**lah-te-RAHL**
left	izquierda (female)	**is-key-ER-da**
	izquierdo (male)	**is-key-ER-do**
leg	pierna	**pi-ERR-nah**
lumbar	lumbar	**loom-BAR**
medial	del centro	**del-SEND-tro**
navel	ombligo	**om-BLEE-go**
near	cerca	**SIR-cah**
neck	cuello	**coo-EH-yo**
organ	órgano	**OR-gah-no**
palm	palma	**PALM-ma**
pelvis	pelvis	**PEL-vis**
posterior	posterior	**post-te-re-OR**
right	derecha	**de-RE-cha**
skull	cráneo	**CRAH-ne-o**
spine	espina	**es-PEE-nah**
superior	superior	**su-pee-re-OR**
tissue	tejido	**te-HEE-do**
toe	dedo del pie	**de-dou-del-pee-EH**

Chapter 3: Integumentary System

This section introduces English and translated Spanish terms and their respective pronunciations that are commonly used in the medical specialty of dermatology.

English	Spanish	Spanish Pronunciation
allergy	alergia	ah-LER-gi-ah
antibiotic	antibiótico	an-tee-be-O-tee-co
biopsy	biopsia	bee-UP-see-ah
black	negra (female)	NE-grah
	negro (male)	NE-groh
blister	ampolla	am-PO-ya
blue	azul	ah-ZOUL
brown	marrón	mar-RON
burn	quemar	kee-MAR
cream	crema	CREE-ma
dermatology	dermatología	der-mah-to-lo-HE-ah
hair	pelo	PEE-lo
infection	infección	in-fec-see-ON
nails	uñas	OO-ny-ahs
pink	rosada (female)	ro-SAH-dah
	rosado (male)	ro-SAH-do
perspiration	perpiración	pers-pee-RAH-see-ON
rash	sarpullido	sar-poo-YEE-do
red	rojo	ROH-ho
small	pequeño	PAY-kay-nyo
skin	piel	pe-EL
ulcer	úlcera	OOL-ce-rah
wound	herida	EH-ree-dah
yellow	amarillo	ah-ma-RE-yoh

Chapter 4: Respiratory System

This section introduces English and translated Spanish terms and their respective pronunciations that are commonly used in the medical specialty of pulmonology.

English	Spanish	Spanish Pronunciation
alveolus	alveolo	al-VE-o-lo
asphyxia	asfixia	as-FEEC-se-ah
asthma	asma	AS-ma
benign	benigno	be-NEEG-no
breathe	respira	res-pe-rah
breathing	respiración	res-pe-rah-see-ON
bronchus	bronquio	BRON-ke-o
chronic	crónico	CRO-nee-co
cough	gripe	GREE-pe
edema	edema	e-DE-mah
epiglottis	epiglotis	e-pe-GLO-tis
influenza	influenza	in-flu-EN-sa
larynx	laringe	lah-RING-heh
lobe	lóbulo	LO-boo-lo
lungs	pulmones	pool-MOH-nes
malignant	maligno	mah-LEEG-no
nose	nariz	nah-REES
nostril	orificio de la nariz	o-re-FEE-see-o de la nah-REES
obstruction	obstrucción	obs-truc-see-ON
pain	dolor	do-LOR
pneumonia	pulmonía	pool-mo-NEE-ah
sinus	cavidad nasal	cah-ve-DAHD nah-SAHL
sputum	esputo	es-POO-to
symptom	sintoma	SIN-to-mah
throat	garganta	gar-GAHN-tah
tonsil	amígdala	ah-MEG-dah-lah
trachea	tráquea	TRAH-ke-ah
voice	voz	vo-ss

Chapter 5: Cardiovascular and Lymphatic Systems

This section introduces English and translated Spanish terms and their respective pronunciations that are commonly used in the medical specialty of cardiology and immunology.

English	Spanish	Spanish Pronunciation
aneurysm	aneurisma	a-ne-oo-REES-mah
artery	arteria	ar-te-REE-ah
atrium	atrio	AH-tree-oh
blood	sangre	SAN-gre
blood clot	coágulo de sangre	co-AH-goo-lo de SAN-gre
blood pressure	presión de la sangre	pre-se-ON de la SAN-gre
capillary	capilar	cah-pe-LAR
catheter	catéter	cah-TE-ter
catheterization	cateterización	cah-te-te-re-sa-see-ON
gland	glándula	GLAN-doo-lah
hardening	endurecimiento	en-doo-re-see-mi-EN-to
heart	corazón	co-rah-SON
heart attack	ataque al corazón	ah-TAH-ke al co-rah-SON
heart rate	ritmo cardíaco	REET-mo car-DEE-ah-co
hemorrhage	hemorragia	eh-mo-RAH-he-ah
lymph	linfático	lin-FAH-te-co
lymph node	nódulo linfatico	NO-du-lo lin-FAH-te-CO
narrow	angosta (female)	an-GOS-ta
	angosto (male)	an-GOS-to
pulse	pulso	POOL-so
rapid	rápida (female)	RA-pi-dah
	rápido (male)	RA-pi-do
rhythm	ritmo	REET-mo
slow	lenta (female)	LEN-tah
	lento (male)	LEN-to
stroke	ataque	ah-TAH-ke
swelling	inflamación	in-flah-MAH-see-ON
valve	válvula	VAHL-voo-lah
varicose vein	vena varicosa	VE-nah va-re-CO-sah
vein	vena	VE-nah
ventricle	ventrículo	ven-TREE-coo-loh
vessel	vaso	VAH-soh
weakness	debilidad	de-be-le-DAHD

Chapter 6: Digestive System

This section is introduces English and translated Spanish terms and their respective pronunciations that are commonly used in the medical specialty of gastroenterology.

English	Spanish	Spanish Pronunciation
antacid	antiácido	**an-te-AH-ci-doh**
appendix	apéndice	**ah-PEN-de-ce**
appetite	apetito	**ah-pe-TEE-to**
belch	eructar	**eh-ruc-TAR**
chew	masticar	**mas-te-CAR**
colon	colon	**COH-lon**
colonoscopy	colonoscopia	**co-lo-nos-co-PE-ah**
constipation	estreñimiento	**es-tre-ny-me-EN-to**
defecate	defecar	**deh-fe-CAR**
diarrhea	diarrea	**de-ah-RE-ah**
digestion	digestión	**de-hes-te-ON**
dyspepsia	dispepsia	**dis-PEP-se-ah**
dysphagia	disfagia	**dis-FAH-he-ah**
esophagus	esófago	**es-SO-fah-go**
gallbladder	vesícula	**ve-SE-cu-la**
gallstone	cálculo biliar	**CAHL-coo-lo bi-le-AR**
glucose	glucosa	**glue-CO-sah**
gums	encia	**en-SE-ah**
hernia	hernia	**ER-ne-ah**
intestine	intestino	**in-tes-TEE-no**
jaundice	ictericia	**ic-te-RE-se-ah**
liver	higado	**EE-gah-do**
mouth	boca	**BO-cah**
pancreas	páncreas	**PAHN-cre-as**
rectum	recto	**REC-to**
sigmoidoscopy	sigmoidoscopia	**sig-mo-e-does-co-PE-ah**
stomach	estómago	**es-TOH-ma-go**
swallow	tragar	**trah-GAR**
teeth	diente	**de-EN-teh**
vomit	vómito	**VO-me-to**

Chapter 7: Urinary System

This section introduces English and translated Spanish terms and their respective pronunciations that are commonly used in the medical specialty of urology.

English	Spanish	Spanish Pronunciation
bladder	vejiga	ve-HE-gah
calculus	cálculo	CAHL-coo-lo
clear	clara (female)	CLAH-rah
	claro (male)	CLAH-ro
cloudy	nublado	noo-BLAH-do
cystoscopy	cistoscopia	se-tos-co-PE-ah
dialysis	diálisis	de-AH-li-sis
diuretic	diurético	de-oo-RE-te-co
dysuria	disuria	de-SU-re-ah
excretion	excreción	ex-cre-se-ON
hematuria	hematuria	eh-mah-TOO-re-ah
kidney	riñón	ree-NYOHN
nocturia	nocturia	noc-TU-re-ah
oliguria	oliguria	o-le-GU-re-ah
protein	proteína	pro-te-E-nah
renal pelvis	pelvis renal	PEL-vis reh-nal
ureter	uréter	u-RE-ter
urethra	uretra	u-RE-trah
urinalysis	urinalisis	u-re-NAH-lee-sis
urinary	urinario	u-re-NAH-re-o
urinary tract infection	infección del tracto urinario	in-fec-se-ON del TRAC-to u-re-NAH- re-o
urinate	orinar	o-re-NAR
urine	orina	o-REE-nah
urology	urología	uh-ro-lo-HE-ah

Chapter 8: Reproductive Systems

This section introduces English and translated Spanish terms and their respective pronunciations that are commonly used in the medical specialties of obstetrics and gynecology (female reproductive system) and urology (male reproductive system; male and female urinary system).

English	Spanish	Spanish Pronunciation
birth	nacimiento	na-se-me-EN-toh
breast	pecho	PE-cho
cervix	cervix	SER-vix
cesarean section	sección de cesárea	sec-se-ON de se-SA-re-ah
chorion	corion	CO-re-on
circumcision	circuncisión	sir-cun-se-se-ON
conception	concepción	con-cep-se-ON
condom	condón	con-DON
dysmenorrhea	dismenorrea	dis-me-no-RE-ah
endometriosis	endometriosis	en-do-me-tri-O-sis
erection	erección	eh-rec-se-ON
genitalia	genitalia	heh-ni-TAH-li-ah
hormone	hormona	or-MOH-nah
hysterectomy	histerectomía	is-te-rec-to-MEE-ah
impotency	inpotencia	in-po-TEN-se-ah
laparoscopy	laparoscopía	la-pa-ros-co-PEE-ah
leukorrhea	leucorrea	le-u-co-RE-ah
mammogram	mamografía	ma-mo-gra-PHI-ah
menopause	menopausia	me-no-PAH-oo-se-ah
menstruation	menstruación	mens-troo-a se-ON
newborn	recién nacida (female)	re-se-EN na-SE-dah
	recién nacido (male)	re-se-EN na-SE-do
ovary	ovario	o-VA-re-o
penis	pene	PE-ne
pregnant	embarazada	em-bah-rah-SA-dah
prostate	próstata	PROS-ta-tah
sexual intercourse	copula coito	COO-pu-la coito
testicle	testículo	tes-TEE-coo-lo
ultrasonography	ultrasonografía	ul-trah-so-no-gra-PHI-ah
uterus	útero	U-te-ro
vagina	vagina	vah-hee-NAH

Chapter 9: Endocrine and Nervous Systems

This section introduces English and translated Spanish terms and their respective pronunciations that are commonly used in the medical specialties of endocrinology and neurology.

English	Spanish	Spanish Pronunciation
adrenal gland	gládula adrenal	GLAN-du-la ah-dre-nal
adrenaline	adrenalina	ah-dre-nah-LEE-nah
brain	cerebro	se-RE-broh
calcium	calcio	CAHL-se-oh
concussion	concusión	con-coo-se-ON
conscious	consciente	cons-se-EN-teh
diabetes	diabetes	de-ah-be-tes
dizzy	mareado	ma-re-ah-do
encephalopathy	encefalopatía	en-ce-fah-lo-pa-TE-ah
epilepsy	epilepsia	eh-pe-LEP-se-ah
fainting	desmayarse	des-ma-YAR-ce
feminine	femenina	fe-mee-NE-nah
goiter	bocio	BO-se-oh
growth	crecimiento	cre-se-me-EN-to
headache	dolor de cabeza	do-LOR de cah-BE-sa
hormone replacement	remplazo de hormonas	rem-PLAH-so de or-MOH-nahs
insulin	insulina	in-su-LEE-nah
iodine	iodo	o-EE-do
masculine	masculino	mas-cu-LE-no
nerve	nervio	NERR-be-oh
pancreas	páncreas	PAN-cre-as
paralysis	parálisis	pa-RA-lee-sis
pituitary	pituitaria	pe-too-e-TAH-re-ah
seizure	asimiento	ah-se-me-EN-to
sensation	sensación	sen-sah-se-ON
spinal cord	espina dorsal	es-pee´-nah dor-SAHL
stroke	ataque cerebral	ah-TAH-ke ce-re-BRAHL
synthesis	síntesis	SIN-te-sis
thyroid	tiroide	te-RO-e-de
unconscious	inconsciente	in-cons-se-en-TEH

Chapter 10: Musculoskeletal System

This section introduces English and translated Spanish terms and their respective pronunciations that are commonly used in the medical specialty of orthopedics.

English	Spanish	Spanish Pronunciation
ankle	tobillo	**to-BE-yo**
arm	brazo	**BRAH-so**
arthritis	artritis	**ar-TREE-tees**
bones	huesos	**oo-EH-sos**
cartilage	cartílago	**car-TEE-lah-go**
collarbone	clavícula	**clah-BE-coo-lah**
fracture	fractura	**frac-TOO-rah**
herniated disk	disco herniado	**dis-coh er-ne-AH-do**
hip	cadera	**ca-DE-rah**
joint	coyunturas	**co-yoon-TOO-rahs**
knee	rodilla	**ro-DEE-yah**
kneecap	rótula	**RO-tu-lah**
ligament	ligamento	**le-gah-men´-to**
movement	movimiento	**mo-be-me-EN-to**
muscle	músculo	**MOOS-coo-lo**
reduction	reducción	**re-duc-se-ON**
rib	costilla	**co-TEE-yah**
sacrum	sacro	**SAH-cro**
shoulder	hombro	**OM-bro**
shoulder blade	lámina del hombro	**LAH-me-nah del OM-bro**
sore	llaga úlcera	**YAH-gah UL-ce-rah**
sprain	torcer	**tor-CER**
sternum	esternon	**es-ter-NON**
stiff	duro	**DU-roh**
support	soporte	**so-POR-teh**
tendon	tendón	**ten-DON**
thigh	muslo	**MUS-lo**
vertebrae	vertebra	**VER-te-brah**
wrist	muñeca	**moo-NYE-cah**
x-ray	rayos-x	**RAH-yos EH-kiss**

Chapter 11: Special Senses: The Eyes and Ears

This section introduces English and translated Spanish terms and their respective pronunciations that are commonly used in the medical specialties of ophthalmology and otolaryngology.

English	Spanish	Spanish Pronunciation
blepharospasm	blefaroespasmo	ble-pha-ro-es-PAS-moh
cerumen	cera de los oídos	CE-rah de los o-EEdos
choroidopathy	coroidopatía	co-ro-e-do-pah-TE-ah
dark	obscuro	obs-COO-ro
deafness	sordera	sor-DEH-rah
diplopia	diplopia	de-plo-PE-ah
eardrum	tímpano del oído	TEEM-pah-no del o-EE-do
ears	oídos	o-EE-dos
eyelid	párpado	PAR-pa-do
eyes	ojos	O-hos
hyperopia	hiperopía	e-per-o-PE-ah
inner ear	oido interior	o-EE-do in-teh-re-OR
iris	iris	EE-ris
light	claro liviano	CLAH-ro le-be-AH-no
macular degeneration	degeneración macular	deh-heh-ne-ra-se-ON ma-coo-LAR
myopia	miopía	me-o-PE-ah
ophthalmoscopy	oftalmoscopía	of-tal-mos-coo-PE-ah
otalgia	otalgía	o-TAHL-he-ah
otitis media	otitis media	o-TEE-tis MEH-de-ah
otoscope	otoscopio	o-tos-CO-pe-oh
otoscopy	otoscopía	o-tos-co-PE-ah
pupil	pupila	poo-PEE-lah
retina	retina	re-TEE-nah
retinitis	retinitis	re-te-NE-tis
sclera	esclera	es-CLE-rah
syncope	síncope	SIN-co-peh
tinnitus	tinitus	tee-NE-tus
vision	visión	be-se-ON

INDEX

Note: An "f" following a page number indicates a figure; a "t" following a page number indicates a table.

A

Abbreviations, 551–557
  body structure, 57
  cardiovascular and lymphatic systems, 176
  digestive system, 202, 237
  ear, 480
  endocrine system, 392
  eye, 480
  integumentary system, 82
  musculoskeletal system, 443
  nervous system, 392
  reproductive system, 338
  respiratory system, 126
  urinary system, 287
Abdomen, quadrants of, 41–42, 42f
Abdominal cavity, 40
Abdominopelvic cavity, 40
Abdominopelvic quadrants, 41–42, 42f, 58
Abdominopelvic regions, 42f, 42–45
Abnormal condition, 103, 201, 225, 234, 257, 258, 414
Above, 31, 33, 201, 208, 364
Above normal, 359, 360, 363, 370, 474
Abrasion, 82
Accessory glands, 326
Accessory organs of digestion, 226–235
Achilles tendon, 440
Achromatopsia, 480
Acidosis, 126
Acne, 82
Acoustic, 474
Acoustic neuroma, 482
Acquired immunodeficiency syndrome (AIDS), 79, 123, 178
Acromegaly, 366
Across, 219, 258, 415
Acute renal failure (ARF), 284
Acute respiratory distress syndrome, 126
Addison disease, 377, 393
Adenitis, 273
Adenocarcinoma, 273
Adenodynia, 273
Adenohypophysis, 365
Adenoids, 101
Adenoma, 67, 273, 359
Adenopathy, 169, 273
Adhesion, 47
Adipectomy, 67
Adipocele, 61
Adipoid, 315

Adipoma, 67, 68
Adipose tissue, 320
Adjective(s), 43, 235, 331
Adrenal, 359, 375
Adrenal cortex, 362f, 368
Adrenal glands, 359, 375–376
Adrenal hormones, 376t, 377–378
Adrenal medulla, 376
Adrenalectomy, 359, 375
Adrenaline, 376, 378
Adrenocorticotropic hormone (ACTH), 362f, 368
Adrenomegaly, 375
Adult respiratory distress syndrome, 126
Aerohydrotherapy, 106
Aerophagia, 103, 106, 209
Aerophobia, 121
Aerotherapy, 106
After, 319, 322
Agglutination, 169
AIDS, 79, 123, 178
Air, 102, 106, 115, 116, 121, 122
Albinism, 75, 77
Albino, 77
Albumin, 263
Aldosterone, 377
Aldosteronism, 377
Alimentary canal, 195
Alopecia, 82
Alveolar, 101
Alveolus(i), 101, 113
Alzheimer disease, 394
Amblyopia, 465
Amniocentesis, 303, 341, 342f
Amnion, 303
Amniotic sac, 303
Amphiarthroses, 424
Anacids, 209
Anacusis, 474, 483
Anaphylaxis, 170
Anastomosis, 50f, 51, 216, 217
Anatomic position, 29
Androgen(s), 327, 377
Androsterone, 327
Anesthesia, 335
Aneurysm, 168, 169f, 177, 388
Aneurysmectomy, 388
Angina pectoris, 165
Angiography, 145, 179
Angioplasty, 172, 180
Angiorrhaphy, 172
Angiorrhexis, 172

Anhidrosis, 67
Anisocoria, 464
Ankylosis, 414, 443
Anorchism, 340
Anorexia, 197
Anosmia, 103
Anoxemia, 127
Answer Key, 505–537
Anterior, 29, 31, 364, 365, 439
Anterolateral, 32
Anteroposterior (AP), 364
Anticoagulants, 167
Antidiuretic hormone (ADH), 362f, 366, 368
Anuria, 281
Anus, 212, 218, 220, 221
Aorta, 145, 150, 157
Aortic aneurysm, 168
Aortic stenosis, 157
Aortic valve, 157, 159
Aortopathy, 157
Aortostenosis, 145
AP, 40
Aphasia, 386
Aplasia, 335
Apnea, 103, 118, 119
Apoplexy, 394
Appendectomy, 211, 238, 238f
Appendicitis, 211, 238
Appendix, 211, 238
Appetite, 197
Arachnoid, 389
Areola, 320
Arm bone, upper, 413, 426
Around, 204
Arrhythmia, 177
Arterial blood gases, 129
Arterial calculus, 155
Arterial hardening, 155
Arterial spasm, 155
Arteriole(s), 157
Arteriolith, 155
Arteriopathy, 155
Arteriorrhaphy, 155
Arteriorrhexis, 155
Arteriosclerosis, 145, 155, 158, 166, 167, 177, 264
Arteriospasm, 155, 158
Arteriostenosis, 146
Artery(ies), 145, 150, 155, 157, 158, 259. *See also specific arteries*
  hardening of, 158

Arthralgia, 424
Arthritis, 414, 424, 444, 445f, 448f
Arthrocentesis, 424, 447
Arthroclasia, 415
Arthrodesis, 415
Arthrodynia, 424
Arthropathy, 424
Arthroplasty, 447
  total hip, 447, 448f
Arthroscopy, 447
Articulate, 424
Articulation, 432
Ascending colon, 217, 218
Ascites, 238
Aspermatism, 331
Aspermia, 327
Asthma, 113, 114f, 118
Astigmatism, 472f, 480
Atelectasis, 102, 126
Atheroma, 145
Atherosclerosis, 166, 167, 177
Athlete's foot, 201
Atlas, 430, 431
Atrial, 162
Atrial flutter, 152
Atrioventricular, 145, 151
Atrioventricular (AV) node, 162
Atrium, 145, 150, 152, 156, 162
Audiometer, 474
Audiometry, 484
Auditory tube, 304, 305, 307, 474, 476
Auricle, 475
Autoexamination, 79
Autografts, 79, 80
Autohypnosis, 79
Axillary nodes, 173
Axis, 430
Azotemia, 257, 258, 282
Azoturia, 282, 287

B

Back, 30, 364
  lower, 44, 436
Backbone, 413, 426, 429, 430, 431f
Backward, 278, 305
Bacterium, 153
Bacteriuria, 283
Bad, 305
Balanitis, 327, 340
Baldness, 82
Balloon valvuloplasty, 181
Barium enema, 240
Barium swallow, 240
Bartholin glands, 301, 317
Basal cell carcinoma, 78, 78f
Basal layer of skin, 65f
Bedsore, 83
Before, 304, 319, 322
Beginning, 305
Behind, 278, 305, 364
Bell palsy, 394
"Belly button," 44
Below, 201, 359, 363, 364, 413, 421, 427
Benign, 272, 273, 334
Benign prostatic hyperplasia, 332

Benign prostatic hypertrophy (BPH), 332
  medical records, 293–295
Bent, 414
Bilateral, 335
Bilateral vasectomy, medical records,
  349–350
Bile, 225, 228
Bile duct, 225, 226, 230
Bile vessel, 225
Biliary duct, 230
Binding, 415
Biopsy, 86, 260
Birth, 304
Black lung, 116
Bladder, 257, 268, 269, 279, 314, 333
Blepharectomy, 470
Blepharedema, 469
Blepharoplasty, 470, 471
Blepharoplegia, 470
Blepharoptosis, 465, 471
Blepharospasm, 464, 470, 471
Blepharotomy, 470
Blind spot, 469
Blood, 127, 156, 209, 305, 312, 372, 375,
  379
Blood clot, 145, 167, 168, 388
Blood condition, 76, 257, 258, 359
Blood flow, through heart, 154–158
Blood urea nitrogen, 288
Blood vessel(s), 145
  renal, 264
  widened, 388
Body, cavities of, 40–41
  cellular level of, 27–28
  levels of structural organization in, 24f
  organization of, 24f, 27–28
  planes of, 30f, 37–40
  structure of, 23–58
    Spanish translations, 570–571
Boil, 82f, 83
Bolus, 205
Bone(s), 374, 413–414, 415, 443–444. *See
  also specific bones*
  structure and function of, 416–422,
  417f
Bone cell, 415
Bone marrow, 385, 387, 414, 418, 421
Bone marrow aspiration biopsy, 179
Bony necrosis, 79
Borborygmus, 238
Bowel movement, 202
Bowman capsule, 276
Bradycardia, 153, 164
Bradyphagia, 153
Bradypnea, 153
Brain, 385, 427
Brain scan, CT, 395
Break, 415
Breast(s), 304, 319–322, 321f, 362f, 369
Breast feeding, 322
Breastbone, 413, 426
Breathing, 103, 113, 118
Bronchial tree, 111
Bronchiectasis, 102, 113
Bronchiole(s), 102, 111, 113
Bronchiolitis, 102

Bronchitis, 113, 114f, 122, 124
Bronchodilators, 129
Bronchopneumonia, 123
Bronchoscope, 102
Bronchoscopy, 129
Bronchospasm, 113
Bronchostenosis, 113
Bronchus(i), 102, 111, 113
Bruise, 83, 83f
Bruit, 177
Bulbourethral glands, 326, 331
Bulla, 85f
Bundle branches, 162
Bundle of His, 162, 165
Bursae, 430
Bursting forth, 304, 312, 319

C

C1-C5, 431–432
Calcaneodynia, 413
Calcaneum, 413, 426
Calcemia, 372, 375, 421
Calcitonin, 371
Calcium, 359, 372, 375
Calculus(i), 155, 225, 230, 231, 232, 258,
  262, 264, 267, 330, 378
Calyx(ces), 274
Cancellous bone, 418
Cancer (CA), 108, 208, 218, 221, 233,
    273, 334
  lungs and, 124
Cancerous, 208, 272, 273, 334
Candidiasis, 338
Capillaries, 158
Carbon dioxide (CO_2), 115, 116,
  155
Carbuncle, 82, 82f
Carcinoma(s), 78, 208, 222, 334
  papillary, 133–135
Carcinosarcoma of esophagus, medical
    records, 246–247
Cardiac, 157, 167
Cardiac catheterization, 179, 180
  medical records, 186–187
Cardiac cycle, 164–168
Cardiac enzyme studies, 179
Cardiography, 179
Cardiomegaly, 145, 165
Cardiorrhaphy, 160
Cardiovascular system, 143–169, 144f
  abbreviations, 176
  diagnostic terms, 179
  pathological terms, 177–178
  Spanish translations, 574
  therapeutic terms, 180–181
  walls of heart, 148–149
Carpal tunnel syndrome, 443
Carpoptosis, 413
Carpus, 413, 426
Cartilage, 111, 419, 436, 437
Cataract, 480
Cataract surgery, 484, 484f
Catheterization, 289
Caudal, 33
Cauterize, 51

Cell(s), 75–78, 280, 388, 415
  body organization and, 27–28
Cellular necrosis, 79
Central nervous system (CNS), 384
Cephalad, 33
Cephalalgia, 426
Cephalodynia, 426
Cephalometer, 427
Cerclage, 344
Cerebral aneurysm, 168
Cerebral infarction, 394
Cerebral palsy, 394
Cerebroid, 389
Cerebrosclerosis, 389
Cerebrospinal, 385
Cerebrospinal fluid analysis, 395
Cerebrovascular, 388
Cerebrovascular accident (CVA), 388,
    394
  medical records, 401–402
Cerebrum, 385, 389
Cervical, 318, 414
Cervical nodes, 173
Cervical vertebra(ae), 430, 431
Cervicitis, 303, 317, 339
Cervicofacial, 430
Cervix, 317, 318
Cervix uteri, 303, 317, 414, 430
Cesarean section (CS, C-section), 324
Chemabrasion, 86
Chemical peel, 86
Chest, 102, 103, 172
Chest radiograph, 48f
Chest x-ray, 129
Child, 415
Childbirth, 305
Chlamydia, 323, 341
Cholangiography, 230
Cholangiole, 225
Cholangitis, 230
Cholecyst, 228, 230, 232
Cholecystalgia, 232
Cholecystectomy, 225, 233
Cholecystitis, 227, 228, 230, 232
Cholecystodynia, 232
Cholecystolith, 229
Cholecystolithiasis, 233
Choledoch, 230
Choledochitis, 230
Choledocholith, 230
Choledocholithiasis, 230, 231f
Choledochoplasty, 230, 233
Choledochorrhaphy, 230
Choledochotomy, 225, 230
Cholelith, 225, 229, 230, 231, 232
Cholelithiasis, 225, 231f, 232
Cholemesis, 228
Chondritis, 111, 419
Chondrocyte, 419
Chondrogenesis, 419
Chondroma, 111, 419
Chondropathy, 111
Chondroplasty, 111
Chondrotomy, 437
Chordae tendineae, 159
Choroid, 464, 467

Choroiditis, 467
Choroidopathy, 464, 468
Chronic obstructive lung disease
    (COLD), 114f, 124
Chyme, 205
Ciliary body, 466–467, 467f
Ciliated epithelium, 105
Circulatory system, 144f, 169–193
Circumcision, 344
Cirrhosis, 227, 238
Clitoris, 301, 317
Closed fracture, 428
Clot(s), 167, 168
Clubfoot, 446, 446f
Clumping, 169
Coccyx, 432
Cochlea, 476
Cochlear implant, 485
COLD, 114f, 124
Colectomy, 217
Colitis, 217, 238
Collecting tubule, 276
Colles fracture, 429
Colon, 211, 215, 217, 219, 221, 222
Colonic polyposis, 238
Colonitis, 222
Colonoscope, 222
Colonoscopy, 211, 221, 221f, 222
Coloposcopy, 342
Color blindness, 480
Colorectal cancer, 238
Colorrhaphy, 218
Colors, combining forms denoting, 75
Colostomy, 211, 218, 218f
Colotomy, 217
Colpalgia, 313
Colpitis, 313
Colpocele, 303
Colpocervical, 317
Colpocystocele, 314
Colpodynia, 313
Colpohysterectomy, 314
Colpopexy, 313
Colpoptosis, 313
Colporrhagia, 314
Colporrhaphy, 314
Colposcope, 303, 317, 318
Colposcopy, 303, 317, 318
Colpospasm, 313
Combining form(s), body structure,
    54–55
  creation of, 5–7
  denoting colors, 75
  digestive system, 200, 211–212, 225
  respiratory tract, 101–102
Combining vowel, 200
Comedo, 83
Comminuted fracture, 429
Common bile duct, 226
Compact bone, 417, 418
Complicated fracture, 429
Compound, 429
Compound nevus, medical record, 90–91
Computed tomography (CT) scan,
    47–48, 48f, 129, 241, 288, 395
Condidiasis, 201

Condition, 196, 235, 257, 327, 370, 464
Conduction pathway, of heart, 162–163,
    163f
Congestive heart failure (CHF), 177
Conjunctivitis, 481
Continence, 283
Contraction, 162, 164, 220
  involuntary, 103, 464
Contracture, 443
Contusion, 83
Convergent strabismus, 481, 481f
Convulsion, 394
Copulatory organ, 326
Coreometer, 464
Cornea, 464, 466, 468
  hard, 70
Corneal grafting, 464
Corneal transplant, 485
Corneitis, 464
Coronal, 38, 39
Coronary artery bypass graft (CABG),
    180, 181f
Coronary artery disease, 166, 166f, 177
Corticosteroids, 129
Coryza, 127
Costalgia, 427
Costochondritis, 436
Cowper glands, 331
Crackle, 127
Cranial, 40
Cranial cavity, 41
Craniotomy, 396, 413
Cranium, 413, 426
Crepitation, 444
Crib death, 128
Crohn disease, 217, 238, 239
Crooked, 414
Cross-eye, 481
Cross-sectional, 39
Croup, 127
Crushing, 258, 267
Cryosurgery, 86
Cryotherapy, 62
Cryptorchidism, 327, 341
C-section, 324
CT scan, 47–48, 48f, 129, 241
Cushing syndrome, 377, 377f, 393
Cusp(s), 159
Cutaneous, 61, 70
Cuticle, 71
Cyanoderma, 75, 77
Cyanosis, 77, 78, 103
Cyst, 83
Cystectomy, 271
Cystic, 228
Cystic duct, 228
Cystic fibrosis, 127
Cystitis, 271, 283
  medical records, 291–292
Cystocele, 257, 269, 269f, 270, 279, 280
Cystolith, 268
Cystolithiasis, 268
Cystolithotomy, 268
Cystoplasty, 271
Cystorrhaphy, 269
Cystorrhexis, 439

Cystoscope, 270, 271
Cystoscopy, 257, 270
Cystourethroscope, 272
Cystourethroscopy, 272
Cystourography, 288
Cytology, 75

D

Dacryadenalgia, 473
Dacryadenitis, 473
Dacryorrhea, 464, 473
Dead, 79
Deafness, 474, 478, 483
Death, 79, 167, 205
Debridement, 86
Decubitus ulcer, 83
Deep vein thrombosis, 177
Deficient, 359, 363, 421
Dentalgia, 204
Dentist, 196, 202, 204
Dentistry, 202
Dentodynia, 204
Deoxygenated, 150
Dermabrasion, 86
Dermatitis, 65, 71
Dermatologist, 61, 65, 69
Dermatology, 69
Dermatoma, 69
Dermatome, 80
Dermatomycosis, 62, 70
Dermatopathy, 69
Dermatophytes, 70
Dermatoplasty, 62, 68
Dermis, 64, 65f, 66
Dermopathy, 70
Descending colon, 217, 218
Destruction, 225, 258, 385, 436
Development, 360
Diabetes, 393
Diabetes mellitus, 379, 380, 381, 393
    medical records, 399–401
    type 1, 380, 393
    type 2, 380, 393
Diabetic coma, 380
Diabetic retinopathy, 481
Diagnosis, 202, 324
Diagnostic procedures, 539–543
Diagnostic terms, 47–51
Dialysis, 258
Diaphoresis, 62, 67
Diaphragm, 40, 120
Diaphysis, 415, 417
Diarrhea, 197, 219, 233, 234
Diarthroses, 424
Diastole, 164
Dictionary, 310
Different, 465
Difficult, 305
Digestion, 197
Digestive system, 195–254, 198f
    abbreviations, 202, 237
    accessory organs of, 226–235
    combining forms, 211–212, 225
    diagnostic terms, 240–241
    pathological terms, 238–240

Spanish translations, 575
    therapeutic terms, 241
Digital rectal examination (DRE), 343
Dilated vein, 328
Dilation, 102, 268
Dilation and curettage (D&C), 344
Dim, 465
Diplopia, 464, 470
Directional terms, 28–34
Discharge, 196, 197, 200, 233, 303, 464, 474
Disease, 196, 258, 304, 329, 427, 436, 464, 465
Dissimilar, 464
Distal, 33, 34, 420
Distal epiphysis, 418
Diuresis, 287
Diuretics, 263
Divergent strabismus, 481f, 482
Diverticula, 239
Diverticular disease, 239, 239f
Diverticulitis, 218
Doppler ultrasonography, 179
Dorsal, 29
Double, 464, 470
Downward, 465
Downward displacement, 258, 413
Drug classifications, 547–550
Dry, 62
Duchenne dystrophy, 446
Duct, 145, 328
Ductus deferens, 326, 331
Dull, 465
Duodenal ulcer(s), 205, 216
Duodenectomy, 214, 216
Duodenorrhaphy, 216
Duodenoscopy, 206, 211, 223
Duodenostomy, 214
Duodenotomy, 215
Duodenum, 211, 213, 214, 215, 216, 226, 229f
Dura matter, 389
Dwarf, 366
Dwarfism, 361, 366
Dysentery, 239
Dysmenorrhea, 319
Dyspepsia, 197, 209
Dysphagia, 197, 209
Dysplasia, 335
Dyspnea, 118, 119
Dysrhythmia, 177
Dystocia, 305
Dysuria, 283, 287

E

E chart, 483
Ear(s), 473–479
    abbreviations, 480
    diagnostic terms, 484
    inner, 477f
    path of vibrations, 477f
    pathological terms, 482–483
    Spanish translations, 580
    structures of, 473, 477f
    therapeutic terms, 485

Ear canal, 475
Earache, 478
Eardrum, 474, 475, 476
Eating, 103, 170, 197, 209
Ecchymosis, 83, 83f
ECG, 164
Echo. *See* Ultrasonography (US)
Echocardiography, 179
Eclampsia, 339
Ectopic pregnancy, 339, 339f
Eczema, 83
Eczematous rash, 83
Edema, 263, 277
Ejaculatory duct, 326
EKG, 164
Electrical, 162
Electricity, 146, 162
Electrocardiogram, 146, 163f, 164
Electrocardiograph, 146
Electrocardiography, 146, 164, 179
Electrodessication, 86
Embolus(i), 177, 388
Emesis, 208
Emmetropia, 472f
Emphysema, 114f, 123, 127
Encephalitis, 385, 387, 427
Encephalocele, 427
Encephaloma, 387, 427
Encephalomalacia, 427
Encephalopathy, 427
End-stage renal disease, 287
Endocardium, 146, 148, 149, 159
Endocrine glands, 367f
Endocrine system, 357–383, 383f
    abbreviations, 392
    diagnostic terms, 395
    pathological terms, 393–394
    Spanish translations, 578
    therapeutic terms, 395
Endometriosis, 340, 340f
Endometritis, 304
Endoscope, 206, 220
Endoscopy, 48, 49f, 206, 220
Enlargement, 165, 170, 197, 225, 235, 264, 332, 359, 375
Enteral, 217
Enterectomy, 217
Enteritis, 217
Enterocele, 279
Enterologist, 202
Enteropathy, 211
Enterorrhaphy, 217
Enterorrhexis, 439
Enteroscope, 222
Enteroscopy, 222
Enuresis, 287
Epidermis, 64, 65f, 66
Epididymides, 335
Epididymis, 326, 331
Epidural space, 389
Epigastric, 43, 208, 209
Epiglottis, 109
Epiglottitis, 127
Epilepsy, 394
Epinephrine, 376, 377
Episiotomy, 304

Epispadias, 341
Epistaxis, 127
Epithelium, ciliated, 105
Epstein-Barr virus, 179
Erythrocyte, 76, 280
Erythrocytosis, 78
Erythroderma, 75
Erythropia, 470
Erythropoiesis, 418, 419
Erythrosis, 78
Erythruria, 280
Esophagitis, 205
Esophagoplasty, 207, 233
Esophagoscope, 196
Esophagoscopy, 206
Esophagotome, 207
Esophagotomy, 207, 208
Esophagus, 196, 203f, 205, 207, 208, 233, 246–247
Esotropia, 481, 482
Estrogen(s), 312, 320, 377
Eupnea, 118, 119
Eustachian tube, 304, 305, 307, 474, 476
Ewing sarcoma, 444
Examination, 222
Excessive, 360, 363, 370, 474
Excision, 116, 167, 225, 303, 304, 320, 327, 328, 359, 414
Excoriations, 85f
Excretory urogram, 288
Exhalation, 120, 121f
Exhale, 115
Exophthalmic, 370
Exophthalmos, 369f, 370, 371, 393
Exotropia, 481, 481f
Expansion, 102, 157
Expiration, 120, 121f
Extracapsular surgery, 485
Extracorporeal shock-wave lithotripsy (ESWL), 234, 285, 285f
Eye(s), 463–472
    abbreviations, 480
    bulging of, 370, 393
    diagnostic terms, 483
    pathological terms, 480–482
    Spanish translations, 580
    structures of, 466–467, 467f
    therapeutic terms, 484–485
Eye tuck, 470
Eyeball, 466
Eyelid(s), 464, 465, 469, 471

F

Fallopian tube(s), 301, 304, 305, 306, 307, 474, 476
False, 305
Farsightedness, 471, 472f
Farthest, 420
Fasting blood sugar, 202
Fat, 68, 315
Fatty plaque, 145
Feces, 218
Female, 303
Female reproductive system. *See* Reproductive system(s), female

Feminization, 377
Femoral, 414
Femur, 414, 417f, 426
Fiberoptic gastroscope, 197
Fibrillation, 177
Fibroid of uterus, 340
Fibroma of uterus, 340
Fibrosis, 69
Fibula, 414, 426
Fibular, 414
"Fight-or-flight" reaction, 378
Fingernail, structure of, 71, 71f
Fingers, bones of, 413, 426
First, 305
Fissure, 85f
Fistula, 239
Fixation, 258, 327, 415
Flat bones, 416, 417
Floating kidney, 265
Flow, 196, 197, 200, 233, 303, 464, 474
Fluid retention, 263
Fluoroscopy, 49
Follicle-stimulating hormone (FSH), 362f, 368
Foot, 415
Foreskin, 333
Forming, 303, 327, 331, 359, 379
Four, 386
Fourth, 322
Fracture(s), and repairs, 428–429
    types of, 428f, 428–429
Front, 30
Frontal, 38
Fungus(i), 62, 70, 71, 122, 201
Furuncle, 82f, 83

G

Galactorrhea, 303
Gall, 225, 228
Gallbladder, 225, 226, 227, 228, 229, 229f, 230, 232, 233
Gallstone, 225, 229, 231, 232
Gametes, 301, 326
Gangrene, 79
Gastralgia, 197, 205
Gastrectomy, 206, 207
Gastric ulcers, 205
Gastritis, 205, 208
Gastroduodenostomy, 216, 217
Gastrodynia, 197, 205
Gastroenteroanastomosis, 216
Gastroenterologist, 202
Gastroenterostomy, 216
Gastroileostomy, 216
Gastrointestinal, 202
Gastrointestinal system. *See* Digestive system
Gastrointestinal tract, 195
Gastrologist, 202
Gastrology, 69, 202
Gastromegaly, 197, 205, 235
Gastroplasty, 207
Gastroscopy, 197, 206, 223
Gastrotome, 207
Genital warts, 341

Genitalia, 301, 317
Giant, 366
Gigantism, 366
Gingivitis, 196, 204
Gingivosis, 204
Gland(s), 169, 196, 200, 273, 358, 365
Glandular disease, 169
Glandular tissue, 320
Glans penis, 327, 333
Glaucoma, 481
Glial cells, 384
Glioma(s), 384, 385
Glomerulitis, 277
Glomerulonephritis, 263, 276, 277, 284
Glomerulopathy, 277
Glomerulosclerosis, 257, 277
Glomerulus(i), 257, 276, 277
Glucagon(s), 378, 379
Glucocorticoid hormone, 376
Glucocorticoids, 376
Glucogenesis, 359, 379, 380
Glucometer, 379
Glucose, 379, 380
Glue, 385
Glycogen, 379, 380
Glycogenesis, 379
Glycogenolysis, 379
Glyconeogenesis, 379
Goiter, 371f
Gonad-stimulating hormone, 327
Gonadotropin(s), 327, 344
Gonads, 326, 327
Gonorrhea, 323, 341
Gout, 444
Graves disease, 369f, 370, 371, 393
Gravida, 322
Greenstick fracture, 429
Growth, 334, 335, 415
Growth hormone (GH), 361, 362f, 365, 368
Gums, 202, 204
Gynecologist, 303, 318
Gynecology (GYN), 318
Gynecopathy, 318

H

Hair, 62, 71
Hair follicle, 66
Hand bones, 413, 426
Hard, 468
Hardening, 62, 69, 257, 264, 277, 439, 465, 467
Hardening of arteries, 177
Head, 426, 427
Hearing loss, complete, 474, 478, 483
    conductive, 483
Heart, 145, 363
    blood flow through, 154–158
    conduction pathway of, 162–163, 163f
    sounds of, 164–168
    structures of, 148, 149f, 150–153, 151f
    valves and cusps of, 159f, 159–160
    walls of, 148–149

Heart attack, 178
Heart condition, 146
Heart failure (HF), 177
Heart valves, 159–160
Heat, 234
Heel bone, 413, 426
Hemangiectasis, 157
Hemangioma, 157
Hematemesis, 209, 313
Hematochezia, 239
Hematologist, 157, 313
Hematology, 157, 312
Hematoma, 312
Hematopathy, 313
Hematosalpinx, 305
Hematuria, 281, 282, 283, 284
Hemiparesis, 386
Hemiplegia, 436, 440
Hemoccult test, 241
Hemophobia, 122
Hemorrhage, 168, 312, 314, 387, 388, 390
　　uterine, 310
Hemorrhoid, 239
Hemosalpinx, 305
Hemothorax, 127
Hepatalgia, 227
Hepatectomy, 227
Hepatic, 228
Hepatic duct, 228
Hepatitis, 225, 226, 227, 235
Hepatitis B, 227
Hepatocyte, 227
Hepatodynia, 227
Hepatolith, 229
Hepatoma, 227
Hepatomegaly, 225, 227, 235
Hepatorrhaphy, 227
Hepatorrhexis, 439
Hepatosis, 232
Hernia(s), 44, 61, 72, 239, 240f, 257,
　　269, 269f, 303, 309, 314, 328, 333,
　　385, 414
Herniated disk, 444, 444f
Herpes genitalia, 341
Heteropsia, 465
Hidden, 327
Hidradenitis, 61
Hidrosis, 66
Hirsutism, 83
Histocompatibility testing, 180
HIV, 178
Hodgkin disease, 172, 178
Holter monitor, 179, 180f
Hordeolum, 481
Horizontal, 38
Hormone replacement therapy (HRT),
　　312, 396
Hormones, 361–363, 362f, 363t
Horny tissue, 70, 464, 468
Human immunodeficiency virus (HIV),
　　178
Humeral, 413
Humerus, 413, 426
Huntington chorea, 394
Hydrocele, 333
Hydrocephalus, 394

Hydronephrosis, 281, 282
Hydrotherapy, 106
Hydrothorax, 127
Hyperbilirubinemia, 239
Hypercalcemia, 372, 375, 421
Hyperemesis, 197, 208
Hyperglycemia, 359, 379, 380, 393
Hyperinsulinism, 379
Hyperopia, 471, 472f
Hyperparathyroidism, 375
Hyperplasia, 335
Hypersalivation, 196, 200
Hypersecretion, 362, 363, 377, 378, 379
Hypertension, 177, 263, 264, 277, 288,
　　378
Hyperthyroidism, 370
Hypertrophy, 360
Hypertropia, 474
Hypocalcemia, 359, 372, 375, 421
Hypochondriac, 43
Hypodermic, 61, 65
Hypogastric, 43
Hypogastric region, 45
Hypoglossal, 196
Hypoglycemia, 379, 380
Hypophysis, 365
Hyposecretion, 362, 363, 377, 378,
　　379
Hypospadias, 287, 341
Hypothyroidism, 393
Hypoxemia, 127
Hypoxia, 103, 127
Hysteralgia, 309
Hysterectomy, 303, 310, 311f
Hysterocele, 307, 311
Hysterodynia, 309
Hysteropathy, 309
Hysteropexy, 310
Hysteroplasty, 311
Hysteroptosis, 310
Hysterosalpingo-oophorectomy, 344
Hysterosalpingography, 342
Hysteroscopy, 310
Hysterospasm, 309
Hysterotome, 324
Hysterotomy, 310, 324

I

IBD, 239
Ichthyosis, 61, 62
Ileectomy, 214
Ileitis, 217
Ileorrhaphy, 216
Ileostomy, 211, 214
Ileotomy, 215
Ileum, 211, 213, 214, 215, 216, 217
Immune, 170
Immunity, 170
Immunocompromised persons, 123
Immunogen, 170
Impacted fracture, 429
Impetigo, 83
Impotence, 341
In, 427
In front of, 304

Incision, 197, 212, 225, 262, 267, 304,
　　324, 413, 436, 437, 474
Incision and drainage (I&D), 86
Incontinence, 283
Increase, 414
Incus, 476
Indigestion, 197
Infarct, 167
Inferior, 31, 32, 33, 39, 40, 154
Inferior vena cava (IVC), 150, 154, 158
Inflammation, 47, 66, 115, 117, 196, 197,
　　199, 204, 211, 217, 219, 225, 230, 232,
　　274, 313, 322, 328, 359, 385, 387, 388,
　　390, 413, 414, 415, 436, 464, 465
Inflammatory bowel disease, 239
Influenza, 127
Inguinal, 43, 44
Inguinal hernia, 44
Inguinal nodes, 174
Inhalation, 120, 121f
Inhale, 115
Inspiration, 120, 121f
Instrument, 268, 307
Instrument for examining, 196, 465, 469
Instrument for measuring, 464, 474
Instrument for recording, 146, 415
Insulin, 378, 379, 380, 393
Insulin-dependent diabetes mellitus
　　(IDDM), 380, 393
Insulinoma, 393
Integumentary structures, 65f
Integumentary system, 59–98
　　abbreviations, 82
　　combining forms for, 94
　　compound nevus, 90–91
　　diagnostic terms, 86
　　pathological terms, 82–85
　　prefixes for, 95
　　psoriasis, 92–93
　　Spanish translations, 572
　　suffixes for, 94–95
　　therapeutic terms, 86
Interatrial septum (IAS), 152, 156
Intercostal muscles, 120, 427
Interior, 440
Interstitial fluid, 169
Interstitial nephritis, 287–288
Interventricular, 146
Interventricular septum (IVS), 152, 156
Intervertebral disk(s), 430
　　degenerative disease of, medical
　　　records, 451–452
Intestine, 211, 213, 217, 269, 279
　　large. *See* Colon
Intraocular, 465
Intraocular lens transplant, 484, 484f
Intravenous, 278
Intravenous pyelogram, 288
Intravenous pyelography (IVP), 277, 278
Intravenous urography, 288
Involuntary contraction, 103, 464
Iridectomy, 485
Iridocele, 468
Iridoplegia, 464
Iris, 464, 467
Irregular bones, 416, 417

Irritable bowel syndrome, 234, 239
Ischemia, 178, 388
Islets of Langerhans, 378

J

Jaundice, 239
Jaw, 201
Jejunal feeding tube, 215
Jejunectomy, 214
Jejunorrhaphy, 211, 216
Jejunostomy, 214
Jejunotomy, 215
Jejunum, 211, 213, 214
Joint(s), 414, 415, 424–425, 443–444
Juvenile warts, 84

K

Kaposi sarcoma, 79, 178
Keratin, 64
Keratitis, 464, 468
Keratoplasty, 464
Keratorrhexis, 468
Keratosis, 61, 70
Keratotome, 468
Keratotomy, 468
Ketosis, 393
Kidney(s), 256, 257, 258, 259–265, 261f,
    264, 362f, 368, 374, 377
Kidney failure, 282
Kidney stone(s), 260, 262f, 267
Killing, 327
Kneecap, 414, 426
KUB, 277, 288
Kyphosis, 444, 445f

L

Labia majora, 301, 317
Labia minora, 301, 317
Labor, 305
Labyrinth(s), 476, 477f
Lacrimal apparatus, 464, 478f
Lacrimal gland, 471
Lacrimal sac, 471, 473
Lacrimation, 464
Lactation, 319, 320
Lactiferous duct, 320
Lactogen, 303
Lamina, 414
Laminectomy, 414
Laparoscopy, 342, 343f
Large intestine, 213
Laryngectomy, 108
Laryngitis, 108, 122
Laryngoscope, 108
Laryngoscopy, 109
Laryngospasm, 109
Laryngostenosis, 109
Larynx, 101, 108, 112
Laser keratotomy, 468
Lateral, 29, 32
Lazy-eye syndrome, 482
Left hepatic duct, 228
Left-sided appendicitis, 239, 239f

Left ventricle (LV), 152
Leg, lower, bones of, 426
Leg bones, 414
Leukemia, 76
Leukocyte(s), 76, 280
Leukocytopenia, 76
Leukocytosis, 78
Leukoderma, 75
Leukopoiesis, 418, 419
Leukorrhea, 280, 340
Linguodental, 201
Lipectomy, 67, 68
Lipocele, 73
Lipocyte(s), 61, 65f, 67, 68
Lipoma, 67
Liposuction, 68
Lithectomy, 284
Lithiasis, 232, 258, 260
Lithotomy, 264
Lithotripsy, 241, 258, 267, 284, 285
Liver, 225, 226, 227, 229, 229f, 232, 235,
    379
Lobar pneumonia, 135–137
Lobectomy, 116, 117
Lobe(s), 116, 117, 320
Lobitis, 117
Lobotomy, 117
Loins, 44, 436
Long bone(s), 416, 417, 417f
Loosening, 225, 258, 385, 436
Lordosis, 444, 445f
Lower back, 44, 436
Lumbar, 43, 432, 433
Lumbar vertebrae, 432
Lumboabdominal, 44
Lumbocostal, 436
Lumbodynia, 432
Lumen, 165, 272
Lung(s), 102, 115, 116, 122
    cancer of, 124
Lung cancer(s), 127
Lunula, 71
Luteinizing hormone (LH), 362f, 366,
    368
LV, 152
Lymph, 170
Lymph capillaries, 172
Lymph cells, 173
Lymph gland, 170
Lymph node(s), 170, 173
Lymph vessel(s), 157, 170, 172
Lymphadenitis, 170, 179
Lymphangiography, 180
Lymphangioma, 170, 172
Lymphatic duct, 172
Lymphatic system, 144f, 150, 169–193,
    173f
    abbreviations, 176
    diagnostic terms, 180
    pathological terms, 178–179
    Spanish translations, 574
Lymphocyte(s), 170, 172, 174
Lymphoid, 172
Lymphoid tissue, 170
Lymphoma, 172
Lymphopathy, 174

Lymphopoiesis, 170, 172
Lymphosarcoma, 179

M

Macular degeneration, 481, 482f
Macule, 85f
Magnetic resonance imaging (MRI), 48f,
    49, 129, 241, 395, 396
Malacia, 72
Male reproductive system. *See*
    Reproductive system(s), male
Malignant, 208, 272, 273, 334
Malignant neoplasms, 334
Malleus, 476
Malnutrition, 208
Mammary glands, 319–322, 321f, 362f
Mammogram, 304
Mammography, 320, 342
Mammoplasty, 320
Many, 258, 282, 305, 360
Mastalgia, 322
Mastectomy, 320, 344
Mastitis, 322
Mastodynia, 322
Mastopexy, 304, 320
Mastoplasty, 320
Matrix, 71
Meal, 225
Measure, 304
Meatus, 257
Mediad, 32
Medial, 32
Median, 38, 39
Mediastinum, 148
Medical record(s), benign prostatic
        hypertrophy, 293–295
    bilateral vasectomy, 349–350
    carcinosarcoma of esophagus, 246–247
    cardiac catheterization, 186–187
    cerebrovascular accident, 401–402
    compound nevus, 90–91
    cystitis, 291–292
    degenerative intervertebral disk
        disease, 451–452
    diabetes mellitus, 399–401
    myocardial infarction (MI), 184–185
    otitis media, 490–491
    papillary carcinoma, 133–134
    postmenopausal bleeding, 347–349
    psoriasis, 92–93
    rectal bleeding, 244–246
    retinal detachment, 488–490
    rotator cuff tear, 453–455
Medical specialties, 559–561
Medical word elements, 497–504
Medullary cavity, 417
Megalocardia, 165
Megalogastria, 205, 206
Megalogastric, 206
Melanin, 66, 77
Melanocyte(s), 66, 76, 77
Melanoderma, 75
Melanoma, 61, 66, 77, 78
Melanosis, 78
Menarche, 305

Méniére disease, 483
Meninges, 385, 389
Meningioma, 385, 389
Meningitis, 389
Meningocele, 385, 389, 395
Meningomyelocele, 395
Menopause, 312, 319
Menorrhagia, 304, 319
Menorrhea, 318, 319
Menses, 304, 305, 318, 319
Menstruation, 304, 305, 318, 319
Metacarpectomy, 413
Metacarpus, 413, 426
Metastasis, 124
Metastasize, 124
Meter, 427
Metrolasty, 311
Microcardia, 165
Microscope, 113
Midsagittal, 38, 39
Milk, 303
Mind, 120
Mineralocorticoids, 377
Mitral valve, 156, 159, 160
Mitral valve murmur, 160
Mitral valve prolapse, 178
Mononucleosis, 179
Mons pubis, 301
Mouth, 196, 199, 200, 201, 206, 214, 216, 217
Movements, body, generated by muscles, 441f
    in pairs, 440t
MRI, 48f, 49, 129, 241
Much, 258, 282, 305, 360
Mucoid, 315, 331
Mucous, 205, 314, 317, 331
Mucus, 205, 314, 317, 331
Multigravida, 322
Multipara, 305
Multiple sclerosis, 394
Murmur, 178
Muscle(s), 421, 435f, 436, 437, 438, 439
    body movements generated by, 441f
    disorders of, 446–447
Muscular dystrophy, 446
Muscular rheumatism, 436
Muscular system, 435–441
Musculoskeletal system, 411–461
    abbreviations, 443
    composition of, 411
    diagnostic terms, 447
    pathological terms, 443–447
    Spanish translations, 579
    therapeutic terms, 447
Musculotendinous rotator cuff injuries, 446
Myalgia, 436, 439
Myasthenia gravis, 446
Mycosis, 70, 201
Myelalgia, 385
Myelitis, 388
Myelocele, 395, 414
Myelogenesis, 422
Myelogram, 422

Myeloma, 388
Myelomalacia, 388, 422
Myocardial infarction (MI), 167, 178
    medical records, 184–185
Myocardium, 148, 149
Myodynia, 439
Myogenesis, 438
Myoma, 121
Myopathy, 121, 436, 439
Myopia, 471, 472f
Myoplasty, 121
Myorrhaphy, 121, 437, 438
Myorrhexis, 436, 437, 439
Myosarcoma, 437
Myosclerosis, 439
Myotomy, 438
Myringoplasty, 485
Myringotomy, 474, 485
Myxedema, 393

N

Nail(s), 62, 72
Nail bed, 71
Nail body, 71
Nail root, 71
Nares, 104
Narrowing, 146, 257
Nasal, 101
Nasal cavity, 106
Nasogastric, 104
Nasogastric intubation, 241
Nasolacrimal duct, 471
Natal, 322
Navel, 44
Nearest, 420
Nearsightedness, 471, 472f
Nebulized mist treatment (NMT), 130, 130f
Neck, 303, 317, 414, 430
Neck of uterus, 303
Necrectomy, 167
Necrophobia, 167
Necrosis, 79, 167, 205
Neonate, 322
Neonatologist, 322
Neonatology, 322
Neoplasms, 334
Nephralgia, 260
Nephrectomy, 260, 265
Nephritis, 260, 284, 287–288
Nephrolith(s), 260, 262, 264, 278
Nephrolithiasis, 260, 262, 264, 267, 284
Nephrolithotomy, 262, 264, 265
Nephrologist, 283
Nephroma, 257
Nephromegaly, 260, 264
Nephron(s), 259, 273, 276f
Nephropathy, 258
Nephropexy, 258, 265, 270
Nephroptosis, 258, 265, 270
Nephrorrhaphy, 265
Nephrosclerosis, 264
Nephroscope, 279
Nephroscopy, 279
Nephrosis, 264

Nephrotic syndrome, 263
Nephrotomy, 265
Nerve(s), 385, 390
Nerve cell, 390
Nervous system, 41, 357, 384–390
    abbreviations, 392
    diagnostic terms, 395
    pathological terms, 394–395
    Spanish translations, 578
    therapeutic terms, 396
Neuralgia, 390
Neuritis, 390
Neuroblastoma, 394
Neurocyte, 390
Neurodynia, 390
Neuroglia, 384, 384f, 390
Neuroglial tissue, 385
Neurohypophysis, 365
Neurolysis, 385
Neuromyelitis, 390
Neuron(s), 384, 384f, 390
Newborn infant, 322
Nipple, 320
Nitrogenous compounds, 258
Nocturia, 282
Node(s), 162, 173
Nodule, 85f
Non-Hodgkin lymphoma, 172, 179
Non-insulin-dependent diabetes mellitus (NIDDM), 380, 393
Noncancerous, 272, 273, 334
Norepinephrine, 378
Nose, 101, 104
Nosebleed, 127
Nostrils, 104
Not, 281, 327, 386, 474
Noun, 235, 331
Nuclear scan, 48f, 49

O

OB-GYN, 318
Obstetrics, 318
Odontalgia, 203
Offspring, 305
Oil gland, 66
Oligomenorrhea, 340
Oligospermia, 331
Oliguria, 277, 282
One half, 386, 436
Onychoma, 72
Onychomalacia, 62, 72
Onychomycosis, 72
Onychopathy, 72
Oophoritis, 323, 324
Oophoroma, 304, 306, 324
Oophoropathy, 307, 382
Oophoropexy, 307
Oophoroplasty, 307
Oophorotomy, 382
Open, 429
Open fracture, 428
Opening, 214, 216, 217, 257
Ophthalmalgia, 469
Ophthalmectomy, 469
Ophthalmodynia, 469

Ophthalmologist, 469
Ophthalmomalacia, 469
Ophthalmoplegia, 469
Ophthalmoscope, 465, 469
Ophthalmoscopy, 469
Optic, 465
Optic disk, 469
Optic nerve, 469
Oral, 196
Oral cavity, 196, 199, 203f
Orchidectomy, 327
Orchidopexy, 382
Orchiopexy, 327, 332
Orchioplasty, 332
Orchiorrhaphy, 332
Origin, 303, 327, 359, 379
Orthodontist, 196, 203, 204
Orthopedics, 415
Orthopnea, 119
Ostealgia, 419
Osteitis, 415, 419
Osteitis deformans, 444, 444f
Osteitis fibrosa cystica, 375
Osteoarthritis, 424
Osteoarthropathy, 425
Osteoarthrosis, 425
Osteoblasts, 418
Osteocyte(s), 415, 418, 419
Osteodynia, 419
Osteogenesis, 418, 420
Osteomalacia, 415, 420
Osteopathy, 419
Osteoporosis, 415, 444, 444f
Osteorrhaphy, 419
Osteosclerosis, 419
Osteotomy, 419
Otalgia, 475, 478
Otitis media, 483
  medical records, 490–491
Otodynia, 475, 478
Otoplasty, 478
Otorrhea, 474
Otosclerosis, 477, 483
Otoscope, 478, 484
Otoscopy, 478, 484
Ova, 301
Ovariorrhexis, 304
Ovary(ies), 301, 306, 323, 362f, 368, 369,
  381–382
Oviducts, 307
Ovulation, 306, 307
Ovum, 307
Oxygen (O$_2$), 103, 115, 116, 155
Oxytocin, 362f, 368

P

P wave, 165
Paget disease, 444, 444f
Pain, 102, 197, 200, 203, 209, 219, 271,
  273, 327, 385, 426, 427, 432, 436, 473,
  478
Painful, 197, 305
Palsy, 394
Pancreas, 225, 226, 229f, 359, 378–381
Pancreatectomy, 233

Pancreatic, 228
Pancreatic cancer, 233
Pancreatic duct, 228
Pancreatic hormone(s), 378, 379, 379t
Pancreatitis, 227, 359
Pancreatolith, 229, 231, 378
Pancreatolithiasis, 232, 378
Pancreatolysis, 225, 378
Pancreatoma, 378
Pancreatopathy, 378
Panhypopituitarism, 393
Papanicolaou (Pap) test, 303, 342
Papillary carcinoma, medical records,
  133–135
Papule, 85f
Para, 323
Paralysis, 106, 386, 436, 440, 464
Paranasal, 104
Parathormone, 374, 374t
Parathyroid glands, 359, 374
Parathyroid hormone (PTH), 374, 374t
Parathyroidectomy, 359
Parital paralysis, 386
Parkinson disease, 394
Parotid gland, 200
Patella, 414, 426
Patellectomy, 414
Patent ductus arteriosus, 178
Pathogens, 323
Pathological, 220
Pathological terms, 47
Pelvic cavity, 40
Pelvic girdle, 426
Pelvic inflammatory disease (PID), 323,
  324
Pelvimetry, 414
Pelvis, 414, 426
Penis, 326, 333
Peptic ulcers, 205
Pericardiectomy, 148
Pericardiorrhaphy, 148
Pericarditis, 148
Pericardium, 148, 149
Perineorrhaphy, 304
Perineum, 304
Periodontics, 197
Periodontitis, 204
Periosteum, 417, 418
Peripheral nervous system (PNS), 384
Pertaining to, 235, 257, 303, 304, 310,
  359, 385, 413, 414, 415, 432, 436, 465,
  474
Pertussis, 127
PET scan, 48f, 50
Petechia, 83
Phacoemulsification, 484f, 485
Phagocyte, 170
Phalanges, 413, 426
Phalangitis, 413
Pharyngitis, 108
Pharyngocele, 108
Pharyngomycosis, 106
Pharyngoparalysis, 106
Pharyngoplasty, 108
Pharyngoplegia, 106
Pharyngospasm, 103

Pharyngostenosis, 108
Pharyngotome, 108
Pharyngotomy, 108
Pharyngotonsillitis, 197
Pharynx, 101, 104, 106, 197, 203f, 205,
  474
Pheochromocytoma, 394
Phimosis, 341
Phlebitis, 145
Phleborrhaphy, 156
Phleborrhexis, 156
Phlebostenosis, 156
Phlebotomy, 156
Photophobia, 481
Photopigments, 469
Phrenology, 120
Phrenospasm, 120
Pia matter, 389
Piles, 239
Pilocystic, 71
Pilonidal, 62
Pineal gland, 381
Pinkeye, 481
Pituitarism, 394
Pituitary gland, 362f, 364
Pituitary hormones, 368t
Plantar warts, 84
Platelet, 388
Pleura(ae), 102, 117, 430
Pleural effusion, 127
Pleuralgia, 102, 117
Pleurisy, 117, 118
Pleuritic, 102
Pleuritis, 117
Pleurocele, 117
Pleurodynia, 117
Pleuropneumonia, 117
Pneumectomy, 102
Pneumocentesis, 116
Pneumoconiosis, 116
Pneumocystis carinii pneumonia, 123
Pneumomelanosis, 116
Pneumonectomy, 115, 116
Pneumonia, 102, 115, 117, 123
  lobar, 135–137
Pneumonocele, 116
Pneumonopathy, 116
Pneumonosis, 116
Pneumothorax, 127, 128f
Poison, 234, 359, 371
Poisoning, 387
Poisonous, 234
Poliomyelitis, 394
Polycystic, 282
Polycystic kidney disease (PKD), 282
Polydipsia, 360, 381
Polyphagia, 381
Polyposis, 240
Polyp(s), 238, 239
Polyuria, 258, 282, 381
Porous, 415
Posion, 280
Positron emission tomography (PET),
  48f, 50, 396
Posterior, 31, 39, 364, 365, 439
Posteroanterior (PA), 364

Posteroinferior, 364
Posterolateral, 32, 364
Posterosuperior, 364
Postmenopausal, 319
Postmenopausal bleeding, medical records, 347–349
Postmenopause, 312
Postnatal, 322
Postprandial, 225
Postural drainage, 129, 130f
Prefixes, 13–15
Pregnancy, 305
Pregnant woman, 305
Premenopausal, 319
Premenopause, 312
Prenatal, 304
Prepuce, 333
Presbycusis, 483
Primigravida, 305, 322
Process of, 464
Process of recording, 234
Proctalgia, 220
Proctitis, 220
Proctodynia, 220
Proctologist, 212
Proctoscopy, 221
Proctospasm, 220
Producing, 303, 327, 331, 359, 379
Progesterone, 312, 320
Progestin, 377
Prolactin, 362f, 368
Prolapse, 258, 413, 465
Prolapsed disk, 444, 444f
Pronunciation, 15
Prostate, 333f
Prostate cancer, 334
Prostate gland, 326, 331, 332
Prostate-specific antigen (PSA) test, 332, 334, 343
Prostatectomy, 334
Prostatic hyperplasia, 333f
Prostatism, 332
Prostatitis, 332, 334, 335
Prostatocystitis, 332
Prostatocystotomy, 333
Prostatomegaly, 332
Protection, 170
Proteinuria, 263, 284
Proximal, 33, 34, 420
Proximal epiphysis, 418
PSA test, 332, 334, 343
Pseudocyesis, 305
Psoriasis, 84, 84f
    medical record, 92–93
Ptyalism, 196, 200
Pulmonary, 157
Pulmonary arteries, 150, 155
Pulmonary capillaries, 113
Pulmonary circulation, 154
Pulmonary function tests, 129
Pulmonary trunk, 150
Pulmonary valve, 155, 159
Pulmonary veins, 150, 156
Pulmonologist, 102
Pupil, 464, 468

Purkinje fibers, 162, 165
Pus, 127, 281
Pustule, 85f
Pyelitis, 277, 278, 279
Pyelogram, 281, 288
Pyelography, 277, 278, 288
Pyelonephritis, 279, 284
Pyelopathy, 274
Pyeloplasty, 257, 278, 281
Pyelostomy, 274
Pyelotomy, 274
Pyloric, 220
Pylorotomy, 197
Pylorus, 197, 220
Pyoderma, 62
Pyonephrosis, 281
Pyorrhea, 281
Pyosalpinx, 340
Pyothorax, 103, 127
Pyuria, 281, 282, 283

Q

QRS wave, 165
Quadriplegia, 386, 440

R

Radiation, 364, 415
Radiation therapy, 421
Radioactive iodine uptake (RAIU) test, 395
Radiograph, 39, 415
Radiography, 48f, 50, 271
Radiologist, 421
Radiology, 40, 421
Radiopharmaceutical, 48f, 49, 50
Radiotherapy, 421
Radius, 415
Rapid, 153
Rapid eating, 153
Raynaud phenomenon, 178
Record(s), 146, 164, 234, 304. *See also* Medical record(s)
Rectal bleeding, medical records, 244–246
Rectalgia, 219
Rectocele, 212, 269, 269f, 270, 279, 280
Rectocolitis, 219
Rectoplasty, 219
Rectospasm, 220
Rectostenosis, 220
Rectovaginal, 219
Rectum, 212, 218, 219, 220, 221, 269, 272, 279
Red, 280, 470
Red blood cells (RBCs), 180, 418
Regional colitis, 217, 238
Regional ileitis, 217
Relating to, 235, 257, 303, 304, 310, 359, 385, 413, 414, 415, 432, 436, 465, 474
Removal, 116, 167, 225, 303, 304, 320, 327, 328, 359, 414
Renal, 257, 263
Renal artery, 259

Renal artery stenosis, 263
Renal biopsy, 260
Renal calculi, 281
Renal cortex, 259, 276
Renal dialysis, 260
Renal disease, 287
Renal failure, 257, 260
Renal hypertension, 263, 288
Renal medulla, 259, 276
Renal pelvis, 257, 274, 277
Renal scan, 288
Renal transplantation, 289
Renal vein, 259
Reproductive system(s), 301–356
    abbreviations, 338
    female, 301–325, 302f, 308f, 309f
        diagnostic terms, 341–343
        pathological terms, 338–340
        therapeutic terms, 344
    male, 326f, 326–336, 330
        diagnostic terms, 343
        pathological terms, 340–341
        therapeutic terms, 344
    Spanish translations, 577
Respiration, 113, 118
Respiratory distress syndrome, acute, 126
    adult, 126
Respiratory system, 99–142
    combining forms of, 101–102
    diagnostic terms, 129
    lower, 100f, 107f, 111–124
    pathological terms, 126–128
    Spanish translations, 573
    structures of, 99, 100f
    therapeutic terms, 129
    upper, 100f, 104–109, 107f
Retina, 465, 467
Retinal detachment, 481
    medical records, 488–490
Retinitis, 467
Retinopathy, 465, 468, 481
Retrograde, 278
Retrograde pyelography, 278, 288
Retroversion, 305, 340
Rheumatic heart disease, 178
Rheumatoid arthritis, 444, 445f
Rheumatoid factor, 447
Rhinitis, 105
Rhinologist, 105
Rhinoplasty, 105
Rhinorrhagia, 105
Rhinorrhea, 101, 105
Rhinotomy, 105
Rhonchi, 128
Ribs, 413, 426, 427, 436
Rickets, 420
Right hepatic duct, 228
Right ventricle (RV), 152
Ringworm, 84
Rinne test, 484
Roentgenology, 421
Rotator cuff, injuries to, 446
    tear of, medical records, 453–455
Rupture, 269, 304, 436, 437, 439
RV, 152

f *indicates figure;* t *indicates table*

S

S1-S5, 433
Sacral vertebrae, 432
Sacrodynia, 432
Sacrospinal, 432
Sacrum, 432, 433
Saliva, 196, 200
Salivary glands, 196, 200
Salpingectomy, 304, 307, 324
Salpingitis, 323, 476
Salpingocele, 307
Salpingopharyngeal, 474
Salpingoplasty, 307
Salpingoscope, 307, 476
Salpingoscopy, 307, 476
Salpingostenosis, 476
Sarcoma, 208
Scabies, 84
Scale, 62
Scan, 48f, 50
Scanty, 331
Scarring, 69
Sciatica, 394
Sclera, 257, 264, 439, 465, 466
    of eye, 62
Scleritis, 465, 467, 468
Scleroderma, 62, 69
Scleromalacia, 468
Sclerosis, 69, 264, 439
Scoliosis, 445f, 446
Scrotum, 329
Sebaceous, 62, 70
Sebaceous gland, 66
Seborrhea, 62
Sebum, 62
Seizure, 394
Self, 79
Semen, 331
Semicircular canals, 476
Seminal fluid, 331
Seminal vesicle(s), 326, 328, 331
Sense organs. *See* Ear(s); Eye(s)
Separation, 225, 258, 385, 436
Sepsis, 47
Septum(a), 152, 153, 156
Sequestrectomy, 447
Sequestrum, 444, 447
Serum, 127
Seven, 432
Sex glands, 327
Sex hormones, 377
Sexually transmitted diseases (STDs),
    323, 341
Shin bone, 414
Shingles, 395
Short bones, 416, 417
Shoulder, rotation and flexion of, 441f
Shoulder joint, injuries to, 446
Sialitis, 200
Sialorrhea, 196, 200
Side, 31, 364
Sigmoid, 219
Sigmoid colon, 212, 217, 221, 222
Sigmoidectomy, 219, 222
Sigmoiditis, 219

Sigmoidoscope, 222
Sigmoidoscopy, 221, 221f, 222, 223
Sigmoidotomy, 212
Simple closed, 429
Single-photon emission computed
    tomography, 50
Sinoatrial (SA) node, 162
Sinus rhythm, 165
Skeletal system, 411–434
    anterior view of, 412f, 425f
Skin, 62, 64–69
    accessory organs of, 70–73
    disease of, 66
    inflammation of, 66
    structure of, 60, 60f, 65f
Skin lesions, 84, 85f
Skin study, 65
Skin test, 86
Skull, 413, 426
Small intestine, 213, 215, 216
Smell, 103
Softening, 415
Somatotropin, 361, 362f, 368
Spanish translations, 563–574
Spasm, 155, 220
Spastic colon, 239
Specialists, 202, 203, 204, 212, 303, 359
Speech, 386
Sperm, 326, 327
Sperm cells, 330
Sperm transporting ducts, 326
Spermatocide, 327
Spermatocyte, 331
Spermatogenesis, 331
Spermatoid, 331
Spermatolith, 330
Spermatozoa, 327, 330
Spermaturia, 331
Spermicide, 327
Spina bifida, 395
Spina bifida cystica, 395
Spina bifida occulta, 395
Spinal, 40
Spinal cavity, 41
Spinal column, 413, 426, 429, 430,
    431f
Spinal cord, 385, 387, 414, 421
Spinal disorders, 444–446
Spine, 385, 432
Spirometry, 129
Spleen, 170
Splenomegaly, 170
Spondylitis, 413, 430
Spondylodynia, 429
Spondylomalacia, 430
Spondylopathy, 430
Spongy bone, 418
Sprain, 446
Squamous, 62
Stapedectomy, 477, 483
Stapedotomy, 483
Stapes, 476
Statins, 180
Steatitis, 61
Stenosis, 220, 263

Sterility, 340
Sternocostal, 413
Sternum, 413, 426
Steroid hormones, 377
Stiffness, 414
Stimulate, 327
Stomach, 104, 197, 203f, 205, 207,
    216
Stomatalgia, 200
Stomatitis, 199, 201
Stomatodynia, 200
Stomatomycosis, 201
Stomatopathy, 196
Stomatoplasty, 206
Stomatosis, 201
Stone(s), 155, 225, 230, 231, 232, 258,
    260, 262, 264, 267, 284, 330, 378
Stool, 218
Stool guaiac, 241
Strabismus, 481f, 482
Straight, 203, 415
Strain, 446
Stratum corneum, 64
Stratum germinativum, 77
Stress test, 179
Stricture, 108, 146, 257
Stridor, 128
Stroke, 178, 388, 394, 471
Structure, 257, 432
Study of, 40, 202, 212, 359
Sty, 482
Subcostal, 413, 427
Subcutaneous, 65, 66, 68, 70
Subcutaneous tissue(s), 65f, 67, 68
    structure of, 60, 60f
Sublingual, 196, 200, 201
Sublingual gland, 200, 201
Submandibular gland, 200
Submaxillary, 201
Sudden infant death syndrome, 128
Sudoresis, 61
Sudoriferous, 70
Sudoriferous gland, 66
Suffixes, 7–13, 21
Sugar, 359, 379
Superior, 33, 40, 375
Superior vena cava (SVC), 150, 154,
    158
Suprarenal, 264, 375
Suprarenal glands, 375–376
Surgical repair, 62, 219, 257, 311, 464,
    474
Suture, 216, 268, 304, 314, 437
Swallowing, 103, 170, 197, 209
Sweat gland, 66, 67
Sweetness, 359
Swelling, 72, 257, 263, 269, 303, 314, 328,
    333, 385, 414
Swimmer's ear, 475
Synarthroses, 424
Synovial fluid, 424
Syphilis, 341
Systemic, 69
Systemic circulation, 154
Systole, 164

T

T wave, 165
Tachycardia, 153, 164
Tachyphagia, 153
Tachypnea, 119, 153
Talipes, 446, 446f
Target organs, 357
Target tissues, 357
TB, 124
Tear(s), 464, 473
Tear gland, 473
Tendinitis, 436, 447
Tendolysis, 436
Tendon, 436, 439
Tendonitis, 436, 447
Tendoplasty, 439, 440
Tendotome, 440
Tendotomy, 440
Tenolysis, 436
Tenotomy, 436
Testalgia, 327
Testectomy, 330
Testicles, 329
Testis(es), 326, 327, 329, 362f, 369,
    381–382
Testitis, 330
Testopathy, 330
Testosterone, 327, 329
Thalamotomy, 396
Therapeutic procedures, 544–546
Thermometer, 234
Thigh bone, 414, 426
Thing, 432
Thirst, 360
Thoracentesis, 120
Thoracic, 172, 432
Thoracic cavity, 40, 119, 119f, 120
Thoracic duct, 172
Thoracic vertebrae, 432
Thoracocentesis, 119, 119f, 120
Thoracodynia, 102
Thoracopathy, 102
Thoracotomy, 119
Threatening, 334
Three, 154
Throat, 101, 104, 106, 197, 205, 474
Thrombectomy, 167, 168
Thrombocyte, 388
Thrombogenesis, 168, 388
Thrombolysis, 145, 167, 168, 388
Thrombolytic therapy, 181
Thrombosis, 167
Thrombus(i), 167, 168, 388
Through, 219, 258, 415
Thymectomy, 381
Thymolysis, 381
Thymoma, 170, 359, 381
Thymopathy, 381
Thymus gland, 170, 359, 381
Thyroid gland, 359, 362f, 369, 370
    in goiter, 371f
Thyroid hormones, 371t
Thyroid-stimulating hormone (TSH),
    362f, 365, 368
Thyroidectomy, 359, 369, 374

Thyroidotome, 371
Thyroidotomy, 371
Thyromegaly, 359, 369
Thyropathy, 369
Thyrotomy, 369
Thyrotoxicosis, 369f, 370
Thyroxine (T$_4$), 370, 371
Tibia, 414, 426
Tibial, 414
Tinea, 84
Tinnitus, 483
Tissue typing, 180
Toes, bones of, 413, 426
Tomography, 51
Tongue, 196, 200
Tonometry, 483, 483f
Tonsils, 101, 197
Tooth (Teeth), 196, 197, 202, 204
Toothache, 203, 204
Torticollis, 447
Total hip arthroplasty, 447, 448f
Toxic, 234
Toxic goiter, 369f, 370
Toxic shock syndrome (TSS), 340
Toxicologist, 359, 371
Toxicology, 234, 371
Toxicopathy, 371
Toxicosis, 234
Toxin, 280
Trachea, 101, 111, 112
Tracheolaryngotomy, 112
Tracheomalacia, 112
Tracheopathy, 112
Tracheoplasty, 112
Tracheostenosis, 112
Tracheostomy, 101, 111, 112f
Tracheostomy tube, 112f
Tracheotomy, 112
Transaortic, 146
Transdermal, 312
Transient ischemic attack, 178,
    395
Transmission, 62
Transverse, 38, 39
Transverse colon, 217, 218
Treatment, 62
Tremor, 394
Trichomoniasis, 341
Trichomycosis, 71
Trichopathy, 62, 71
Trichosis, 71
Tricuspid valve, 154, 159
Triiodothyronine (T$_3$), 371
Troponin I, 179
Tubal ligation, 344
Tube, 304, 305, 307, 474, 476
Tubercles, 124
Tuberculosis (TB), 124
Tumor(s), blood, 312
    connective tissue, 437
    digestive system, 208
    fatty, 68
    kidney, 257
    nervous system, 384, 385
    ovarian, 304, 306

skin, 85f
thymus gland, 359
types of, 334
urinary tract, 273
Turning, 305, 474
Twitching, 103, 220, 464
Two, 154
Tympanic membrane, 474, 475, 476
Tympanoplasty, 474, 485
Tympanostomy, 485
Type 1 diabetes, 380, 393
Type 2 diabetes, 380, 393

U

Ulcer, 85f, 205, 216, 240
Ulcerative colitis, 239
Ultrasonography (US), 48f, 51, 179, 234,
    241, 285, 342–343
Ultrasound. *See* Ultrasonography (US)
Umbilical, 43, 44
Umbilical region, 44
Umbilicus, 44
Under, 359, 363, 413, 421, 427
Unequal, 464
Upon, 208
Upper, 33
Upper GI series, 240
Upper GI tract endoscopy, 206
Uremia, 257, 258, 282, 288
Ureter(s), 257, 267, 268
Ureteralgia, 268
Ureterectasis, 267, 268
Ureteritis, 267
Ureterocystoscope, 268
Ureterocystoscopy, 268
Ureterolith(s), 267, 268, 278
Ureterolithiasis, 267
Ureterolithotomy, 267
Ureteromegaly, 267
Ureteropyeloplasty, 278
Ureterorrhaphy, 269
Ureterostenosis, 257
Urethra, 257, 267, 271, 272, 279,
    326
Urethral stricture, 272
Urethralgia, 271
Urethrectomy, 271
Urethritis, 271
Urethrocele, 258, 279, 280
Urethrocystitis, 272
Urethrodynia, 271
Urethropexy, 271
Urethroplasty, 271
Urethrorectal, 272
Urethroscope, 272
Urethroscopy, 272
Urinalysis, 288
Urinary, 257
Urinary bladder, 267, 268
Urinary incontinence, 283
Urinary meatus, 267
Urinary system, 255–300, 256f, 261f
    abbreviations, 287
    diagnostic terms, 288

pathological terms, 287–288
Spanish translations, 576
therapeutic terms, 289
Urinary tract infection (UTI), 271, 272, 273, 281
Urination, 258, 283
excessive, 381
Urine, 257, 258, 280, 281
Urogenital, 336
Urogram, 288
Urography, 288
Urologist, 280, 283
Urology, 280
Urotoxin, 280
Urticaria, 84
Uterine hemorrhage, 310
Uterine retroversion, 305
Uteropexy, 310
Uteroplasty, 311
Uteroscopy, 310
Uterovaginal, 303
Uterus, 301, 303, 304, 306, 309, 310, 311, 318, 324, 362f, 368
neck of, 414

V

Vagina, 219, 301, 303, 306, 313, 314, 317
Vaginal, 314, 318
Vaginal hysterectomy, 314
Vaginitis, 313
Vaginocele, 303
Vaginoplasty, 313
Vaginoscope, 313
Vaginotomy, 313
Valve(s), 154, 155, 156, 157, 159–160
Valvuloplasty, 181
Varicocele, 328
Varicose veins, 178
Vas deferens, 145, 328, 331, 335
Vascular, 145, 157
Vasectomy, 328, 335, 336f
Vasectomy reversal, 335, 336, 336f
Vasospasm, 145

Vasovasostomy, 335, 336, 336f
Vein(s), 145, 150, 156, 157, 259, 328. *See also specific veins*
Vena cava(ae), 150, 154, 158
Venereal disease, 323, 341
Venereal warts, 84
Venosclerosis, 156
Venospasm, 156
Venotomy, 156
Venous, 145
Ventricle(s), 146, 150, 151, 152, 155, 156
Ventricular, 152
Ventriculotomy, 151
Venule, 157
Vertebra(ae), 413, 426, 429, 430
Vertebral, 413
Vertebral column, 413, 426, 429, 430, 431f
Vertebrectomy, 429
Vertebrocostal, 430
Vertebrosternal, 430
Vertigo, 483
Vesicle, 85f
Vesicocele, 257
Vesicoenteric, 269
Vesiculitis, 328
Vessel(s), 145, 172, 328
blood, 145
Vestibule, 476
Villi, 213
Virilism, 377
Vision, 464, 465, 470
Visual acuity test, 483
Visual examination, 211, 221, 257, 303
Vitamin D deficiency, 420
Vitiligo, 84
Voice box, 101, 108
Voiding cystourography, 288
Volvulus, 240
Vomiting, 197, 208, 209, 228
Vulva, 301, 304, 317
Vulvitis, 317
Vulvopathy, 304, 317
Vulvouterine, 317

W

Wall-eye, 481f, 482
Wart, 84
Water, 106, 333
Wheal, 85f
Wheezes, 129
White, 280
White blood cells, 180, 418
White blood count (WBC), 76
White of eye, 257, 264
Whooping cough, 127
Widening, 388
Wilms tumor, 288
Windpipe, 101, 111
Within, 427, 465
Without, 281, 327, 331, 386, 474
Without formation, 335
Woman, 303, 322
Womb. *See* Uterus
Word building, 10–12
Word elements, 3–15, 25–27, 36–37
Word roots, 3–5
Wrist bones, 413, 426
Writing, 234, 304
Wryneck, 447

X

Xanthemia, 76
Xanthocyte, 76
Xanthoderma, 75
Xanthoma(s), 75, 76
Xanthopia, 470
Xanthosis, 78
Xeroderma, 62, 72, 75
X-ray(s), 364, 415, 421
chest, 129

Y

Yeasts, 70
Yellow, 470